CONTENTS

Foreword

The Case of the Month has been a feature of the *British Journal of Radiology* since 1986. According to the guidelines for authors, cases of the month "... report recognized but rare abnormalities, or are teaching cases with points of general interest that might be seen at an examination". Most of the cases combine the two descriptions of interesting patients and important differential diagnoses. The purpose is therefore to inform and to interest the reader.

The readers of this anthology may fall into two categories. Firstly, radiologists in training who are preparing for the FRCR or other higher specialist examinations should find useful nuggets of information to carry with them into the examination. Secondly, consultant radiologists may find these cases, which cover the broad spectrum of imaging, both challenging and diverting.

The choice of cases is that of the Editor. Some comments, for which the Editor takes entire responsibility, are added, mainly with the aim of updating key references and to reflect modern trends in imaging practice. A list, categorizing the questions in relation to body systems, is to be found towards the back of the book. An index is also provided for ease of subject reference.

The main acknowledgment must go to all those authors who, over the years, have contributed cases of the month in order to educate and entertain their radiological colleagues. The distinctly international flavour of the cases is an enduring feature. I am grateful to the BIR Publications Department staff, especially Tim Hogan, Julia Rodd and Julie Richardson, for all their expertise and hard work in producing this book. I also wish to thank Philip Shorvon for his perceptive advice and support.

G H Whitehouse
Editor

A tightening of the belt

[1]R CHAUDHURI, [2]I MALIK and [1]J B BINGHAM

[1]Department of MRI, Division of Radiological Sciences, UMDS and [2]Department of Medicine, Guy's Hospital, St Thomas Street, London SE1 9RT, UK

A 65-year-old man presented with a 2 week history of an aching pain in the right loin, radiating to the back of both thighs. This pain occurred within walking 25 yards and was relieved by rest. His symptoms had started after changing a car tyre and, consequently, he attributed them to this. He had, however, also been dyspnoeic. On further questioning he had noted feeling bloated and had loosened his trouser belt by two notches. A provisional diagnosis of spinal stenosis or intermittent claudication was made and he was referred for MRI of the lumbar spine. T_1 weighted spin echo images in the right parasagittal plane and at the level of the lumbosacral disc space are shown in Figures 1 and 2. The images show that although there was evidence of minor disc disease the lumbar canal was of normal dimensions. Because of an additional finding an MR angiogram was obtained and this is shown in Figure 3. What do the three MR images show (Figures 1–3) and what is the diagnosis? How could you confirm your diagnosis?

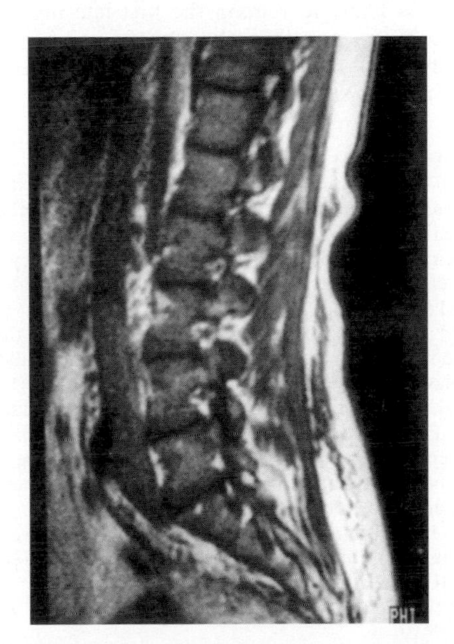

Figure 1. T_1 weighted spin echo image through the lumbar spine in a right parasagittal plane.

Based on the case of the month originally published in Br J Radiol 1994;67:663–4.

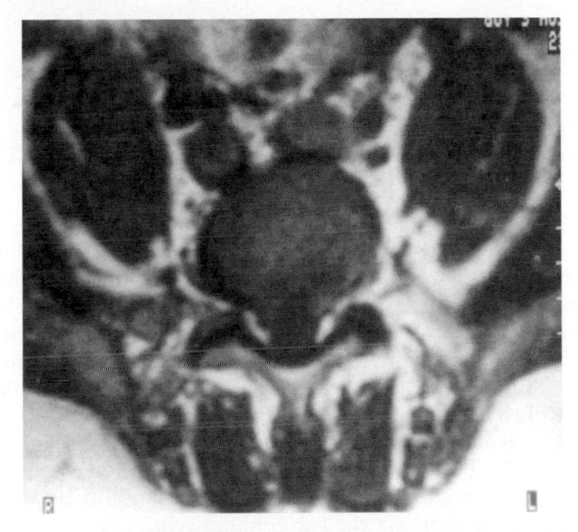

Figure 2. T_1 weighted spin echo axial image at the level of the lumbosacral disc space.

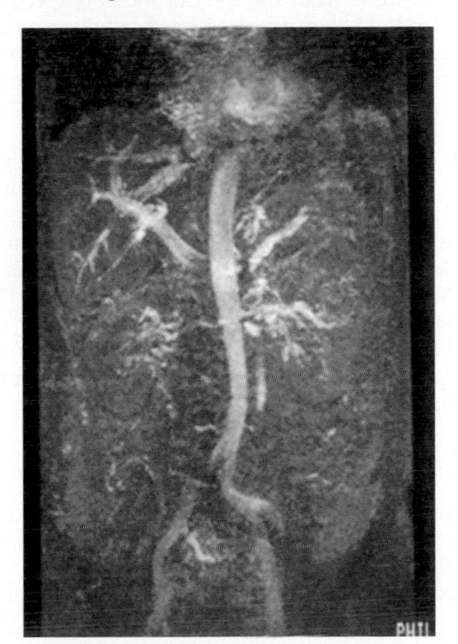

Figure 3. 2D MR angiogram of the abdominal vessels. The maximum intensity projection is shown which is a summation of all individual slices obtained from the scan.

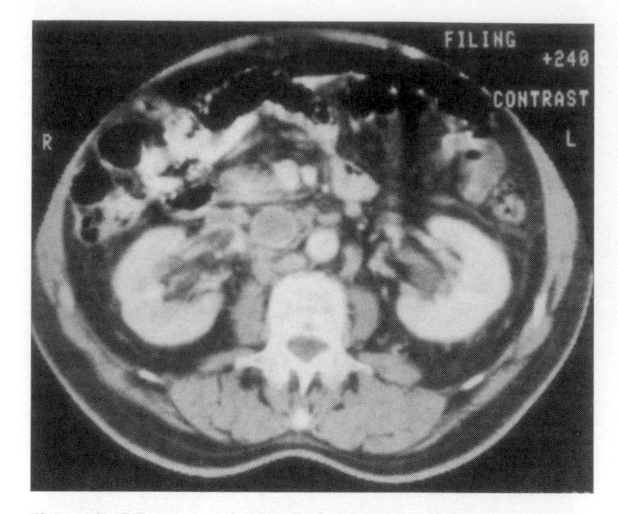

Figure 4. CT scan at the level of the renal veins.

Figure 1 showed that the normal flow void in the inferior vena cava (IVC) was replaced by homogeneous signal, also visible in the iliac veins (Figure 2) compatible with thrombus. MR angiography was performed using a 2D time-of-flight technique which displayed flowing blood as bright signal and vessels containing no or very low flow as dark. The major arteries as well as the portal and splenic veins were well seen but there was no signal from the IVC, iliac, femoral or the right renal veins. There was some flow in the left renal vein and there was collateralization via the left gonadal vein.

A diagnosis of inferior vena caval and iliac vein thrombosis, extending from the level of the portal vein down to the femoral veins, was confirmed by ultrasound (US) and CT. Contrast enhanced CT (Figure 4) demonstrated a distended cava with an enhancing rim, with thrombus extending into the right renal vein. No intraabdominal masses were visualized.

A V/Q scan showed evidence of small pulmonary emboli. The patient was anticoagulated and made good clinical progress. However, 1 year after presentation there was persistent thrombosis of the IVC and right iliac and femoral veins. He had an elevated sedimentation rate (57 mm h^{-1}) and mild hyperglycaemia. Despite extensive investigation, an underlying cause of the thrombosis did not become apparent and this must be considered a case of primary idiopathic inferior vena cava thrombosis.

IVC thrombosis may be primary (in 14%) or can occur secondary to many conditions including extension or external pressure from retroperitoneal tumours, especially of the kidney (about 30% of cases); it can also be secondary to intraabdominal sepsis, surgery or trauma, hypercoagulable states, or external pressure from aortic aneurysms or diseases of the liver [1, 2]. While once a postmortem diagnosis, it has become progressively easier to diagnose radiologically, and can often be medically or surgically treated.

IVC thrombosis can be imaged using US, CT or vena cavography. US is the simplest, safest and most widely available technique. US is the preferred method for demonstrating the cranial extent of thrombus and may also show the cause of obstruction [3]. Its disadvantages are that extrahepatic collaterals are poorly seen and bowel gas artefact may impair the study.

CT outlines tumour thrombus more reliably if it traverses the caval wall and displays the other abdominopelvic structures well. Neither US nor CT is accurate in determining invasion of the caval wall by tumour if thrombus is limited to the lumen and neither can distinguish blood clot from tumour thrombus [3].

Percutaneous vena cavography is invasive and carries the small risk of dislodging thrombus. Sometimes, the caudal extent of thrombus cannot be demonstrated because of preferential flow into collateral vessels, and a combined femoral and brachial approach would be needed to determine accurately both cranial and caudal extent.

MR demonstrates well the upper and lower extent of intravenous thrombus, using spin echo and gradient echo sequences, both with and without gadolinium-DTPA enhancement [4–6]. Other organs can be evaluated. Recent articles suggest that blood clot can be reliably differentiated from tumour thrombus, and that it is possible to identify invasion of the caval wall. In the future, while US is likely to remain the first-line investigation for inferior vena cava thrombosis, MRI and MR angiography promise to become more important in equivocal cases. [*See also Soler et al [7], ED*]

References

1. Missal ME, Robinson JA, Tatum RW. Inferior vena cava obstruction: clinical manifestations, diagnostic methods and related problems. Ann Intern Med 1965;62:133–61.
2. Siqueira-Filho AG, Kottke BA, Miller E. Primary inferior vena cava thrombosis: report of nine cases. Arch Intern Med 1976;136:799–802.
3. Didier D, Racle A, Etievent JP, Weill F. Tumour thrombus of the inferior vena cava secondary to malignant abdominal neoplasms: US and CT evaluation. Radiology 1987;162:83–9.
4. Hricak H, Amparo E, Fisher MR, et al. Abdominal venous system: assessment using MRI. Radiology 1985;156:415–22.
5. Hansen ME, Spritzer CE, Sostman HD. Assessing the patency of mediastinal and thoracic inlet veins: value of MR imaging. AJR 1990;155:1177–82.
6. Gehl H-B, Bohndorf K, Klose K-C. Inferior vena cava tumour thrombus: demonstration by Gd-DTPA enhanced MR. JCAT 1990;14:479–81.
7. Soler R, Rodriguez E, Lopez MF, et al. Eur J Radiol 1995;19:101–6.

A case of obstructive jaundice

[1]J F GRIFFITH, [1]S K BERA and [2]D E LOFT

Departments of [1]Radiology and [2]Medicine, Walsgrave Hospital, Coventry CV2 2DX, UK

A 33-year-old man presented with upper abdominal pain and progressive jaundice of 2 months' duration. 5 months earlier, he had jumped from the third floor of a psychiatric hospital sustaining multiple fractures of his face, cervical and lumbar spines and lower limbs. On examination, he was mildly icteric and was moderately tender in the epigastrium. Dark stools were present per rectum. Liver function tests were deranged in a cholestatic pattern. Endoscopic retrograde choledochopancreatography (ERCP) confirmed haemobilia and demonstrated extrinsic compression of the proximal common bile duct and left intrahepatic duct (Figure 1). Ultrasound demonstrated dilated intrahepatic bile ducts with a large inhomogenous mass at the hilum (Figure 2). CT was subsequently performed (Figures 3a and b).

What is the diagnosis and what investigation would you recommend to confirm this?

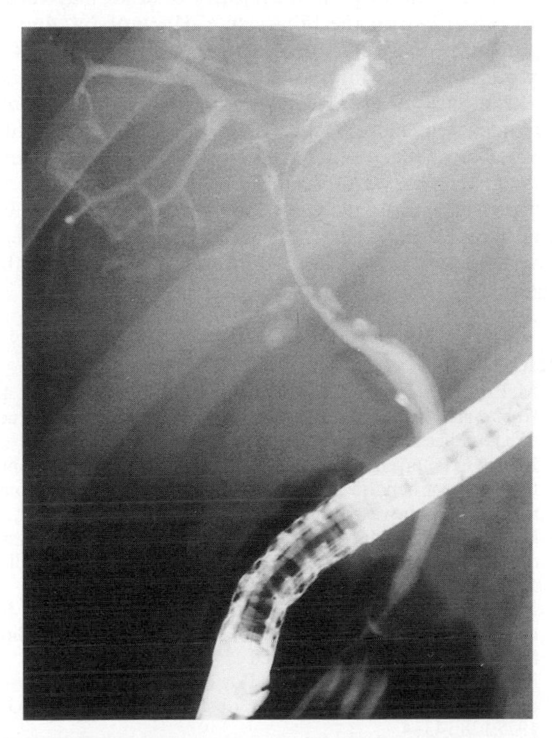

Figure 1. Endoscopic retrograde choledochopancreatography.

Based on the case of the month originally published in Br J Radiol 1997;70:107–8.

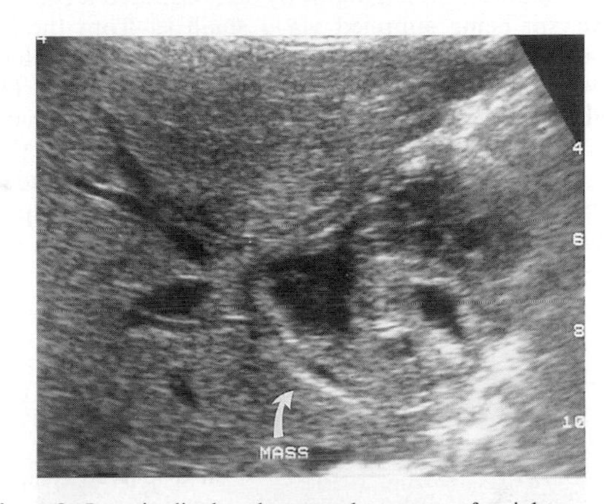

Figure 2. Longitudinal ultrasound scan of right upper quadrant.

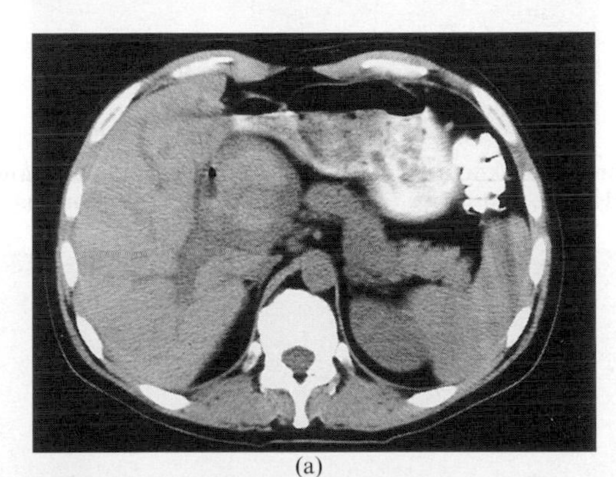

(a)

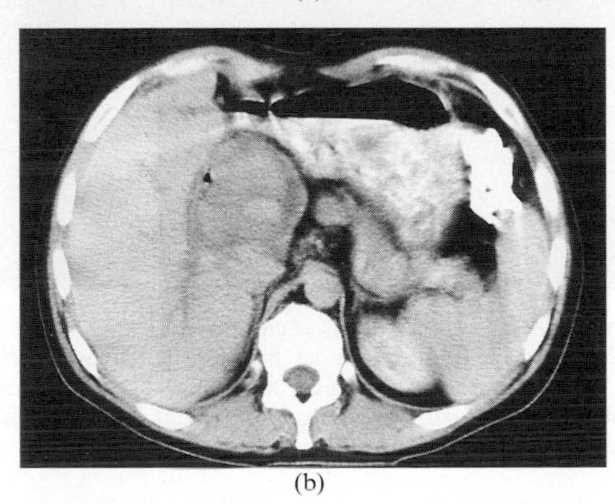

(b)

Figure 3. (a) Pre-contrast and (b) post-contrast enhanced CT scans.

The diagnosis was post-traumatic pseudoaneurysm of the left hepatic artery leading to haemobilia and obstructive jaundice.

Doppler ultrasound is the recommended investigation (Figure 4). This showed pulsatile flow present eccentrically within the mass confirming its vascular nature. Luminal enhancement was present on contrast enhanced CT (Figure 3b) which also demonstrated compression of the left portal vein and duodenum. Selective hepatic digital subtraction angiography demonstrated a pseudoaneurysm being supplied via a small jet from the left hepatic artery (Figure 5). The parenchymal phase showed the area occupied by thrombus (arrowed). The right hepatic artery was occluded and replaced by collaterals. Venous phase confirmed that the left portal vein branch was also occluded. Embolization was undertaken. However, attempted catheter advancement to the origin of the aneurysm was unsuccessful and resulted in dissection and occlusion of the left hepatic artery stump. Subsequent arteriography via the coeliac axis showed no filling of the aneurysm with supply to the small left lobe being maintained via collaterals. Liver function tests soon returned to normal. A repeat ultrasound was recommended but was refused by the patient.

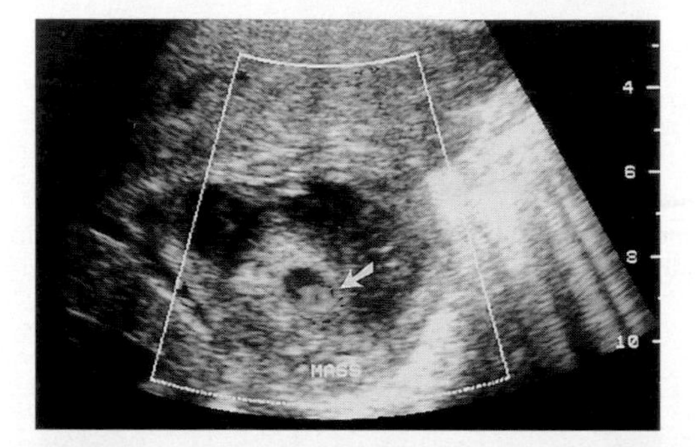

Figure 4. Black and white print of colour Doppler ultrasound showing flow in lumen (arrowed) surrounded by thrombus.

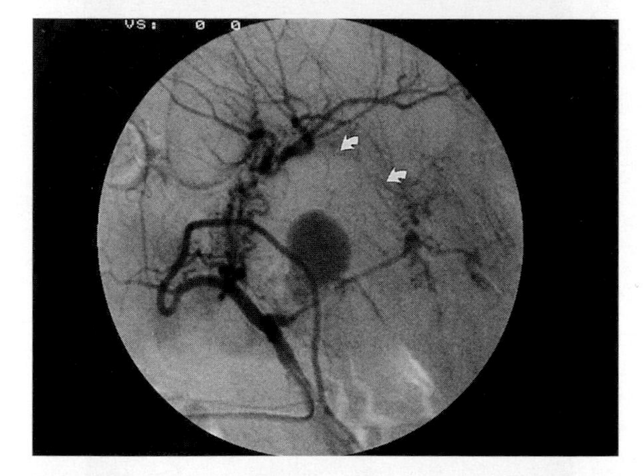

Figure 5. Digital subtraction angiogram showing lumen of pseudoaneurysm filling via a jet from the left hepatic artery. Note the surrounding avascular area representing thrombus (arrowed). The proximal segment of the right hepatic artery is replaced by collaterals.

The triad of upper abdominal pain (70% of cases), gastrointestinal haemorrhage (60%) and jaundice (50%) is seen in 30% of cases with hepatic pseudoaneurysm formation [1] and, particularly with the prior history of trauma, should give a strong clue to the diagnosis. Trauma is nowadays the most common aetiological factor for development of hepatic pseudoaneurysms [2]. This can be blunt or penetrating non-iatrogenic trauma or iatrogenic following hepatobiliary surgery, liver biopsies or percutaneous interventional procedures [2, 3]. In this case, with the absence of any direct abdominal trauma, an acceleration–deceleration type injury sustained during the fall is likely to have damaged the hepatic artery bifurcation leading to thrombosis of the right hepatic artery and partial avulsion of the left hepatic artery with pseudoaneurysm formation. Less common aetiologies are atherosclerosis [1, 4] and mycotic aneurysms [5].

Jaundice is most commonly due to extrinsic biliary compression although in a minority of cases may result from blood clot in the biliary tree. Haemobilia, due to rupture into the biliary tree, is normally torrential if it presents soon after injury. Haemobilia occurring late, *i.e.* weeks, months or even years after injury usually presents with recurrent melaena [2]. Occasionally, rupture into the portal system occurs with portal hypertension and variceal bleeding [2]. Colour Doppler ultrasound clearly defines the nature and size of the pseudoaneurysm [3]. Angiography helps map the vascular anatomy particularly as a prelude to selective arterial embolization, the treatment of choice in most cases [2].

References

1. McEwan-Alvarando G, Villarreal HR, Broders AC Jr, et al. Aneurysm of the hepatic artery. An unusual case of obstructive jaundice. Am J Dig Dis 1967;12:509–14.
2. Rosch J, Petersen BD, Hall LD, Ivancev K. Interventional treatment of hepatic arterial and venous pathology: a commentary. Cardiovasc Interven Radiol 1990;13:183–8.
3. Hutchinson CE, Mackinlay JY, Buckels JA. Pseudoaneurysm of transplant hepatic artery: a late presentation. Br J Radiol 1993;66:158–60.
4. Mehnert PJ, Freeman LM. Obstructive jaundice caused by hepatic artery aneurysm demonstration by radionuclide imaging techniques. J Nucl Med 1971;12:761–2.
5. Mojab K, Lim LT, Esfahani F, Portela L. Mycotic aneurysm of the hepatic artery causing obstructive jaundice. AJR 1977;128:143–4.

A painful red eye

A C DOWNIE, D C HOWLETT and A K BANERJEE

Department of Radiology, St Thomas' Hospital, Lambeth Palace Road, London SE1 7EH, UK

A 31-year-old Gurkha living in Nepal was referred with a 4 month history of worsening redness, swelling and pain affecting both eyes, mainly the right. On examination he was pyrexial and had gross right-sided proptosis and periorbital oedema. Visual acuity was normal.

The initial diagnosis was of cavernous sinus thrombosis, complicated by a Group B Streptococcal orbital cellulitis and septicaemia, the latter having been cultured from his blood. He failed to show any improvement on appropriate antibiotic therapy. Further investigations included CT and MRI of the orbits (Figure 1). Biopsies were also taken from the right ethmoid sinus and post-nasal space.

What do the images show? What is the differential diagnosis? Dramatic improvement rapidly followed a single form of intervention. What was it?

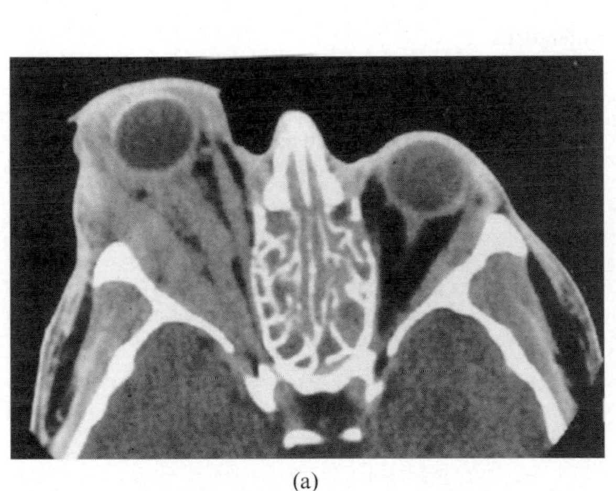

(a)

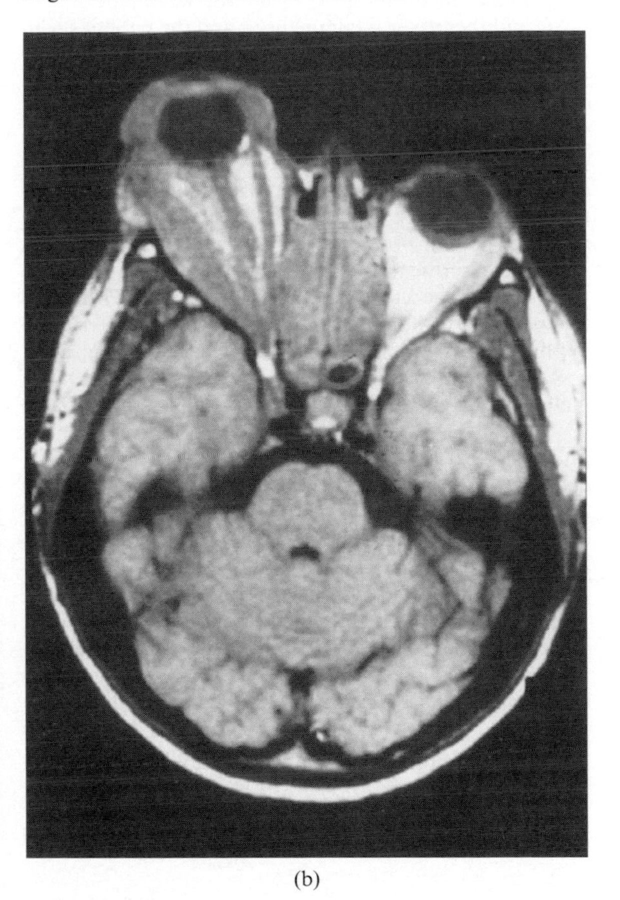

(b)

Figure 1. (a) Axial CT scan of the orbits. (b) Axial MRI scan of the orbits.

Based on the case of the month originally published in Br J Radiol 1995;68:1131–2.

Axial CT showed severe right-sided proptosis and extensive soft tissue behind the orbit involving the optic nerve and extraocular muscles, predominantly on the right. In addition there was soft tissue in the ethmoid sinuses.

Axial T_1 weighted MRI scans through the orbit again demonstrated the right-sided proptosis with extensive peri- and retro-orbital soft tissue replacing the bright signal of normal retrobulbar fat (compare the other eye). Coronal MRI demonstrated normal cavernous sinuses.

The differential diagnosis of an orbital mass includes orbital pseudotumour, lymphoma, primary or metastatic orbital tumours, sarcoidosis, Wegener's granulomatosis, thyroid ophthalmopathy, cavernous sinus fistula and local inflammation [1].

The histology showed a chronic inflammatory infiltrate including plasma cells, lymphocytes and histiocytes with no evidence of malignancy, and a diagnosis of granulomatous orbital pseudotumour was made.

Steroid therapy was commenced and the patient's condition improved dramatically, as demonstrated by the repeat CT scan performed 7 days later (Figure 2).

Orbital pseudotumour is an idiopathic inflammatory condition of the orbit for which no other local or systemic cause can be found [1]. It usually presents with an acute painful proptosis, with or without diplopia. It was first described by Birch-Hirschfield [2]. The same pathological process can be seen in the superior orbital fissure or cavernous sinus where it may give rise to painful ophthalmoplegia or Tolosa-Hunt syndrome.

Radiological features seen in orbital pseudotumour include an orbital mass (which often enhances with intravenous contrast medium), infiltration of retrobulbar fat, proptosis, extraocular muscle enlargement, apical fat oedema, muscle tendon and sheath enlargement, and optic nerve thickening [1]. The absence of bony erosion or paranasal sinus involvement favours pseudotumour, although both can occur in this condition, and intracranial extension has also been reported occasionally.

Where extraocular muscle thickening is present, the main differential diagnosis is thyroid ophthalmopathy. In the latter condition the muscles, usually inferior and medial rectus, show fusiform enlargement with sharply defined borders, whereas in pseudotumour the infiltration is irregular and poorly defined, and involves the tendinous insertions into the globe.

It has been claimed that the CT features can reliably differentiate pseudotumour from other conditions and

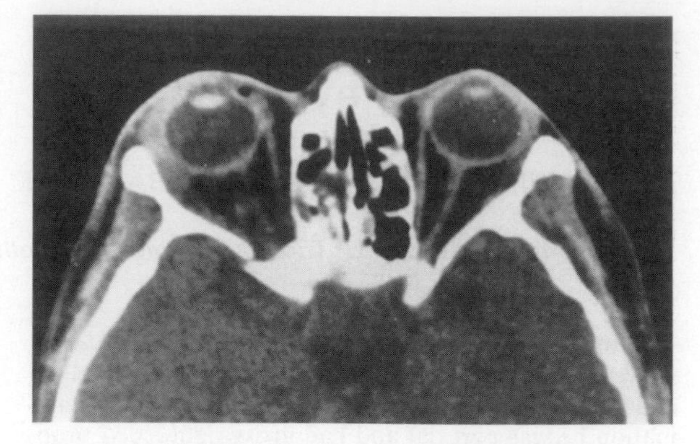

Figure 2. Axial CT scan of the orbits 7 days later.

that biopsy is hazardous [3]. However, this is doubtful largely because lymphoma in particular is often indistinguishable from pseudotumour without biopsy, and both conditions may be steroid responsive initially but require different management [4]. To complicate this further, lymphoma may also arise in histologically proven pseudotumour.

Histology of the lesion varies from a mixture of polymorphs, granulation tissue, plasma cells and histiocytes to a predominantly lymphocytic form which may in its chronic form be pre-malignant.

Traditionally, the condition is said to respond dramatically to steroids. However, the diffuse and extensive variety in particular may respond poorly or relapse, requiring immunosuppressive therapy or radiotherapy, and may result in a "frozen orbit". [*See also Hardman et al [5] for a description of MR findings in orbital pseudotumour, ED*]

References

1. Flanders AE, Mafee MF, Rao VM, Choi KH. CT characteristics of orbital pseudotumours and other orbital inflammatory processes. JCAT 1989;13:40–7.
2. Birch-Hirschfield A. Zur diagnostik und pathologie der orbitaltumoren. Deutsche Ophthalmologische Gesellschaft 1905;32:127–35.
3. McNicholas MMJ, Power WJ, Griffin JF. Idiopathic inflammatory pseudotumour of the orbit: CT features correlated with clinical outcome. Clin Radiol 1991;44:3–7.
4. Westacott S, Garner A, Moseley IF, Wright JE. Orbital lymphoma *versus* reactive lymphoid hyperplasia: an analysis of the use of computed tomography in differential diagnosis. Br J Ophthalmol 1991;75:722–5.
5. Hardman JA, Halpins FS, Mars S, et al. MRI of idiopathic orbital inflammatory syndrome using fat saturation and Gd-DTPA. Neuroradiol 1995;37:475–8.

A clinical red herring

C R MURCH and A J NEWMAN TAYLOR

Royal Brompton National Heart and Lung Hospital, Sydney Street, London SW3 6NP, UK

A previously healthy 16-year-old schoolboy was admitted to hospital with a 4-month history of increasing shortness of breath, which had followed a sore throat. 2 months later, he was short of breath after climbing stairs and hills, and was unable to participate in sports. He had no previous medical history other than migrainous headaches. Both of his parents had had sarcoidosis, although neither had received treatment. At the time of his hospital admission he seemed a fit young man without abnormal physical signs. His chest radiograph raised the possibility of prominent hila but CT showed no enlarged hila or mediastinal lymph nodes. He was discharged from hospital and remained stable for 2 months after which he became increasingly short of breath over a period of 2 days. He was referred and admitted to this hospital.

On examination at this time, he was cyanosed both centrally and peripherally; he had a pulse rate of 120/min and a blood pressure of 120/60 with a fourth heart sound and a raised jugular venous pressure. He had end inspiratory crackles audible over the bases of both lungs.

Investigations showed him to be hypoxic with a respiratory alkalosis (pO_2 7.20 kPa (54 mmHg), pCO_2 1.93 kPa (14 mmHg), pH 7.55, HCO_3 12.6 mmol l^{-1}) breathing 28% oxygen. Lung function tests showed a mixed mild obstructive and restrictive defect without response to inhaled bronchodilator with reduced carbon monoxide transfer. The serum angiotensin converting enzyme was normal. Bronchoscopy was normal and bronchoalveolar lavage had a normal cell count. His ECG showed "p" pulmonale, right axis deviation with tall *R* waves and ST depression between V1 and V4, changes consistent with right ventricular hypertrophy.

His chest radiograph at the time of this admission with enlargement of the right base is shown in Figures 1 and 2. What radiological abnormalities are present and what is the most probable diagnosis?

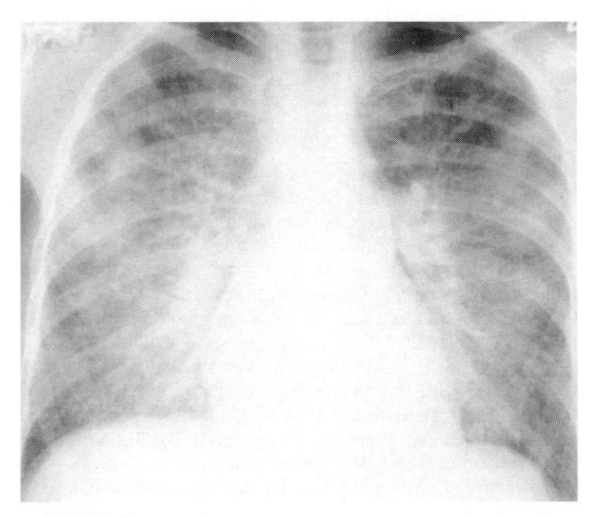

Figure 1. PA chest radiograph.

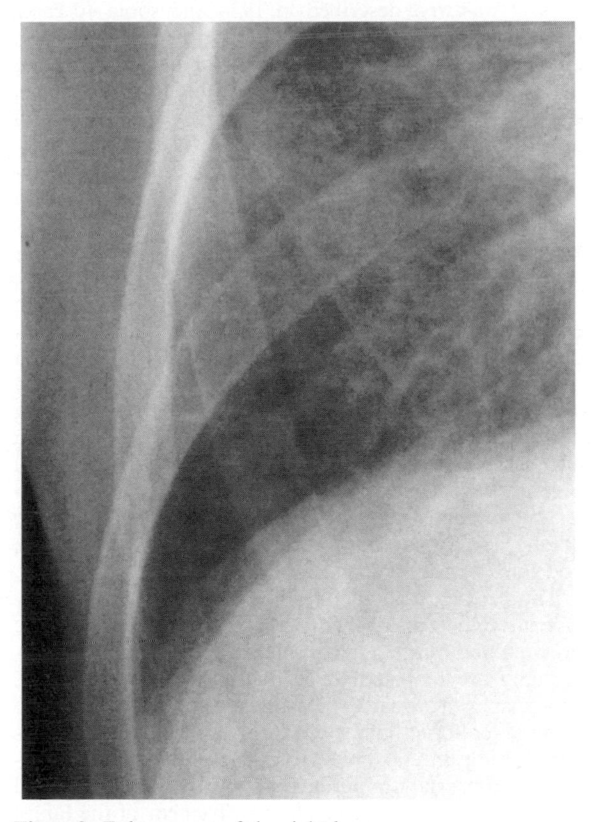

Figure 2. Enlargement of the right base.

Based on the case of the month originally published in Br J Radiol 1991;64:637–8.

His hypoxia became more severe despite increasing concentrations of inspired oxygen. On the third day of his admission the patient arrested and died.

At post-mortem there was patchy congestion of the lungs with septal oedema and dilated lymphatics. Haemosiderin was present within the alveolar septa, macrophages and in elastic tissue. Medium sized pulmonary arteries were hypertrophied. Almost all pulmonary veins showed partial or complete occlusion by intimal fibroelastic tissue. Multiple lumina within veins suggested recanalization of organizing thrombus. There was marked right ventricular hypertrophy. The findings were those of pulmonary veno-occlusive disease (PVOD).

The chest radiograph showed enlargement of the proximal pulmonary arteries with fine hazy shadowing throughout both mid and lower zones, mainly centrally within the lungs, sparing the periphery, best seen in the left lung. Interstitial (Kerley "B") lines were present at the bases (Figure 2).

The diagnosis of PVOD is suggested by the combination of pulmonary oedema and pulmonary arterial hypertension in the absence of mitral valve disease. PVOD was first described in 1934 and some 40 cases have since been reported. It predominantly occurs in children and young adults, the youngest recorded case being an infant of 8 weeks and the oldest a woman of 67 years. More than one half of reported cases have been aged below 20 years.

This case demonstrates the features of PVOD very well. Progressive exertional dyspnoea is a constant symptom variably accompanied by cyanosis, orthopnoea, syncope, dizziness, clubbing and haemoptysis. On examination, crackles in the lungs owing to pulmonary oedema and signs of pulmonary arterial hypertension may be found. Hypoxia, hypocapnia and respiratory alkalosis are also typical. The chest radiograph showing pulmonary arterial hypertension, pulmonary oedema and septal lines, without evidence of raised left atrial pressure associated with ECG changes of right ventricular hypertrophy and "strain", are characteristic. The diagnosis may be confirmed by cardiac catheterization and lung biopsy.

The cardiac catheter findings of marked pulmonary arterial hypertension with a normal capillary wedge pressure and pulmonary oedema on the plain chest radiography are reported to be diagnostic of PVOD [1]. This paper advocates measuring the wedge pressure using a balloon floatation catheter, as measurements taken using an end hole catheter are unreliable in pulmonary arterial hypertension owing to peripheral arterial occlusion. The patchy involvement of the lungs, present in this case, is a frequent finding [2] and can be offset by taking repeated readings in different segments of lung.

Histological examination of the lungs shows narrowing or occlusion of pulmonary veins and venules by intimal fibrosis. Recent thrombus in various stages of organization occurs occasionally but recanalization is frequently seen, causing eccentricity of the lumen and the presence of intraluminal fibrous septa. Larger pulmonary veins may be involved and venous arterialization may occur. Patches of oedema, haemorrhage (where haemosiderin is often present) and interstitial fibrosis may also occur in the lungs [3]. Interstitial pneumonitis and hypertrophy of mucous glands and goblet cells have also been reported [4].

The aetiology of PVOD is unknown and may result from a variety of causes. Pulmonary venous endothelium contains less plasminogen activator than endothelium elsewhere in the circulation. It is postulated that any inhibition of this may result in a greater tendency to thrombosis. An infective agent, such as a virus, is believed by many to be the cause, although none has yet been isolated. Many of the patients describe a flu-like illness prior to the onset of symptoms. In addition, some of the histological changes, interstitial pneumonitis and mucous cell hypertrophy are also found during infections [4]. Several cases of PVOD occurring in siblings have been described and this would suggest a genetically determined predisposition [3]. At least three cases have been associated with Raynaud's disease. All were women, aged between 46 years and 67 years, the oldest group of patients with this disease. In one of these patients immune complexes were identified in the alveolar wall, possibly activating clotting factors or platelets [5]. This patient was treated with azothioprine with improvement in her disease. With the exception of this one patient, treatment with corticosteroids, anticoagulants, antibiotics and vasodilator drugs have all failed to alter the invariably fatal outcome of this disease.

The patient presented here, on initial assessment, was diagnosed as suffering from sarcoidosis, owing largely to his strong family history and absence of physical signs to suggest otherwise. Subsequently, this diagnosis became untenable; however, correct diagnosis at an earlier stage of the disease is unlikely to have altered the final outcome. [*An interesting case report on this subject is by Cassart et al [6], showing CT findings, ED*]

References

1. Rambihar VS, Fallen EL, Cairns JA. Pulmonary veno-occlusive disease: antemortem diagnosis from roentgenographic and hemodynamic findings. Can Med Assoc J 1979;120:1519–22.
2. Thadani U, Burrow C, Whitaker W, Heath D. Pulmonary veno-occlusive disease. Q J Med New Series XLIV 1975; 173:133–59.
3. Hasleton PS, Ironside JW, Wittaker JS, Kelly W, Ward C, Thompson GS. Pulmonary veno-occlusive disease. A report of four cases. Histopathol 1986;10:933–44.
4. Wagenvoort CA. Pulmonary veno-occlusive disease. Entity or syndrome? Chest 1976;69:82–6.
5. Sanderson JE, Spiro SG, Hendry AT, Turner-Warwick M. A case of pulmonary veno-occlusive disease responding to treatment with azothioprine. Thorax 1977;32:140–8.
6. Cassart M, Gevenois PA, Kramer M, et al. Pulmonary veno-occlusive disease: CT findings before and after single-lung transplantation. AJR 1993;160:759–60.

A pain in the neck

M E MURRAY and C HERON

Department of Radiology, St George's Hospital, Blackshaw Road, London SW17 0QT, UK

A 29-year-old woman presented with persistent neck pain for 1 week, following a road traffic accident in which she had sustained a whiplash injury. On examination, all movements of the neck were slightly restricted by pain, but there was no local tenderness and neurological examination was normal. Anteroposterior, lateral and left oblique radiographs of the cervical spine are shown and certain features marked with arrows (Figures 1–3).

What is your provisional diagnosis and how would you confirm it?

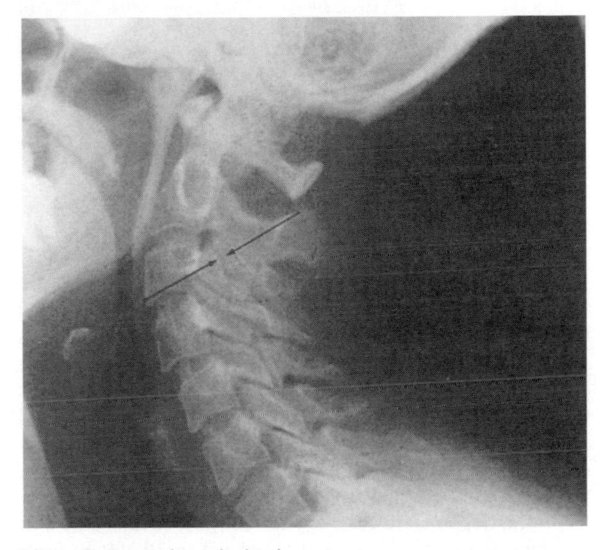

Figure 2. Lateral cervical spine.

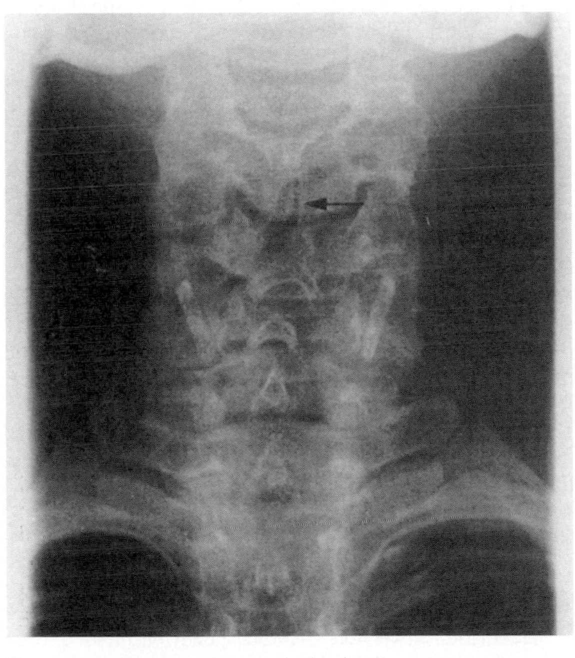

Figure 1. Anteroposterior cervical spine.

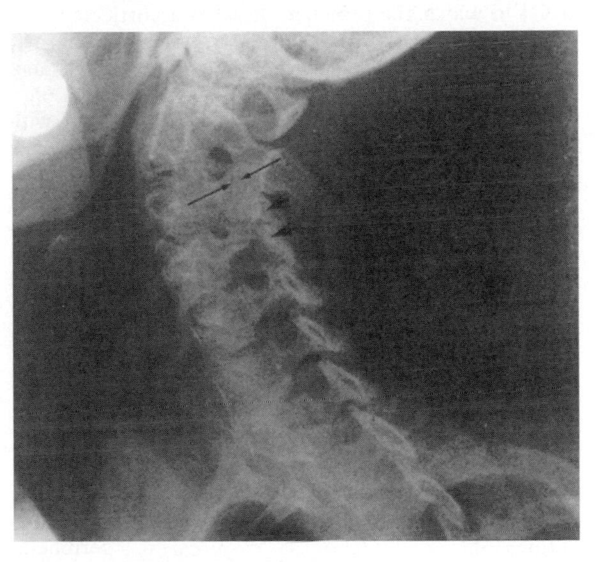

Figure 3. Left oblique cervical spine.

Based on the case of the month originally published in Br J Radiol 1995;68:931–2.

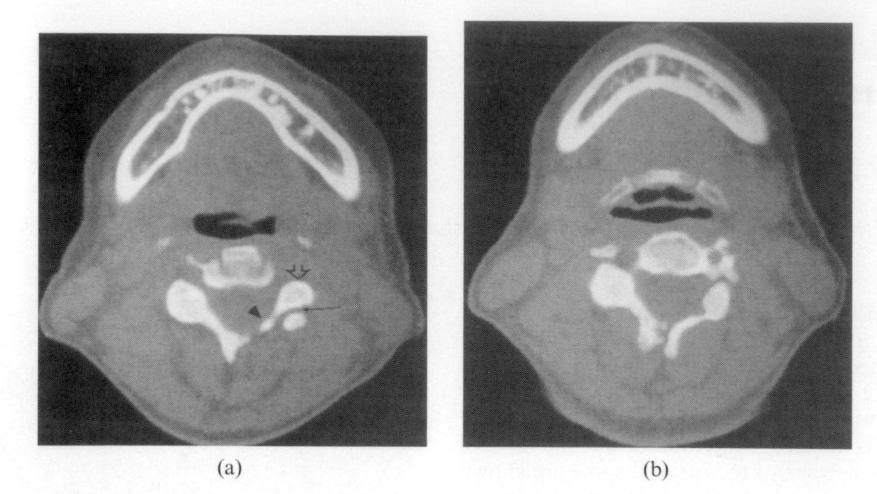

(a) (b)

Figure 4. (a) Axial scan through the body of C3. (b) Axial scan through the body of C4.

Figure 1 is of the anteroposterior cervical spine and showed spina bifida occulta of C4 (arrow). Figure 2 shows the lateral cervical spine. The arrows outline a vertical cleft with well corticated margins separating the superior and inferior facets of C3. The articular masses at C3 and C4 were deformed. The left oblique cervical spine is shown in Figure 3. The vertical cleft is again outlined (long arrows) and lies behind the left pedicle of C3. The left laminae at C3 and C4 (short arrows) were hypoplastic, as were the pedicles at these levels. The exit foramen between C3 and C4 appeared small. These findings are characteristic of unilateral cervical spondylolysis at C3 in which the principal defect is a corticated cleft within the articular pillar between the superior and inferior facets (the equivalent of the pars interarticularis in the lumbar spine).

Cervical spondylolysis is frequently associated with spina bifida occulta, hypoplastic pedicle and dysplastic lamina at the same level with or without dysplastic posterior elements in adjacent vertebrae [1]. This diagnosis was confirmed with axial CT through C3 and C4 (Figure 4).

Figure 4a is an axial scan through the body of C3 and the well corticated cleft in the articular pillar is clearly seen (long arrow). The left lateral mass and lamina (open arrow and arrowhead, respectively) are hypoplastic. Figure 4b is an axial scan through the body of C4. There is spina bifida occulta and the left lateral mass and lamina are again hypoplastic. The unilateral hypoplastic posterior elements at C3 and C4 have allowed a degree of axial rotation giving the impression of a small left exit foramen between these vertebrae, as seen on the oblique radiograph.

Cervical spondylolysis is an uncommon finding, first described in 1951 [2]. The commonly associated findings of dysplastic posterior elements and spina bifida occulta favour a congenital origin. There appears to be a spectrum of congenital anomalies affecting the cervical spine which includes another unusual but well recognized defect: absence of the cervical pedicle, which is itself associated with dysplasia of the ipsilateral lamina and transverse process [3]. It has been postulated that spondylolysis occurs when two chondrification centres on one side of the neural arch fail to fuse into a single ossification centre and that the absent pedicle occurs when there is total failure of development of one chondrification centre [4]. There are two reported cases of spondylolysis combined with absent pedicle [2, 5].

Cervical spondylolysis has been described at all levels except C7 [1] and may be unilateral as in this case or bilateral in which case spondylolisthesis may occur. It may also affect two levels simultaneously. Forsberg et al [1] report seven cases of cervical spondylolysis which were originally misdiagnosed as unilateral facet dislocation or fracture of the articular pillar. Features in favour of congenital spondylolysis include: (1) Absence of soft tissue swelling and of neurological signs. (2) Well corticated, smooth spondylolytic defect. (3) The presence of associated features such as spina bifida occulta and hypoplastic posterior elements at the same or adjacent levels.

Awareness of this condition and its typical associated features on both plain film and CT will reduce the potential for misdiagnosis and inappropriate treatment.

References

1. Forsberg DA, Martinez S, Vogler III JB, Wiener MD. Cervical spondylolysis: imaging findings in 12 patients. AJR 1990;154:751–5.
2. Perlman R, Hawes LE. Cervical spondylolisthesis. J Bone Joint Surg 1951;33A:1012–3.
3. Wiener MD, Martinex S, Forsberg DA. Congenital absence of a cervical spine pedicle. AJR 1990;155:1037–40.
4. Schwartz AM, Wechsler RJ, Merric DL, et al. Posterior arch defects of the cervical spine. Skeletal Radiol 1982;8:135–9.
5. Gehweiler JA, Martinez S, Clark WM, et al. Spondylolisthesis of the axis vertebra. AJR 1977;128:682.

Executive distress

R NOVELL, G STANSBY and R DICK

Academic Department of Surgery and Department of Radiology, The Royal Free Hospital School of Medicine, London NW3, UK

A 35-year-old sales executive presented with a history of abdominal discomfort and distention of 2 months duration. Systematic enquiry revealed an increased frequency of bowel action and vague dyspepsia over the same period. Examination showed a poorly defined mass extending from the periumbilical region to the right iliac fossa. Abdominal ultrasound demonstrated ascites but was unhelpful in further characterizing the mass. CT of the abdomen was then performed (Figures 1 and 2). What does this show and what diagnosis would account for these appearances?

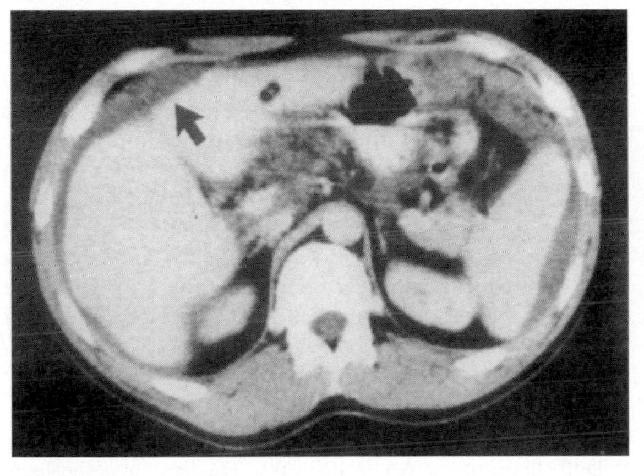

Figure 1. CT.

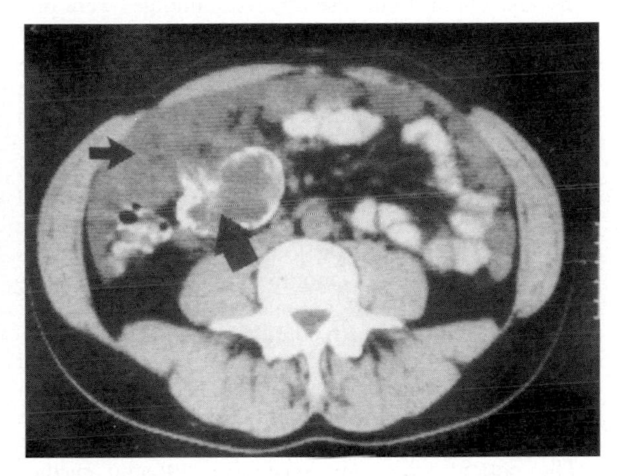

Figure 2. CT.

Based on the case of the month originally published in Br J Radiol 1991;64:67–8.

The upper cut of the CT scan, at the level of the lower border of T12, showed a soft tissue mass of low attenuation adjacent to the left lobe of the liver. Indenting or "scalloping" of the liver margin by the mass was seen (Figure 1, arrow). On the lower cut, at the level of L4, a rim of soft tissue of similar density to the extrahepatic mass was seen anterior to the small bowel which contained oral contrast material. Posterior to the mass, and continuous with it, was a calcified cystic structure 5 cm in diameter (Figure 2, arrow). A large volume of ascites was present.

The patient underwent laparotomy 5 days later. At operation the peritoneal cavity was filled with mucoid ascites. Multiple nodules of tumour extended over the entire visceral and parietal peritoneum. The anterior mass shown on CT proved to be a multiloculated semicystic tumour involving the omentum and ascending and transverse colon. Four discrete cystic nodules were present in the mesentery of the terminal ileum. The largest measured 5 cm in diameter and was calcified, corresponding to the CT appearances. An extended right hemicolectomy and omentectomy were performed and the abdomen repeatedly lavaged with distilled water.

Histology showed a moderately differentiated mucinous adenocarcinoma involving the omentum and serosal peritoneum. No intrinsic abnormality of the ileal, colonic or appendiceal mucosa was found. The mesenteric cysts were found to consist of smooth muscle, lined by columnar epithelium. Three contained mucus and cellular debris only, but the fourth contained invasive adenocarcinoma identical to that in the resected mass. The final diagnosis was pseudomyxoma peritonei in association with mucinous adenocarcinoma arising in an enteric duplication cyst.

The patient was commenced on systemic chemotherapy with mitomycin C and 5-fluorouracil postoperatively; this was later changed to oral chlorambucil. He has returned to work and remains well 21 months following surgery. Repeated ultrasound scans have shown no evidence of recurrent tumour.

Ileal duplication cysts are a rare congenital anomaly. They are usually asymptomatic but may be complicated by recurrent abdominal pain, perforation or bleeding, particularly if lined by heterotopic gastric mucosa [1]. Intussusception may occur if the cyst is closely associated with the bowel wall, and such cysts tend to present early in life. They are occasionally, as in this case, multiple [2]. Malignant change in a duplication cyst is a very uncommon event [3, 4].

Pseudomyxoma peritonei is characterized by massive gelatinous ascites and "studding" of the visceral and parietal peritoneum by mucinous nodules. It most commonly arises from neoplasms of the ovary and appendix [5], although a few reported cases have arisen from true mucocoele of the appendix. Very uncommonly it may be associated with other adenocarcinomas of gut origin. There has been one previous report of pseudomyxoma in association with heterotopic gastric mucosa from ileal duplication cysts [1]. The presentation is characteristically insidious, and the diagnosis most frequently made at operation. Common symptoms are abdominal discomfort and distension, and a mass is often palpable abdominally. Plain abdominal radiographs may show characteristic "eggshell" calcification surrounding encysted mucinous collections. CT typically demonstrates ascites, low attenuation areas with calcified margins, and displacement or compression of the abdominal viscera. Visceral invasion is not seen [6].

Pseudomyxoma spreads exclusively by the transcoelomic route and appears to have little or no tendency to metastasize to distant sites. The natural history of the disease varies widely and patients may remain relatively asymptomatic for many years, but the eventual prognosis is poor with a 10-year survival of under 20% [5]. Surgery is usually palliative, although a favourable response has been reported with radical surgery combined with intraperitoneal chemotherapy [7], with five out of seven patients apparently disease free after 2–4 years.

References

1. Duffy G, Enriquez AA, Watson WC. Duplication of the ileum with heterotopic gastric mucosa, pseudomyxoma peritonei and nonrotation of the midgut. Gastroenterol 1974;67:341–6.
2. Forshall I. Duplications of the intestinal tract. Postgrad Med J 1961;37:570–89.
3. Orr MM, Edwards AJ. Neoplastic change in duplications of the alimentary tract. Br J Surg 1975;62:269–74.
4. Smith JHF, Hope PG. Carcinoid tumour arising in a cystic duplication of the small bowel. Arch Pathol Lab Med 1985;109:95–6.
5. Fernandez R, Daly J. Pseudomyxoma peritonei. Arch Surg 1980;115:409–14.
6. Lee HH, Agha FP, Weatherbee L, Boland CR. Pseudomyxoma peritonei: radiologic features. J Clin Gastroenterol 1986;8:312–6.
7. Sugerbaker PH, Kern K, Lack E. Malignant pseudomyxoma peritonei of colonic origin; natural history and presentation of a curative approach to treatment. Dis Colon Rectum 1987;30:772–9.

A painful knee

A M DAVIES and N EVANS

Department of Radiology, Royal Orthopaedic Hospital, Birmingham, UK

A 37-year-old Asian woman presented with a 10 month history of periodic pain in the lateral aspect of the right knee, becoming more severe over the past 2 weeks. Plain radiography is shown (Figure 1). A bone scan showed a solitary, uniform focus of increased activity corresponding to the abnormality on the radiographs. CT was performed (Figure 2). All routine laboratory investigations were normal.

What is the differential diagnosis and what is the most likely diagnosis in this patient?

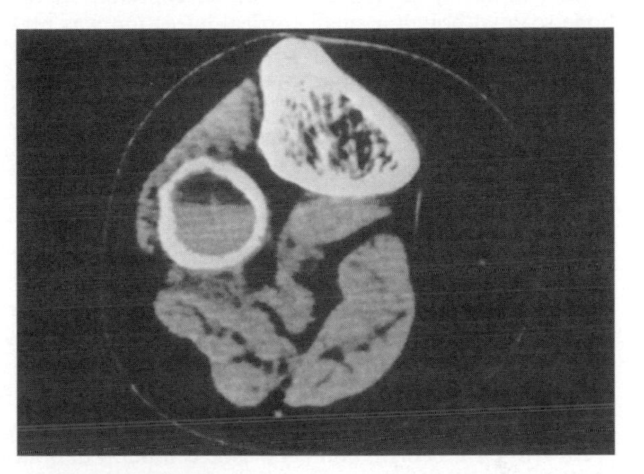

Figure 2. Axial CT scan through the proximal tibia and fibula.

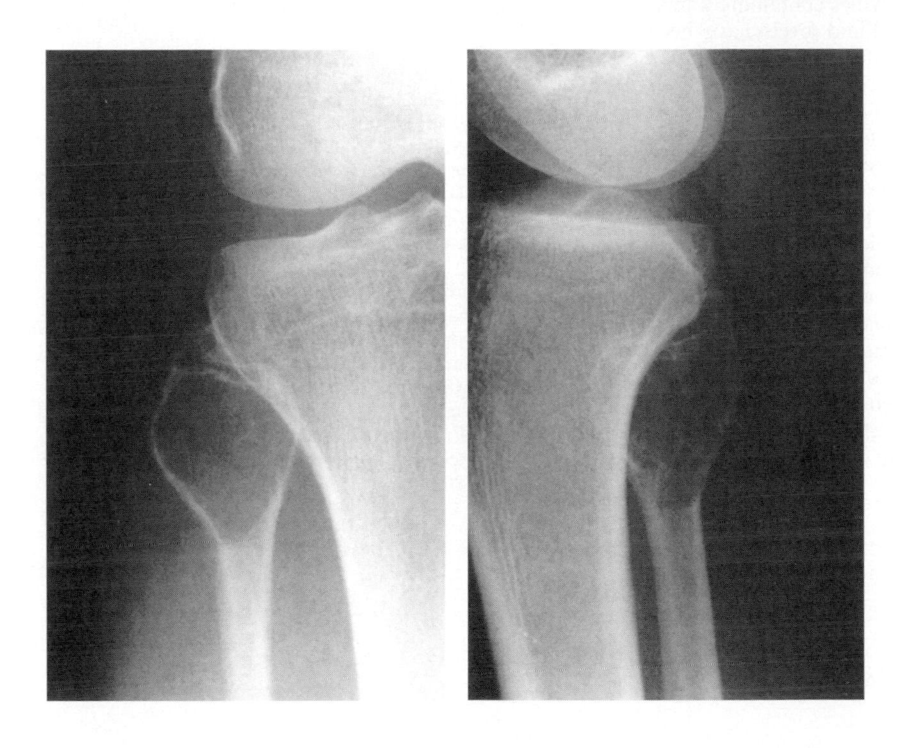

Figure 1. (a) Anteroposterior and (b) lateral radiographs of the head of the fibula.

Based on the case of the month originally published in Br J Radiol 1989;62:1103–4.

Plain radiography showed an expansile, lytic lesion in the head of the fibula, which had a well defined margin with a small cortical infraction posteriorly. CT demonstrated the expansile nature of the lesion.

The differential diagnosis of an expansile, lytic lesion in the head of the fibula includes a giant cell tumour, aneurysmal bone cyst, simple bone cyst, enchondroma and a brown tumour.

The patient was rather old to present with a simple bone cyst and little activity would be expected on the bone scan, although a small cortical infraction was present. The absence of calcification within the matrix of the tumour made an enchondroma less likely and, although the ethnic origin of the patient should alert one to the possibility of metabolic bone disease, the normal laboratory investigations and bone density excluded a brown tumour.

It was impossible in this case to distinguish on the plain radiographs between a giant cell tumour and an aneurysmal bone cyst. CT, however, showed a fluid level within the tumour, which is a diagnostic feature of an aneurysmal bone cyst (ABC), and was subsequently confirmed histologically in this case.

An ABC is a benign, non-neoplastic condition of bone consisting pathologically of varying amounts of vascular and fibrous tissue surrounding cavities containing a mixture of blood and serous fluid. Fluid levels have been described as a characteristic CT feature of an ABC [1, 2] and are presumed to represent sedimentation of blood within the cystic cavities. The fluid levels may be single in unilocular lesions, as in this case, or multiple in multilocular lesions, as illustrated in a different patient in Figure 3. To demonstrate the fluid level the examination must be performed in a plane perpendicular to the fluid level and the patient should remain motionless for at least 10 min prior to scanning to allow the contents of the cavity to settle [1]. Similar appearances have been described in ABCs imaged with magnetic resonance [3, 4].

Although typical of an ABC, the presence on CT of a fluid level within a bone lesion should not be considered pathognomonic as it has also been described in a telangiectatic osteosarcoma [1], a malignant tumour that also has a large vascular element, but does not have a well defined margin.

Figure 3. Large multilocular lesions in the right iliac bone of a 10-year-old boy showing multiple, small fluid levels within the individual loculi.

The precise aetiology of an ABC is unknown but it is now accepted that a significant proportion of cases, probably in excess of one-third, arise in pre-existing bone lesions. These include fibrous dysplasia [5], giant cell tumour, non-ossifying fibroma, chondroblastoma and osteosarcoma. It is therefore important to appreciate that the identification of a fluid level on CT may be due to a secondary ABC [5], although the underlying primary lesion may not be visible radiographically. [*See the excellent review article by Kransdorf and Sweet [6], ED*]

References

1. Hudson TM. Fluid levels in aneurysmal bone cysts: a CT feature. AJR 1984;142:1001–4.
2. Hertzanu Y, Mendelsohn DB, Gottschalk F. Aneurysmal bone cyst of the calcaneus. Radiology 1984;151:51–2.
3. Hudson TM, Hamlin DJ, Fitzsimmons JR. Magnetic resonance imaging of fluid levels in an aneurysmal bone cyst and in anticoagulated human blood. Skeletal Radiol 1985;13: 267–70.
4. Beltran J, Simon DC, Levy M, Herman L, Weis L, Mueller CF. Aneurysmal bone cysts: magnetic resonance imaging at 1.5 T. Radiology 1986;158:689–90.
5. Diercks RL, Sauter AJM, Mallens WMC. Aneurysmal bone cyst in association with fibrous dysplasia. J Bone Joint Surg 1986;68B:144–6.
6. Kransdorf MJ, Sweet DE. Aneurysmal bone cyst: concept, controversy, clinical presentation and imaging. AJR 1995;164:573–80.

The changing mediastinum

[1]D H REED and [2]S MORGAN

Departments of [1]Radiodiagnosis and [2]Radiotherapy, Addenbrooke's Hospital, Cambridge CB2 2QQ, UK

A 73-year-old man presented with cough and shortness of breath. He was a non-smoker and had no history of previous respiratory problems. 12 months previously a right occipital lobectomy was performed for a Grade IV astrocytoma. At that time his chest radiograph was normal (Figure 1). He had received a post-operative course of cranial irradiation and dexamethasone 2 mg twice daily was commenced. On examination his chest was clear. In view of his symptoms a chest radiograph was requested (Figures 2, 3).

What do the radiographs show and what is the differential diagnosis? How can the problem be resolved?

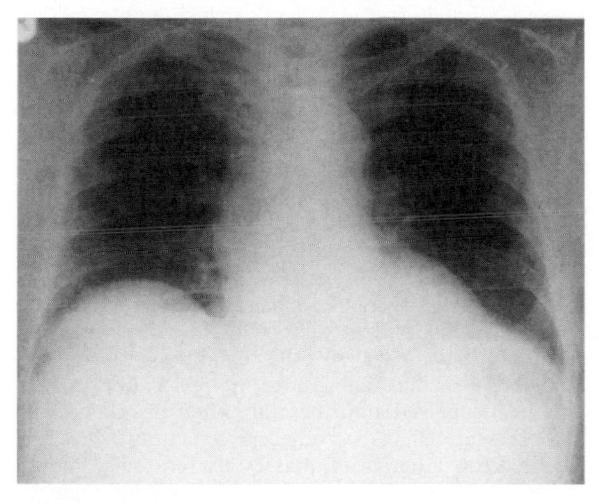

Figure 1. Normal posteroanterior chest radiograph taken 1 year previously.

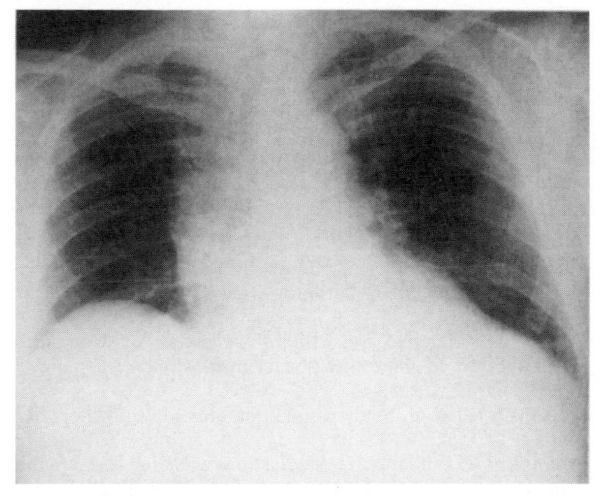

Figure 2. Posteroanterior chest radiograph.

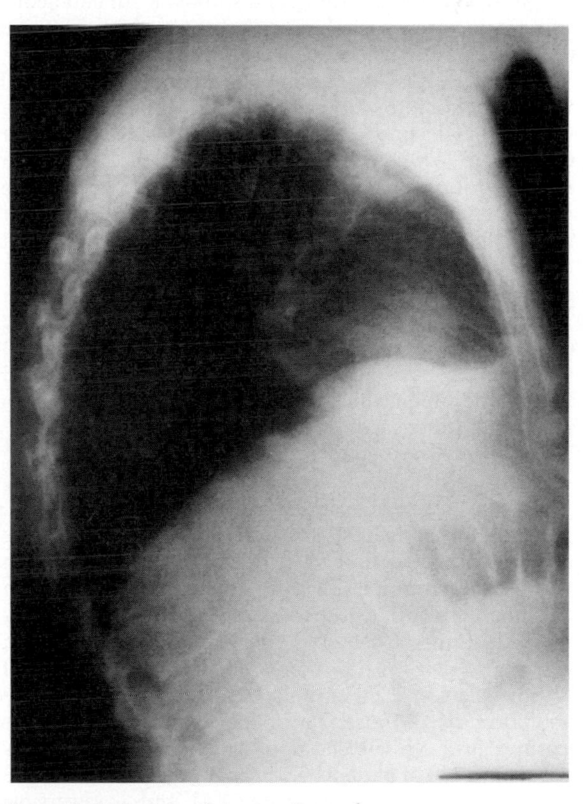

Figure 3. Right lateral chest radiograph.

Based on the case of the month originally published in Br J Radiol 1988;61:695–6.

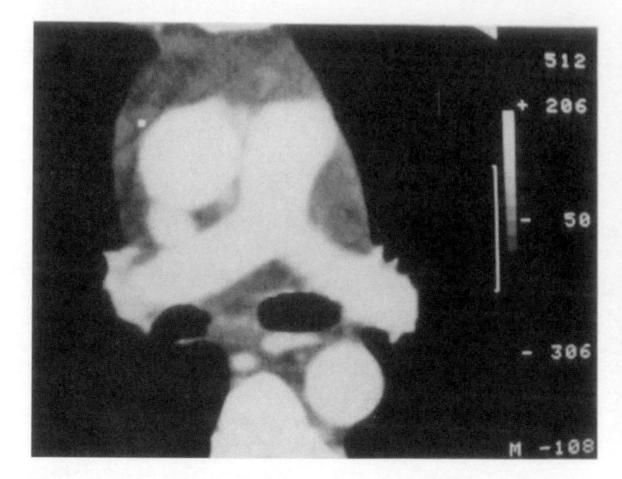

Figure 4. CT of the mediastinum at the level of the bifurcating main pulmonary artery. Fat envelopment of the mediastinal structures is demonstrated. The cursor position shows a Hounsfield number of −108 (level −50, window 512).

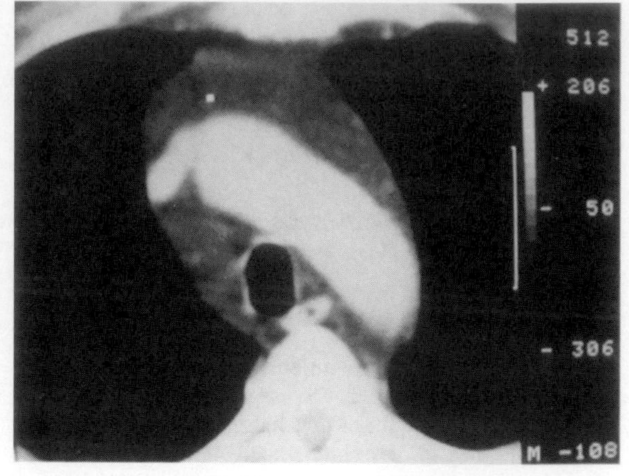

Figure 5. CT at the level of the aortic arch showing fat envelopment (level −50, window 512).

In retrospect, the original radiograph of the chest still appeared to be normal. The recent chest radiograph showed mediastinal widening with a large right paratracheal soft tissue mass. There were prominent epicardial fat pads. The lateral radiograph showed a subcutaneous soft tissue mass posterior to the upper thoracic spine and a crush fracture of a lower dorsal vertebra.

The differential diagnosis of the smooth mediastinal widening should include: widespread lymphadenopathy, mediastinal haemorrhage, mediastinitis, and excess fat deposition. The history of high dose glucocorticoid administration, the presence of epicardial fat, the "buffalo hump", collapsed vertebrae and the absence of a discreet mediastinal mass on the lateral radiograph would lead one to suspect mediastinal lipomatosis secondary to steroid therapy.

Thoracic CT is the next investigation of choice (Figures 4, 5). This demonstrates that the mediastinal widening is due entirely to excess fat (mean −108 Hounsfield units) which is smoothly contoured and surrounds all other mediastinal structures.

Fat is a normal constituent of the mediastinum [1]. Mediastinal lipomatosis refers to the pathological state of excess fat deposition which occurs in association with Cushing's syndrome [2] or simple obesity [3]. In Cushing's syndrome the mediastinal lipomatosis represents another facet of the centripetal fat deposition which also gives rise to the well known appearances of "moon" facies, "lemon-on-sticks" physique and the "buffalo hump". Indeed, our patient demonstrated these features in a classical fashion. Mediastinal lipomatosis occurs in 15% of patients given enough steroids to cause features of Cushing's syndrome [4] and is reversible following steroid cessation.

The radiographic signs of mediastinal widening in conjunction with large epicardial fat pads, retrosternal fat, paravertebral fat, a buffalo hump or supraclavicular fat together with an awareness of the relevant history should allow the diagnosis to be made. CT is useful if diagnostic doubt remains. In mediastinal lipomatosis, a smoothly-contoured diffuse envelopment of the mediastinal structures is seen, as in this patient. Displacement or compression of the airway, oesophagus and major vessels is unusual. In this patient there is slight side-to-side narrowing of the trachea. In other conditions causing low attenuation mediastinal lesions, more localized masses may be recognized, and these are often associated with local pressure effects on adjacent structures. Causes of localized low attenuation masses are teratoma, lipoma, thymolipoma, liposarcoma or fat in a diaphragmatic hernia.

Spread of gliomas beyond the central nervous system is rare [5] but in other malignancies, mediastinal involvement is much more common and its detection has major therapeutic and prognostic implications. The accurate assessment of the mediastinum in cancer patients on steroid therapy is therefore of great importance if the correct diagnosis is to be made.

References

1. Heitzman ER. The mediastinum. In: Radiologic correlations with anatomy and pathology. St Louis: CV Mosby, 1977;16:22–3.
2. Bein ME, Manaiso AA, Mink JH, Hansen GC. Computed tomography in the evaluation of mediastinum lipomatosis. JCAT 1978;2:379–83.
3. Lee WJ, Fattel G. Mediastinal lipomatosis in simple obesity. Chest 1976;70:308–9.
4. Santini LC, Williams JL. Mediastinal widening (presumable lipomatosis) in Cushing's syndrome. New Engl J Med 1971;284:1357–9.
5. Brander WL, Turner DR. Extracranial metastases from a glioma in the absence of surgical intervention. J Neurol Neurosurg Psychiatr 1975;38:1133–5.

The case of the bulging Bulgarian

Z HALPERN, M AVERBUCH, J PAPO, R SHILO and Y LEVO

Departments of Medicine "T" and Radiology, Ichilov Hospital, Tel Aviv Medical Center, Tel Aviv, Israel

A 67-year-old Jewish male born in Bulgaria was admitted because of progressive swelling of the abdomen and both legs. The patient gave a history of recurrent orogenital ulceration, arthralgia and pustular dermatitis for the past 10 years. The relevant physical examination revealed severe oedema of both legs with trophic skin changes and ulcerating stasis dermatitis. He had marked distension of the superficial abdominal veins. There was no evidence of liver disease or ascites. Routine laboratory tests as well as barium examination of the gastrointestinal tract, a chest radiograph and a liver and spleen scan were all normal.

An ultrasound examination (Figure 1) and CT (Figure 2) of the upper abdomen were performed and are illustrated.

What is the clinical diagnosis and what do the investigations show?

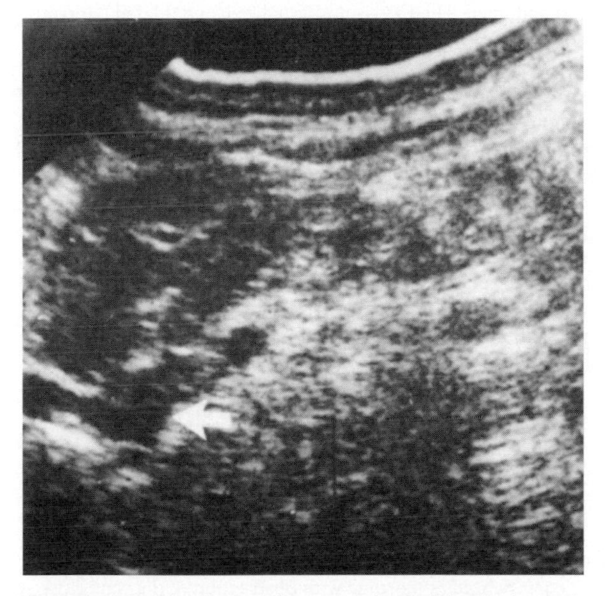

Figure 1. A longitudinal, right parasagittal abdominal scan in the region of the liver.

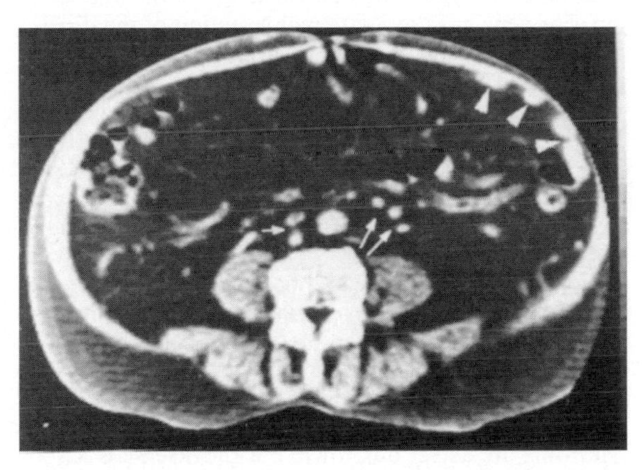

Figure 2. A transverse CT section adjacent to the lower pole of the kidneys, after intravenous contrast medium.

Based on the case of the month originally published in Br J Radiol 1986;59:187–8.

Since Behcet in 1937 described a triad of orogenital ulceration and ocular lesions, a number of additional features have been recognized as part of the complex now known as Behcet's syndrome [1]. These include erythema nodosum, pustular dermatitis, arthritis, neurological disorders and recurrent thrombophlebitis.

The ultrasound study clearly demonstrated complete obstruction of the inferior vena cava (IVC) (arrow) in the presence of a normal liver and spleen, and the absence of ascites. CT showed the non-visualization of the IVC and the superficial subcutaneous (arrowheads) and deep periaortic and paravertebral venous network (long arrows) bypassing the occlusion.

Bilateral femoral venography (Figure 3) showed the collateral venous pathways.

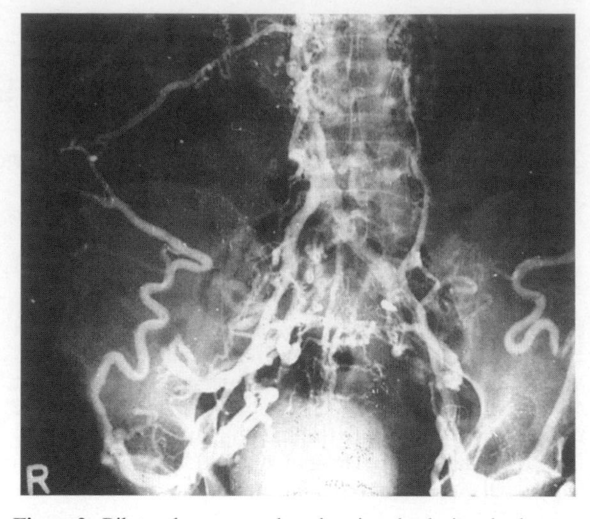

Figure 3. Bilateral venography showing both inguinal areas and abdomen. The IVC is not visualized, and dilated paravertebral and abdominal wall venous collaterals are demonstrated.

Vascular involvement such as recurrent superficial or deep thrombophlebitis is relatively common in Behcet's syndrome [1]. In contrast, obstruction of the inferior or superior vena cava is a rare manifestation of the disease, and only very few cases have been reported in recent years [2, 3]. The true incidence of caval thrombosis is yet to be determined. However, a relatively higher incidence among Jews has been suggested. Until recently the only way of documenting major vein occlusion was by venography. This procedure is obviously associated with all the possible complications of an invasive technique. In Behcet's syndrome the problems associated with venography are greatly increased because of the widespread nature of the vascular involvement. Moreover, the procedure might enhance vascular injury and thrombosis due to the particular vulnerability of the vascular system and the increased coagulability which characterize Behcet's disease. The aetiology and pathogenesis of this syndrome are as yet unknown, but the disease is associated with enhanced chemotaxis of leucocytes and inflammatory response and with decreased fibrinolytic activity [1]. It is well known that relatively severe skin lesions may follow a needle-puncture of the skin in Behcet's disease (the "pin-prick" sign).

In view of these possible risks of venography in Behcet's disease, the need for alternative, non-invasive, imaging techniques is apparent.

In the patient presented here, ultrasound and CT proved to be extremely useful and accurate in establishing the diagnosis of IVC occlusion [*as would MRI, ED*]. We believe that these techniques should replace venography in patients with the presumptive diagnosis of IVC obstruction, especially in Behcet's disease where invasive procedures are contraindicated. Some patients with IVC obstruction will develop the syndrome of hepatic venous hypertension (Budd–Chiari) in which ascites is usually present and which may be associated with Behcet's syndrome. In some of these patients and particularly in those having a web in the IVC, cavography and balloon dilatation may be helpful [4].

References

1. Chajek T, Fainaru M. Behcet's disease. Report of 41 cases and a review of the literature. Medicine 1975;54:179–96.
2. Enoch BA, Costillo-Olivares JL, Khoo TCL, Grainger RG, Henry L. Major vascular complications in Behcet's syndrome. Postgrad Med J 1968;44:453–9.
3. Kansu E, Ozer FL, Akalin E, Guler Y, Zileli T, Tanman E, et al. Behcet's syndrome with obstruction of the vena cava. A report of seven cases. Q J Med 1972;41:151–68.
4. Jeans WD, Bourne JF, Read AE. Treatment of hepatic vein and inferior vena caval obstructions by balloon dilatation. Br J Radiol 1983;56:687–9.

A curious cause of a paediatric abdominal mass

D C HOWLETT, P N MALCOLM and L M MACDONALD

Department of Radiology, St Thomas' Hospital, Lambeth Palace Road, London SE1 7EH, UK

A 4-year-old West Indian girl presented with a 4 day history of fever and upper abdominal pain. On examination she was unwell with a temperature of 39.5°C. She had "beetroot red" palms and the mucous membranes of her mouth and eyes were infected. Small left cervical lymph nodes were palpable. Cardiovascular and respiratory examinations were unremarkable. She was noted to have a tender mass in her right flank accompanied by guarding, but no frank peritonism.

The results of the laboratory investigations were as follows: white-cell count of 18.4×10^9 l^{-1}; liver function tests showed a mild hepatitic picture; and Paul-Bunnell test, hepatitis serology and urinalysis were all negative.

A chest radiograph was normal. An abdominal radiograph (Figure 1) was followed by an ultrasound scan (Figure 2) and then by CT (Figure 3).

What is the abdominal mass? What is the diagnosis and what further investigation should be performed?

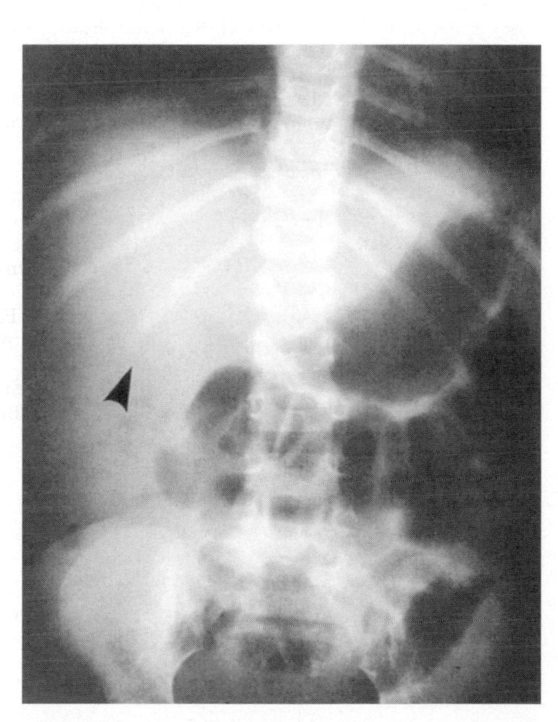

Figure 1. Plain supine abdominal radiograph.

Based on the case of the month originally published in Br J Radiol 1996;69:1075–6.

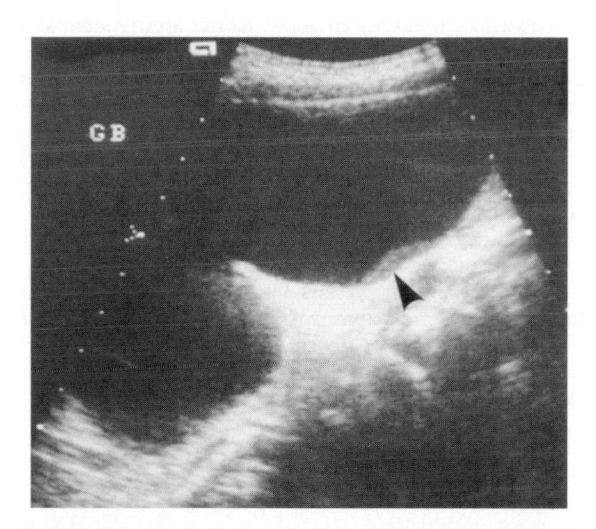

Figure 2. Longitudinal ultrasound scan through the right side of the abdomen.

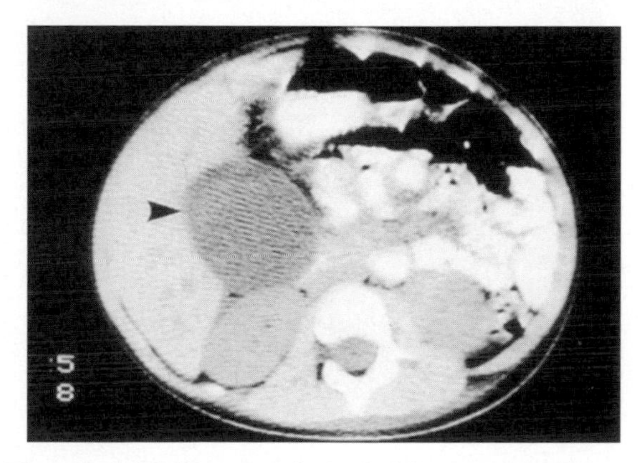

Figure 3. Axial CT scan at the level of the porta hepatis.

The abdominal radiograph showed a soft tissue mass in the right side of the abdomen (Figure 1, arrow). The initial diagnosis was that of an intussusception following a viral illness. Ultrasound of the abdomen showed a large, thin-walled, hypo-echoic mass in the right flank containing a small amount of echogenic debris. The liver, kidneys, spleen and pelvic organs were unremarkable. There was no evidence of either biliary calculi or biliary tree dilatation (Figure 2).

A CT scan confirmed the presence of a thin-walled cystic mass extending from the right subcostal region into the pelvis (Figure 3). No abdominal lymphadenopathy was seen.

The cystic structure represents a huge, distended gallbladder. The diagnosis is Kawasaki disease (mucocutaneous lymph node syndrome) complicated by acute hydrops of the gallbladder. The child should have an echocardiogram to exclude the cardiac abnormalities common in this condition. This was performed soon after admission and was normal.

Kawasaki disease is an acute, febrile multisystem vasculitis. It is rare, with an incidence of one per 100 000 population per year. It occurs in childhood with a peak incidence between 1 and 2 years of age and is more common in males.

The aetiology of the disease is unclear. Recent work has postulated a role for the exotoxin produced by B-haemolytic streptococci. This is thought to act as a superantigen that stimulates the immune system activation associated with the illness [1].

Affected children present with a fever and cutaneous manifestations are prominent [2]. These include a maculopapular rash over extensor surfaces and erythema of palms and soles. Cervical lymphadenopathy and conjunctivitis also occur.

Cardiovascular complications are relatively common. Coronary artery dilatation or aneurysm formation has been reported in up to 40% of patients [3]. Aneurysm formation occurs most frequently in the proximal segment of the left coronary artery. Coronary artery thrombosis occurs in less than 10% of aneurysms which measure 9 mm or more. Pericardial effusion and myocarditis also occur. Other manifestations include a polyarthritis, aseptic meningitis, hepatitis and pneumonitis.

Gallbladder hydrops in association with Kawasaki disease has been well described and often settles with conservative treatment. It is characterized by a massively distended gallbladder and no evidence of stones, inflammation or a congenital anomaly [4]. The cause is unclear, although transient oedema of the cystic duct, or compression of the cystic duct by enlarged lymph nodes may both play a role.

Treatment of Kawasaki disease involves aspirin and high dose gammaglobulin. The use of gammaglobulin early in the illness is thought to reduce the incidence of cardiovascular complications making early recognition of the disease important [5].

References

1. Akiyoma T, Yashiro K. Probable role of streptococcus pyogenes in Kawasaki disease. 1993;152:82–92.
2. Ducos MH, Taieb A, Sarlangue J, et al. Manifestations cutanees de la maladie de Kawasaki. A propos de 30 observations. Ann Dermatol Venereol 1993;120:589–97.
3. Casey F, Craig B, Shanks D, et al. Kawasaki disease—the Northern Ireland experience. Irish J Med Sci 1993;162: 397–400.
4. Hayden KC, Swischuk LE. Liver, gallbladder and bile ducts. In: Paediatric ultrasonography (1st edn). London: Williams & Wilkins, 1987:186–8.
5. Leung DY. Kawasaki disease. Current Opin Rheumatol 1993;5:41–50.

A curious case of pelvic calcification

[1]D J GRIER and [2]G N A SIBLEY

Departments of [1]Clinical Radiology and [2]Urology, Bristol Royal Infirmary, Marlborough Street, Bristol BS2 8HW, UK

A 48-year-old woman complained of chronic dysuria, urinary frequency and incontinence. 20 years previously invasive carcinoma of the cervix had been treated by Wertheim's hysterectomy and radiotherapy (cobalt-60). Between 5200 and 6000 rads tumour dose were administered over 36 days with no immediate complication.

A colostomy was performed 2 years later for colonic obstruction due to a stricture of the rectosigmoid. She subsequently developed bilateral ureteric strictures which required an ileal interposition, the distal end of the ileal segment being anastomosed to the bladder dome. Both of these episodes were ascribed to fibrosis secondary to radiotherapy.

Multiple urine cultures showed persistent growths of proteus and coliform organisms, and urinary pH was frequently raised. During this time there had been several episodes of metabolic acidosis and renal calculi had been treated with lithotripsy. 10 years after this a pneumonectomy was performed for an anaplastic bronchial carcinoma. Her general health was good with no evidence of recurrence of either tumour to date.

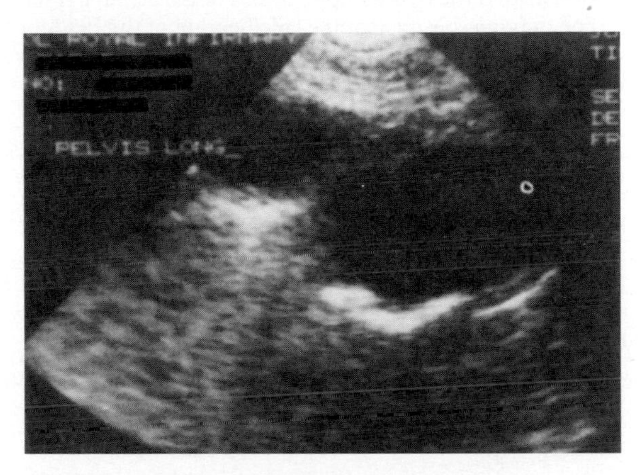

Figure 2. Longitudinal ultrasound scan of the pelvis.

The following investigations were performed in the investigation of her urinary tract (Figures 1–3).

What is the most likely cause for these appearances? What is the most appropriate management?

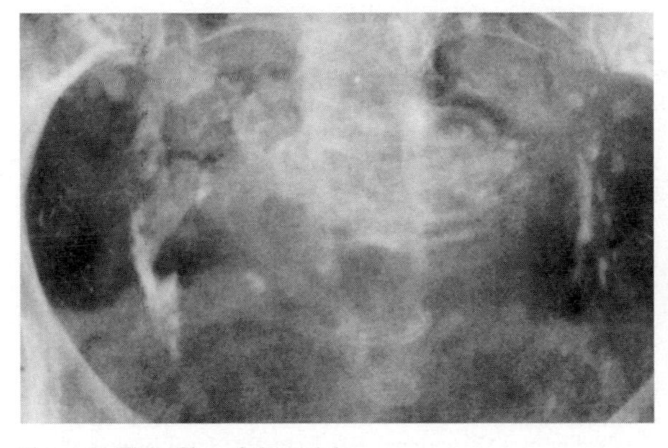

Figure 1. Plain film of the pelvis.

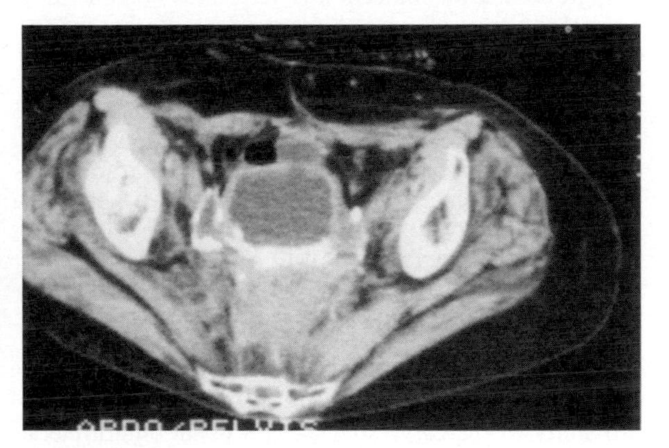

Figure 3. CT of the pelvis.

Based on the case of the month originally published in Br J Radiol 1992;65:945–6.

The plain radiograph (Figure 1) showed extensive calcification within the pelvis. Ultrasound (Figure 2) demonstrated an echogenic posterior bladder wall with distal acoustic shadowing. CT (Figure 3) confirmed extensive calcification, thickening and deformity of the posterior and lateral bladder wall, and also showed paravesical calcification.

Cystoscopy showed a calcareous slough on the posterior bladder wall, some of which could be scraped away only with difficulty. Intravenous urography (Figure 4) demonstrated the overall appearance of the urinary tract.

The diagnosis is dystrophic calcification of the bladder wall due to alkaline encrusting cystitis. In this condition there is deposition of urinary phosphate on the bladder wall, a process facilitated by chronic inflammation and fibrosis of the bladder wall and alkaline urine in which phosphate is less soluble. Infection with proteus spp. is implicated in the aetiology, as it is a urea splitting organism leading to raised urinary pH. This patient had persistent urinary growths of proteus and other organisms. Management of this condition is by acidification and sterilization of the urine. Occasionally cystoscopic removal of adherent calcareous slough is required [1].

This patient has since undergone an ileal conduit urinary diversion in view of persistent infection and troublesome incontinence.

Radiographically visible calcification of the urinary bladder (other than calculi) is rare. Recognized causes include transitional cell carcinoma, schistosomiasis, tuberculosis and cyclophosphamide cystitis [2].

Visible bladder wall calcification in association with non-granulomatous infection is very rare. There is only one other report of a case 6 years after radiotherapy for carcinoma of the cervix [3].

Alkaline encrusting cystitis was a common diagnosis before the widespread use of antibiotics, usually affecting women of childbearing age. Typical symptoms were of dysuria, suprapubic pain and often haematuria. An increased incidence of this condition was noted in patients undergoing radiotherapy for bladder tumours [1]. Injury to the bladder wall as a result of radiotherapy, leading to inflammation, necrosis and fibrosis, in the presence of alkaline urine was felt to favour deposition of urinary phosphate.

That the calcification in this case predominantly affected the posterior bladder wall is probably due to its proximity to the cervix. The region of the interureteric ridge of the bladder wall is considered the most vulnerable site for damage. Further, its vascular supply may have been compromised by the Wertheim's hysterectomy.

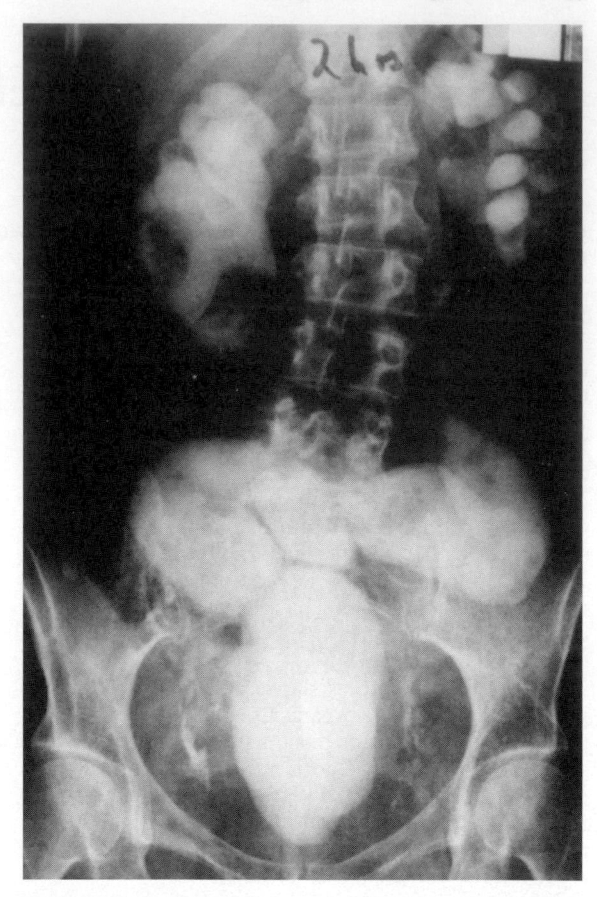

Figure 4. Intravenous urogram; delayed film showing bilateral hydronephroses and ileal interposition.

As this patient has had several complications secondary to pelvic radiotherapy, it is not surprising that the radiological appearances of encrusting cystitis are so florid. Recognition of this condition is helpful because prompt treatment of urinary tract infection, particularly proteus, and acidification of the urine at an early stage may prevent, or even reverse, progression.

References

1. Jamieson RM. The treatment of phosphatic encrusted cystitis (alkaline cystitis) with nalidixic acid. Br J Urol 1966;38:89–92.
2. Gross BH. Bladder and ureteral calcifications. Semin Roentgenol 1979;14:261–2.
3. Harrison RB, Stier FM, Cochrane JA. Alkaline encrusting cystitis. AJR 1978;130:575–7.

A pensioner's plight

[1]J M FIELDS, [2]A B HAWTHORN, [1]I ZAMMIT-MAEMPEL and [1]N THOMAS

Departments of [1]Diagnostic Radiology and [2]General Medicine, North Manchester General Hospital, Manchester, UK

A 69-year-old man was admitted for investigation of a swollen, painful left leg present for 1 year. He had suffered three episodes of rigors. 4 years previously he had had a Dacron aortic bifurcation trouser graft inserted, from below the renal arteries to both common femoral arteries, for a dissecting abdominal aortic aneurysm. On examination there was a generalized increase in size of the left leg which was warmer than the right leg. There was a small effusion in the left knee joint. In view of these symptoms and his past medical history, plain radiographs of the left ankle (Figure 1) and subsequently dynamic CT of the abdomen (Figure 2) were performed. What are the abnormal findings and what is the diagnosis?

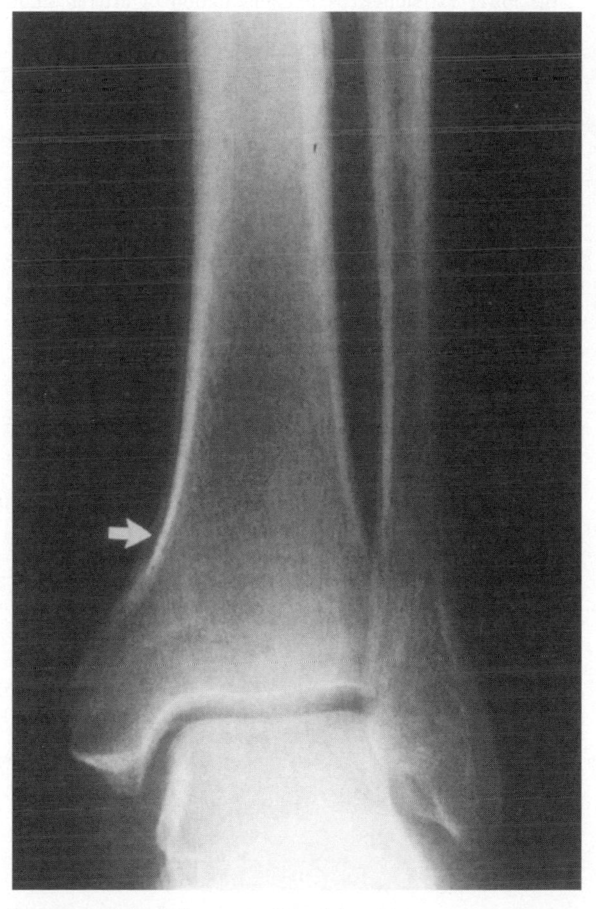

Figure 1. Plain radiograph of the left ankle.

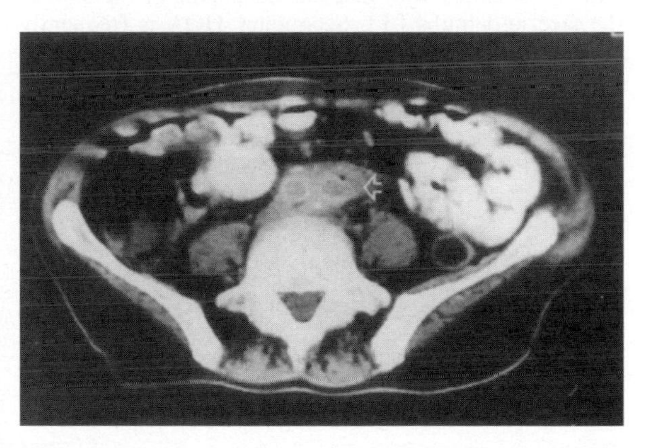

Figure 2. CT scan just below the level of bifurcation of the aortic graft.

Based on the case of the month originally published in Br J Radiol 1994;67:511–2.

The plain radiograph of the left ankle showed a marked periosteal reaction along the metadiaphyseal region of the distal tibia and fibula. Similar findings were noted on the radiograph of the left knee.

The CT scan showed an ill defined rim of soft tissue (arrow) encasing the calcified Dacron graft. On subsequent slices this was seen to extend along the left distal limb of the graft. Within this soft tissue rim are small pockets of air.

The patient developed septicaemia, recurrent buttock abscesses and vasculitic lesions of the left foot. Blood cultures grew *Streptococcus milleri* and *Proteus*. At laparotomy the graft was found to be infected and was replaced. The final diagnosis was secondary hypertrophic osteoarthropathy (HOA) of the left leg resulting from an infected Dacron aortic trouser graft.

HOA is characterized by the presence of periosteal new bone formation, digital clubbing and arthritis. Hereditary HOA is known as pachydermoperiostosis and is associated with marked thickening of the skin of the face and limbs [1]. Secondary HOA is frequently associated with lung pathology, bronchogenic and pleural tumours, lung abscesses and cystic fibrosis [2]. Other causes include cirrhosis of the liver, inflammatory bowel disease, lymphoma, patent ductus arteriosus and bacterial endocarditis. Both humoral and neurogenic theories have been proposed to explain the development of HOA, the pathogenesis of which is still a mystery [3]. HOA secondary to an infected Dacron aortofemoral graft is rare; there have been nine cases reported in the literature [1, 4]. Six of the cases had periostitis in both legs, in the remainder periosteal reaction was confined to one leg. In all patients there were clinical features of infection associated with symptoms of HOA. Patients presented between 3 and 4 years after insertion of their Dacron grafts [4]. Angiographic findings of tortuous arteries with decreased transit time of contrast medium indicate increased blood flow through the affected limb [4].

The finding of periosteal reaction in patients with arterial prostheses may be a presenting manifestation of graft sepsis. Dynamic CT is an accurate method of assessing this, as demonstrated in this case.

References

1. Walter RD, Resnick D. Hypertrophic osteopathy of a lower extremity in association with arterial graft sepsis. AJR 1981;137:1059–61.
2. Sorin SA, Askari A, Rhodes RS. Hypertrophic osteopathy of the lower extremities as a manifestation of arterial graft sepsis. Arth Rheum 1980;23:768–70.
3. Stein HB, Little HA. Localised hypertrophic osteopathy in the presence of an abdominal aortic prosthesis. Can Med Assoc 1978;118:947–8.
4. Angelena H, Williams DM, Zelenock GB, Braunstein EM. Unilateral hypertrophic osteopathy in a patient with an infected axillary-axillary bypass graft. Radiology 1987; 162:573–4.

The dyspeptic disco dancer

[1]R J PECK, [1]K NG and [2]A LI

Departments of [1]Diagnostic Radiology and Organ Imaging, and [2]Surgery, Prince of Wales Hospital, Shatin, NT, Hong Kong

A 25-year-old woman who enjoyed regular visits to the local disco, presented early in 1987 with hepatomegaly and a mass arising from the pelvis. She was otherwise fit and normal.

7 years previously she had developed painless jaundice. Laparotomy at another hospital showed a mass in the pancreatic head and a Whipple's operation was performed. Histology at that time was said to be carcinoma of the pancreas, and she and her parents were informed of the poor prognosis. However, she remained well for the next 3 years before returning to the same hospital because of recurrent nocturnal epigastric pain and an epigastric mass. Obstruction by recurrent tumour was diagnosed but at laparotomy widespread metastases were found in the liver. The stomach was not obstructed but an anastomotic ulcer was found.

It was considered that she had an "inoperable tumour" and further surgery was not performed. Her family doctor treated her with ranitidine which gave good symptomatic relief. The presence of multiple hepatic metastases, with histology similar to that found previously, was taken to suggest an advanced stage of the disease with a poor prognosis, although she had already survived 3 years.

Despite the poor prognosis she remained fit and well for the next 4 years enjoying an active social life until she noticed a lower abdominal mass, which led to her admission to hospital.

Figures 1 and 2 are CT scans of upper and lower abdomen (post-biopsy). Can you explain the apparent contradiction between the history and the clinical progress?

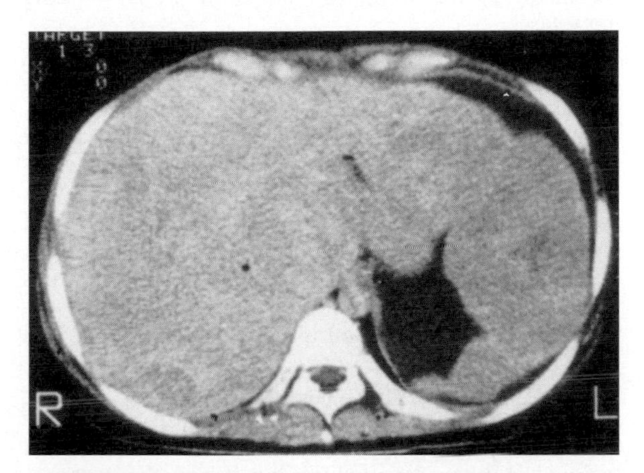

Figure 1. CT of upper abdomen.

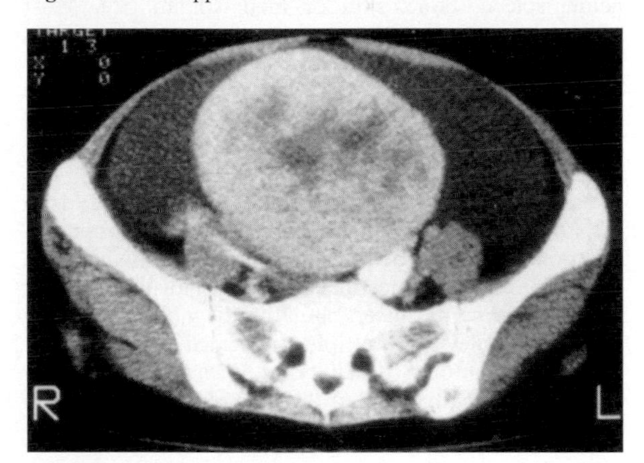

Figure 2. CT of lower abdomen.

Based on the case of the month originally published in Br J Radiol 1988;61:417–8.

The striking feature of this woman's history was the long course and apparent relative benignity of the disease, especially with an initial diagnosis of carcinoma of the pancreas. The history of anastomotic ulceration following a Whipple's operation is the clue which suggests that the lesion may be a gastrinoma. The CT scans show a large mass in the lower abdomen and multiple hepatic nodules. The fluid within the abdomen is haemorrhage secondary to the biopsy. The definitive diagnosis was reached by biopsy of the mass and the liver which showed the histology to be gastrinoma, both probably being metastases.

In 1955, Zollinger and Ellison [1] described the syndrome of upper gastrointestinal ulceration, increase of gastric acid secretion and non-β islet-cell tumours (gastrinomas) of the pancreas. Gastrinomas represent approximately 20% of all islet-cell neoplasms. 90% of gastrinomas are found within the pancreas, 5% in the proximal duodenum and the remainder in various sites including hilum of spleen and stomach. Pancreatic gastrinomas may be single or multiple and measure from 2 mm to 20 cm.

Two-thirds of gastrinomas are histologically or biologically malignant. One-half to two-thirds of patients with gastrinomas have metastases, most commonly in regional lymph nodes and liver, but also involving peritoneum, spleen, bone, skin or mediastinum [2]. Most patients present with the symptoms of peptic ulceration, the majority involving the stomach and first part of the duodenum. Multiple ulcers tend to occur also in the distal duodenum and jejunum. Diarrhoea, steatorrhoea and vitamin B12 malabsorption are other presenting features.

Barium studies may show prominent mucosal folds in the stomach, duodenum and, sometimes, the jejunum. In addition, there may be large amounts of fluid within the stomach and small intestine. Ulcers are indistinguishable from simple peptic ulcers, but the diagnosis should be suspected if they are multiple, or located distally.

Islet-cell tumours of all types that are hormonally active are typically small at the time of presentation and are frequently not seen on CT [3], being indistinguishable from solid adenocarcinoma, although calcification has been noted in malignant islet-cell tumours, a finding almost never seen in adenocarcinoma. The smaller islet-cell tumours are usually isodense with pancreas but larger tumours may have low attenuation areas of necrosis [4]. Demonstration of functioning islet-cell tumours by CT has been reported in between 30% and 70% of cases. CT has not been shown to be useful in detecting ectopic primary tumours but metastatic deposits from pancreatic and ectopic tumours may be detected even when the primary tumour is not seen.

Angiography and, in particular, venous sampling have both been shown to be more sensitive than CT in the detection of primary islet-cell tumours. There have also been reports of successful intraoperative tumour localization by ultrasound [5]. The definitive diagnosis of Zollinger–Ellison syndrome, however, depends upon the demonstration of an increased serum gastrin level by radioimmunoassay.

Mortality in Zollinger–Ellison syndrome is lowest after gastrectomy because overwhelming ulcer disease rather than malignant tumour invasion is the more common cause of death [2]. As this patient demonstrates, the original Whipple's operation with resulting loss of gastric secretory cells probably explains her limited gastrointestinal symptoms, and she is now mainly troubled by her abdominal mass.

The planned treatment is debulking or removal of the pelvic tumour and administration of streptozotocin for the hepatic metastases.

References

1. Zollinger RM, Ellison EH. Primary peptic ulceration of the jejunum associated with islet cell tumours of the pancreas. Ann Surg 1955;142:709–28.
2. Braunwald E, Isselbacker KJ, Petersdorf RG, Wilson JD, Martin JF, Fauci AS. Harrison's principles of internal medicine (11th edn). New York: McGraw-Hill, 1987:1250–2.
3. Lee JKT, Sagel SS, Stanley RJ. Computed body tomography. New York: Raven Press, 1983:221.
4. Moss AA, Gamsu G, Genant HK. Computed tomography of the body. Philadelphia: WB Saunders, 1983:749–51.
5. Ruechert KF, Klotter HJ, Kummerle F. Intra-operative ultrasonic localisation of endocrine tumours of the pancreas. Surgery 1984;96:1045–7.

Recurrent abdominal pain in a young man

M B MATSON, A G HATRICK and D C HOWLETT

X-ray Department, 2nd Floor Tower, Guy's Hospital, Guy's and St Thomas' NHS Trust, London SE1 9RT, UK

A 34-year-old Caucasian man initially presented with a 3-week history of generalized abdominal pain but no other symptoms. He had no relevant medical history and was on no medication. He appeared well and physical examination was unremarkable. Chest and plain abdominal radiographs were normal. The patient then proceeded to a barium enema examination (Figure 1). He then underwent laparotomy and a surgical procedure.

2 years later, the patient presented with vague upper abdominal discomfort but no other symptoms. Physical examination was again unremarkable. Routine blood tests and chest and abdominal radiographs were normal. A CT scan of the abdomen was performed following oral contrast administration. Two of the CT sections are shown; one at the level of L1 in the suprarenal region and one through the lower poles of the kidneys (Figures 2 and 3).

What abnormal features are shown on the barium enema and CT? What operation had been performed? What is the underlying diagnosis?

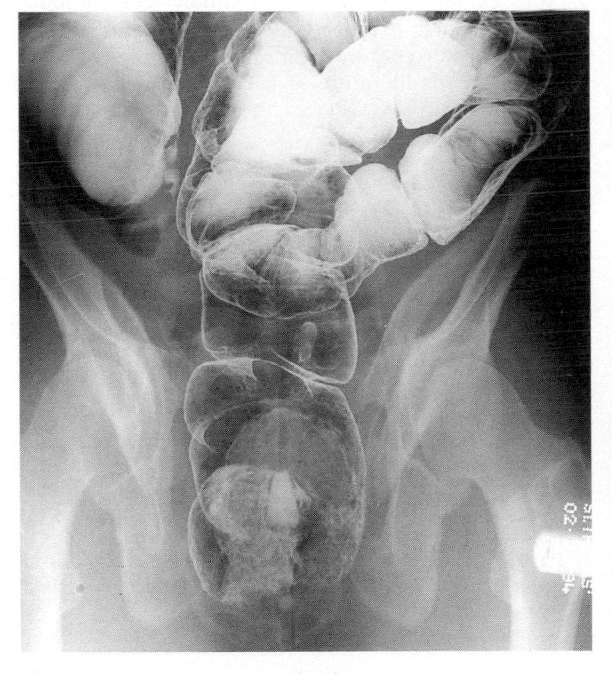

Figure 1. Barium enema examination.

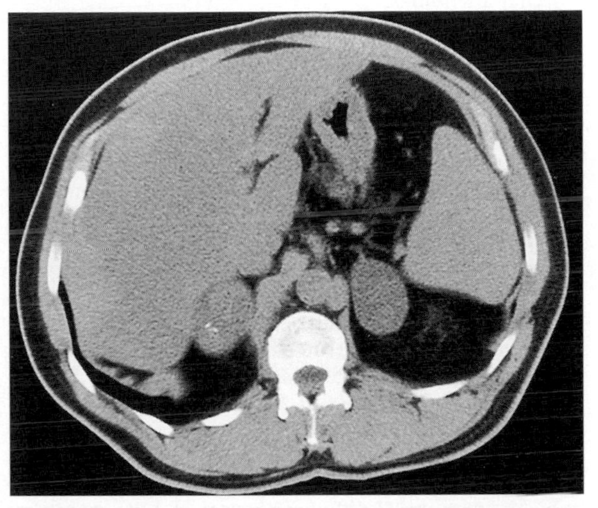

Figure 2. CT at the level of L1 in the suprarenal region.

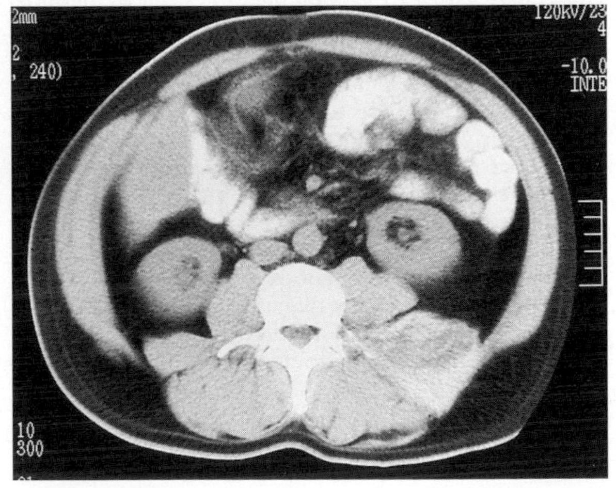

Figure 3. CT through the lower poles of the kidneys.

Based on the case of the month originally published in Br J Radiol 1998;71:1105–6.

The barium enema (Figure 1) demonstrated multiple polyps in the rectum and sigmoid colon. These were shown on biopsy to be adenomas. A total colectomy with ileoanal pouch formation was performed. The CT scan 2 years later showed bilateral soft tissue masses in the adrenal glands, with some flecks of calcification in the right adrenal mass (Figure 2). The lower CT section showed a heterogeneous mass in the left quadratus lumborum muscle (Figure 3). The radiological diagnosis of desmoid tumour was confirmed by percutaneous biopsy.

Urinary and serum assays for catecholamines were negative and the patient proceeded to biopsy of the right adrenal gland mass. Histology revealed this to be a benign, non-functioning adrenocortical adenoma.

The final diagnosis was familial adenomatous polyposis with associated desmoid tumour and bilateral adrenal adenomas.

Familial adenomatous polyposis is caused by a genetic abnormality of the adenomatous polyposis coli (APC) gene located on chromosome 5q21. There is an autosomal dominant inheritance although up to 20% of patients do not have a history of familial adenomatous polyposis, suggesting spontaneous mutation of the disease gene in these patients. This condition is characterized by the presence of hundreds or thousands of adenomatous polyps in the large bowel. Gardner, in 1953, described a syndrome consisting of multiple cutaneous lesions occurring simultaneously with hereditary polyposis and osteomatosis. Gardner's syndrome also has a genetic defect at the same locus on the 5q21 chromosome, and the colonic polyposis is due to germline mutations of the APC gene. This has led to the conclusion that the two disorders are different phenotypic expressions of different clusters of APC mutations [1]. Mutations in certain regions of the APC gene are associated with extracolonic features such as desmoid tumours, while mutations in other regions correlate with severity of the colonic disease. The identification of the APC gene allows children from families with familial adenomatous polyposis to be screened for gene mutation in their early teens. Those positive for the mutation can be offered elective colectomy, while those who do not carry the gene mutation can be spared the previous practice of regular check colonoscopies.

Since Gardner's first description, extracolonic manifestations in familial adenomatous polyposis are now recognized to be the rule rather than the exception [2]. Nearly all patients have polyps in the upper gastrointestinal tract and periampullary carcinoma of the duodenum is the commonest cause of death in patients treated by colectomy and ileorectal anastomosis. Jejunal and ileal polyps have also been reported. Other extracolonic manifestations include papillary thyroid carcinoma, multiple epidermal cysts, medulloblastoma, pancreatic carcinoma and hypertrophy of the retinal pigment epithelium [3].

About 10% of patients with familial adenomatous polyposis will develop desmoids, benign fibromatous lesions occurring most commonly in the abdominal wall and mesentery [4, 5]. Their development has been linked with previous surgery, oral contraception and pregnancy. The anterior abdominal wall lesions usually present as a clinical mass, but imaging is useful for ingrowing tumours which can displace abdominal and pelvic organs. The mesenteric desmoid tumours most commonly arise at the base of the small bowel mesentery and are more aggressive in their behaviour. CT shows them as irregular, infiltrative and non-enhancing masses with an attenuation of about 45–60 Hounsfield units. The paraspinal muscles are a less common site of desmoids, which may present with back pain.

Adrenal adenomas are a rare association of familial adenomatous polyposis. A case of bilateral adrenal adenomas in a familial adenomatous polyposis patient was reported in the early 1950s. The number of reported cases is now in double figures, but is likely to increase as CT scanning becomes more widely used. Adrenal carcinomas, first described in 1967 in a patient with Gardner's syndrome, are even rarer with only two cases described in the literature [6]. Nevertheless, biopsy of any adrenal mass is advised in patients with familial adenomatous polyposis.

References

1. Rustgi AK. Hereditary gastrointestinal polyposis and non-polyposis syndromes. N Engl J Med 1994; 331:1694–702.
2. Jagelman DG. Extracolonic manifestations of familial polyposis coli. Cancer Genet Cytogenet 1987; 27:319–25.
3. Harned RK, Buck JL, Olmsted WW, Moser RP, Ros PR. Extracolonic manifestations of the familial adenomatous polyposis syndromes. AJR 1991;156:481–5.
4. Gurbuz AK, Giardiello FM, Petersen GM, Krush AJ, Offerhaus GJA, Booker SV, et al. Desmoid tumours in familial adenomatous polyposis. Gut 1994;35:377–81.
5. Magid D, Fishman EK, Jones B, Hoover HC, Feinstein R, Siegelman SS. Desmoid tumours in Gardner syndrome: use of computed tomography. AJR 1984;142:1141–5.
6. Painter TA, Jagelman DG. Adrenal adenomas and adrenal carcinomas in association with hereditary adenomatosis of the colon and rectum. Cancer 1985;55:2001–4.

Radio-opaque hemithorax in a neonate

M F CREAGH, L M MACDONALD and D C GARVIE

Departments of Radiology and Paediatrics, St Thomas' Hospital, London SE1 7EH, UK

A 1-day-old male infant, delivered by Caesarean section at term to a 20-year-old primigravida, presented with an apnoeic episode associated with hypoxia and cyanosis. The chest radiograph at presentation is shown (Figure 1). Treatment with antibiotics and oxygen was commenced, and the baby gradually improved over the subsequent 10 days. A repeat chest radiograph was unchanged in appearance. An ultrasound examination of the liver (Figure 2) and a perfusion scan of the chest (Figure 3) were performed.

What abnormalities have been shown and what is your differential diagnosis?

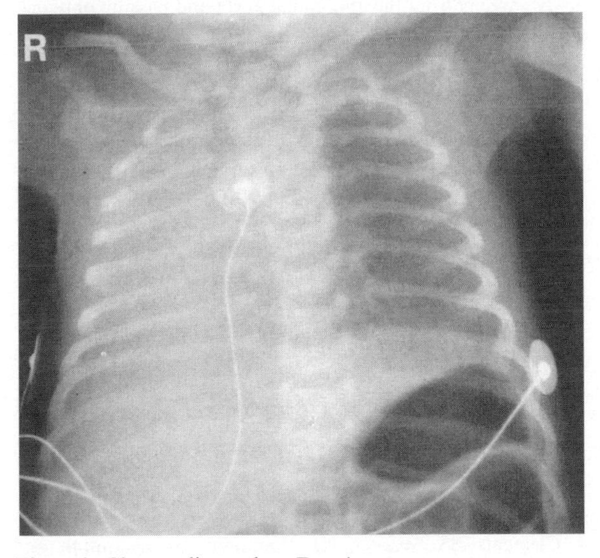

Figure 1. Chest radiograph at Day 1.

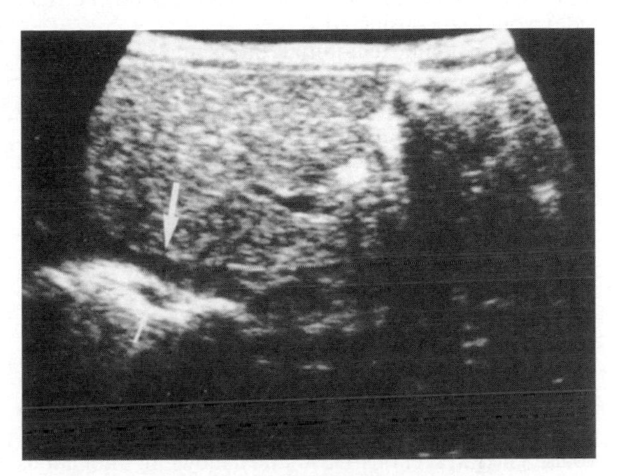

Figure 2. Longitudinal section through the liver. Large arrow, inferior vena cava.

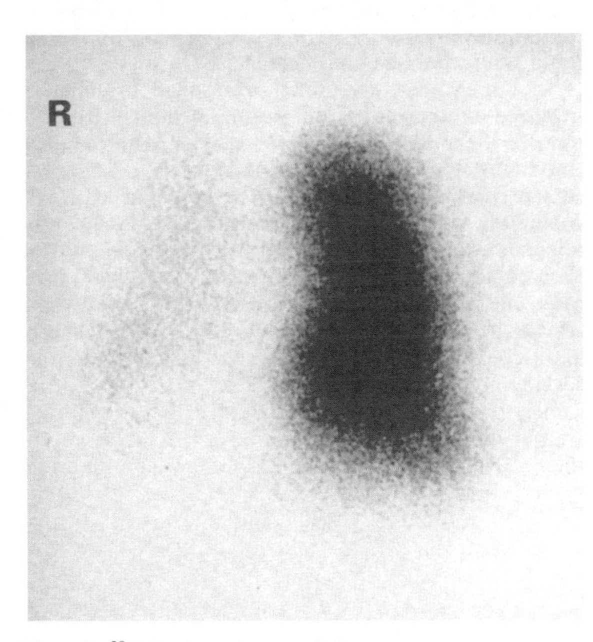

Figure 3. $^{99}Tc^{m}$-microsphere perfusion scan.

Based on the case of the month originally published in Br J Radiol 1989;62:951–2.

The differential diagnosis includes collapse/consolidation of the right lung secondary to infection, obstruction of major bronchi by mucus plugs or aspiration of meconium or fluid. Congenital abnormalities such as complete lobar agenesis and pulmonary sequestration, although rare, are definite possibilities. If there was less evidence of mediastinal shift, the differential diagnosis would be enlarged to include causes of pleural fluid collections. Thus, hydrothorax, pyothorax, haemothorax and chylothorax (commoner in males and on the right side) would be considered.

In our patient, the initial ultrasound examination showed an aberrant vessel passing obliquely from the region of the aorta, behind the inferior vena cava and traversing the right hemidiaphragm (small arrow, Figure 2). A $^{99}Tc^{m}$-microsphere perfusion scan showed hypoperfusion of the right lung via the pulmonary circulation. The definitive diagnosis was made by an intravenous digital subtraction angiogram (DSA) (Figure 4), using a peripheral injection incorporating the limb muscle compression technique [1]. With this technique, contrast medium is injected into a superficial hand or foot vein and is held in the deep venous system by application of tourniquets. By simultaneous release of tourniquets and limb compression, a satisfactory bolus of contrast medium can then be propelled into the central veins. The intravenous DSA study shows an anomalous artery arising from the abdominal aorta and passing above the right hemidiaphragm.

The diagnosis in this case was pulmonary sequestration.

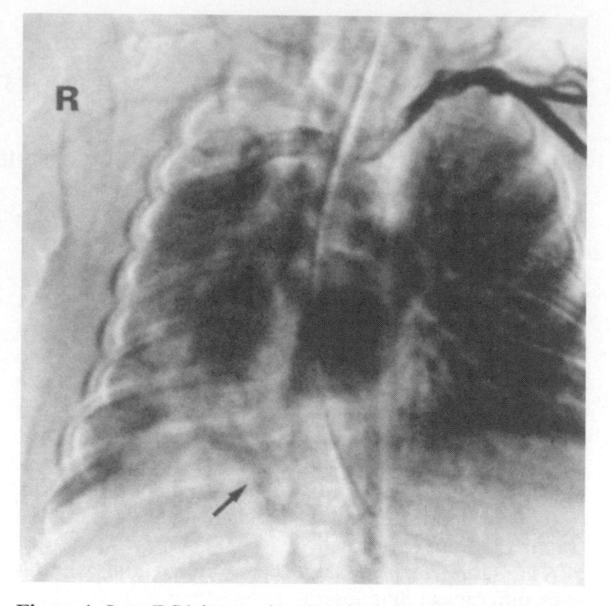

Figure 4. Late DSA image showing the anomalous artery (small arrow) arising from the abdominal aorta and passing obliquely above the right hemidiaphragm.

Pulmonary sequestration is part of the broad spectrum of congenital bronchopulmonary-vascular malformations. The term was first used to describe a "disconnected bronchopulmonary mass or cyst with an anomalous systemic artery supply" [2]. Subsequently, cases were discovered that did not correspond to the original description and hence the term "sequestration spectrum" was coined [3]. More recently, Clements and Warner [4] have attempted to apply a unifying concept to all congenital lung lesions on the basis of abnormal development of the four principal lung constituents, namely tracheo-bronchial airway, lung parenchyma, arterial supply and venous drainage. Their scheme provides a theoretical explanation as to how a single insult, occurring during early lung development *in utero*, can produce such diverse congenital abnormalities as pulmonary sequestration, the "scimitar" syndrome, cystic adenomatoid malformation and congenital lobar emphysema.

Our patient underwent embolization of the anomalous vessel and remains well.

References

1. Lea Thomas M, Hicks P. Limb muscle compression: an alternative technique for intravenous digital subtraction angiography. Br J Radiol 1987;60:123–5.
2. Pryce OM. Lower accessory pulmonary artery with intralobar sequestration of lung: a report of seven cases. J Pathol 1987;58:457–67.
3. Sade RM, et al. The spectrum of pulmonary sequestration. Ann Thorac Surg 1974;18:644–55.
4. Clements BS, Warner JO. Pulmonary sequestration and related congenital bronchopulmonary-vascular malformation: nomenclature and classification based on anatomical and embryological considerations. Thorax 1987;42:401–8.

Not so pseudo

C J WAKELEY, V N CASSAR-PULLICINO and I W MCCALL

Department of Diagnostic Imaging, Robert Jones & Agnes Hunt Orthopaedic Hospital, Oswestry, Shropshire, UK

A 9-year-old boy presented in the Casualty Department complaining of a painful neck. The previous night his brother had jumped on his head causing forced flexion of his cervical spine. The patient had restricted active and passive neck movements without neurological symptoms or signs. Figure 1 shows lateral views in flexion and extension of his cervical spine on admission to hospital.

Describe the radiological appearances. What is your diagnosis?

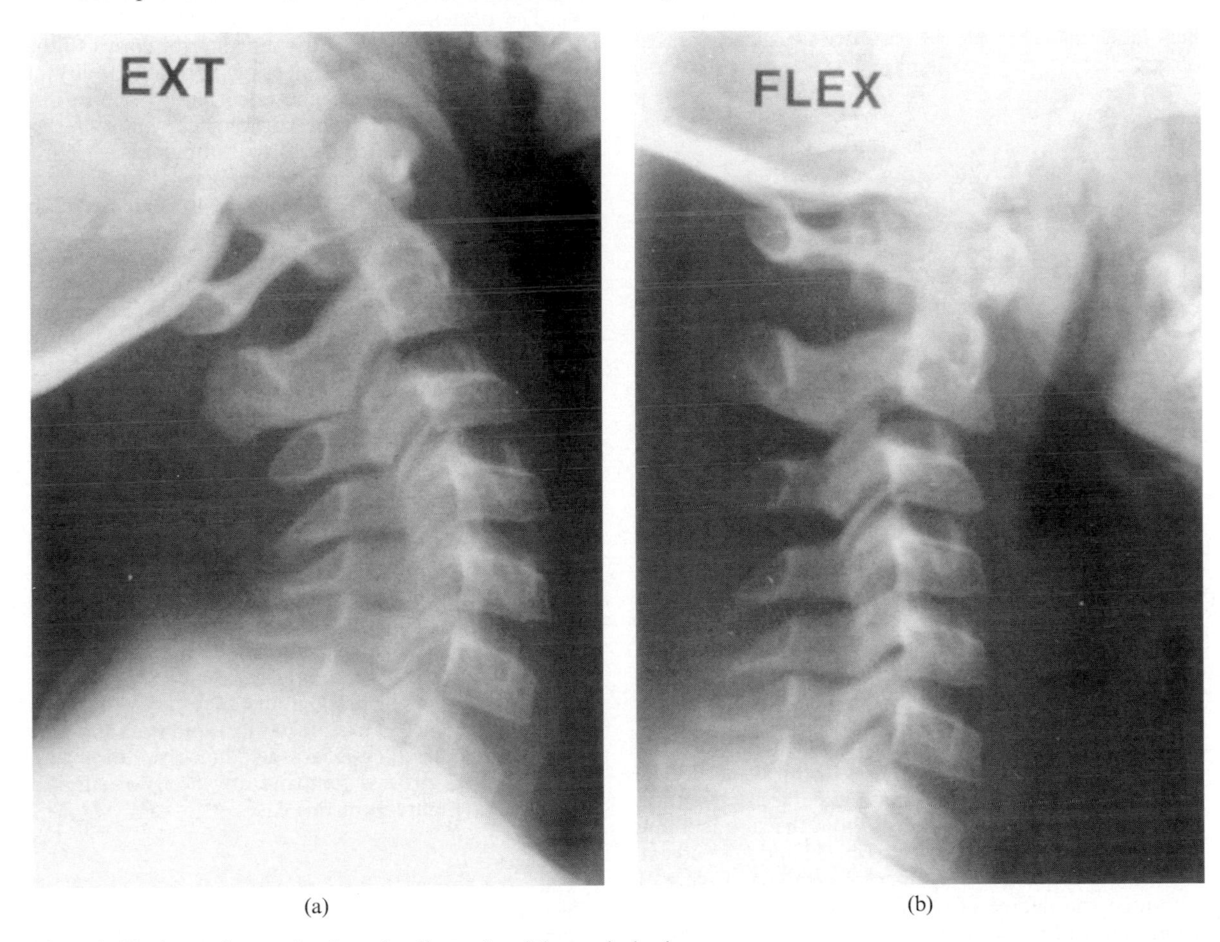

(a) (b)

Figure 1. Flexion and extension lateral radiographs of the cervical spine.

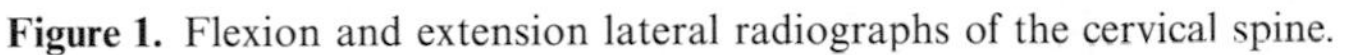

Based on the case of the month originally published in Br J Radiol 1991;64:375–6.

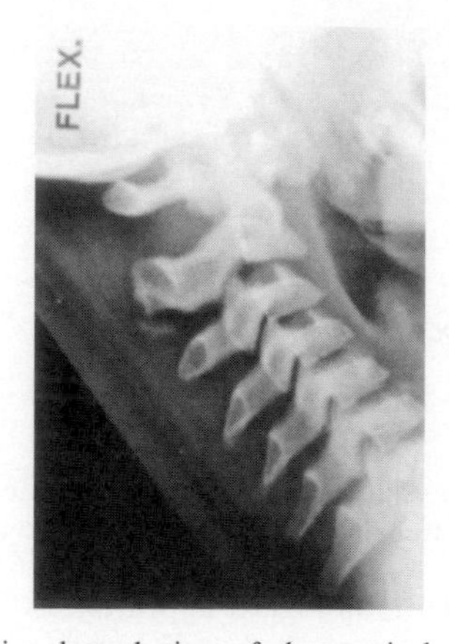

Figure 2. Flexion lateral view of the cervical spine. Pseudosubluxation of C2/C3 with intact posterior cervical line. New bone formation in the interspinous space at C2/C3.

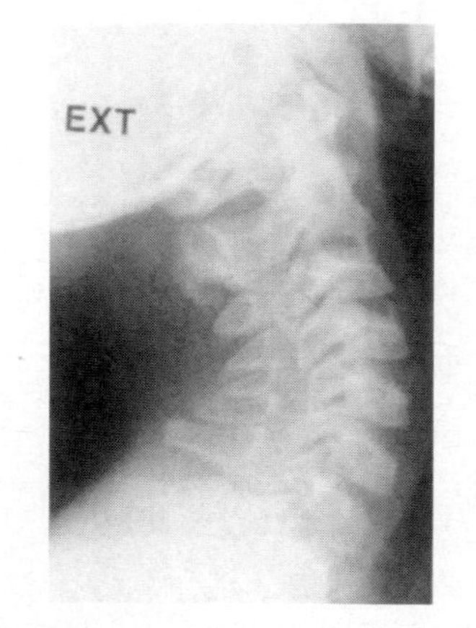

Figure 3. Post-traumatic new bone formation and incorporation with spinous process of C2.

The radiological features were consistent with physiological C2/3 pseudosubluxation. Rapid resolution of his neck pain allowed the patient's early return home. A month later, the radiographic appearances were unchanged and the patient was entirely asymptomatic, participating fully in sports activities including heading footballs! He remained symptom-free with a normal range of neck movements, but radiographs 3 months later showed soft tissue ossification in the supraspinous and interspinous ligaments between C2 and C3, indicating healing of posterior ligamentous trauma (Figure 2). Although the degree of C2/C3 angulation and subluxation were within the accepted normal range, this patient had clearly sustained disruption of the posterior ligamentous complex at the same level.

Physiological anterior displacement of C2 on C3 in children is a well recognized feature. Its misinterpretation in some cases has led to prolonged and unnecessary treatment. This phenomenon is most commonly encountered prior to the age of 8 years [1, 2]. The frequency and degree of displacement diminishes with age, and most authors report an upper age limit of 14 years [3, 4]. A few cases, however, have occurred between 17 and 21 years of age [5]. The main fulcrum for motion of the cervical spine in the sagittal plane is at the C2/C3 level in children and the C5/6 level in adults. Apart from the anterior wedging of the upper cervical vertebral bodies and the horizontal alignment of the apophyseal joints normally present at this level, the hypermobility has been ascribed to the increased ligamentous laxity associated with underdevelopment of neck musculature in the young. On flexion, the posterior arch of C2 moves forward with the body of C2 and, in so doing, aligns itself in a straight line fashion with the posterior arches of C1 and C3. This alignment is normal and constitutes the basis of the posterior cervical line [4]. The posterior cervical junction will pass through (or less than 1 mm in front of) the anterior cortex of the spinolaminal line of C2, indicating normal stability at this segment. This helpful line is currently used to distinguish physiological from pathological anterior displacement and is seen to be normal in our case.

The degree of normal motion through the C2/C3 apophyseal joints between full flexion and full extension can be striking with a "step-off" of up to 4 mm [4]. The underlying factors that predispose to the physiological C2/C3 variant must also make this level the most vulnerable in a forced flexion injury and predispose to posterior ligamentous disruption. The presence of ligamentous ossification in this patient indicates that serious injury was sustained to the posterior osteoligamentous complex of C2 and C3, and false comfort was derived from the radiographic criteria discussed above. Posterior ligamentous damage is serious, predisposing to spinal instability. The previous literature on C2/C3 pseudosubluxation has been notable by the minimal radiographic follow-up, which was deemed unnecessary in view of the asymptomatic state of the patients. Given a history of trauma, our case indicates that the presence of pseudosubluxation should not be taken as synonymous with absence of any significant injury, and children with injuries to the neck should be treated symptomatically for whatever soft tissue injury that may be present, despite the presence of pseudosubluxation. Radiographic evidence of increased ossification and incorporation with the C2 spinous process removed any need for surgical intervention (Figure 3) in this case.

References

1. Townsend EH, Rowe ML. Mobility of the upper cervical spine in health and disease. Paediatrics 1952;10:567–72.
2. Jacobson G, Bleecker HH. Pseudosubluxation of the axis in children. AJR 1959;82:472–81.
3. Cattell HS, Filtzer DL. Pseudosubluxation and other normal variations in the cervical spine in children. J Bone Joint Surg 1965;47A:1295–309.
4. Swischuk LE. Anterior displacement of C2 in children: physiologic or pathologic? Radiology 1977;122:759–63.
5. Harison RB, Keats TE, Winn HR, Riddervold HO, Pope TL. Pseudosubluxation of the axis in young adults. J Can Assoc Radiologists 1980;31:176–7.

Fit and ... well

R D THOMAS and A J GOULD

Department of Radiology, Poole General Hospital, Longfleet Road, Poole, Dorset BH15 2JB, UK

Previously fit and well, a 65-year-old man awoke at 3 am with searing interscapular pain. The general practitioner administered morphine and referred him urgently to hospital. On arrival he was pale and sweaty with a mild tachycardia and he refused to move his arms. Physical examination was otherwise unremarkable and, of note, his blood pressure was normal. He was considered likely to have suffered a myocardial infarction, although an electrocardiogram (ECG) showed only the tachycardia. A chest radiograph was considered normal by the admitting clinicians.

The "arrest team" was called 2 h after admission and found the patient cyanosed and having a grand mal epileptic attack. He recovered spontaneously.

He continued to complain of severe pain between his shoulders to the extent that the admitting junior staff tentatively diagnosed acute myalgia and requested urgent ESR. Concern that the pain may represent an aortic dissection prompted a request for mediastinal CT. The chest radiograph was not available to the radiologist supervising the CT, from which three images are reproduced (Figure 1). Is there any evidence of an aortic dissection? What is your diagnosis?

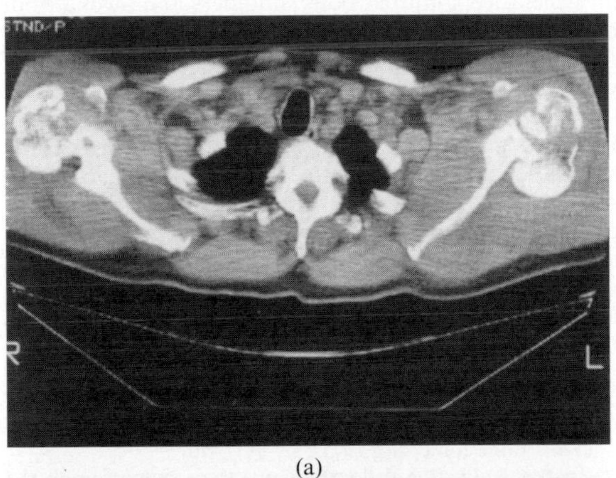

(a)

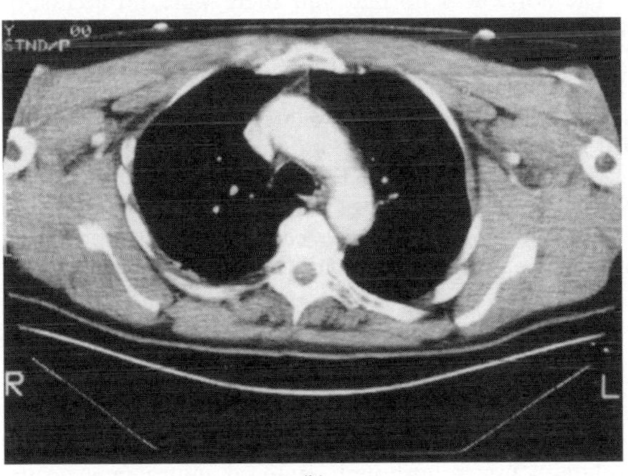

(b)

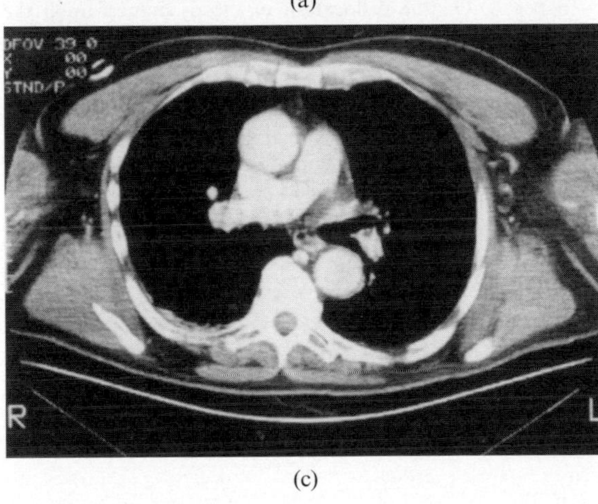

(c)

Figure 1. Three representative slices from CT of the mediastinum: (a) is unenhanced, (b) and (c) are enhanced.

Based on the case of the month originally published in Br J Radiol 1992;65:1145–6.

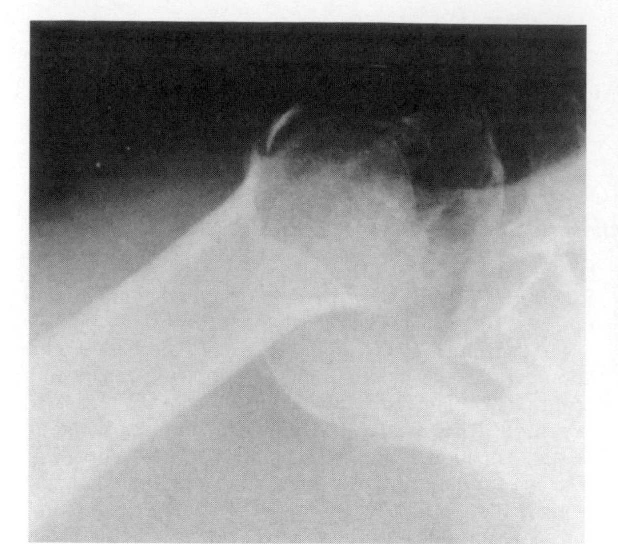

Figure 2. Axial radiograph of the right shoulder.

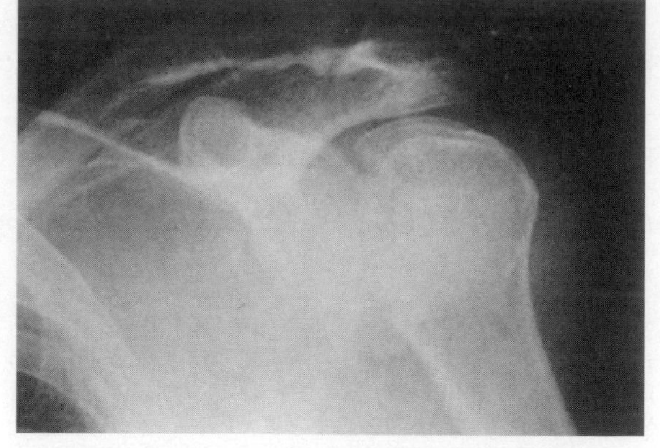

Figure 3. Anteroposterior radiograph of the left shoulder.

The aorta was normal and there were no accessory findings (such as pleural fluid) to suggest a dissection. The shoulders, however, were seen to be fractured (Figures 2 and 3). Plain radiographs of the shoulders are illustrated and show bilateral posterior fracture-dislocation. This is an uncommon event. Dislocation of the shoulders is usually in an anterior direction. Posterior dislocation accounts for perhaps 15% [1] and occurs as a result of violent muscle contraction, the posterior muscle groups being stronger than the anterior.

Bilateral posterior fracture-dislocation of the shoulders is usually accounted for by two aetiologies: epileptic fits and electric shock, typically historically, electroconvulsive therapy. Trauma more commonly results in a unilateral injury, although bilateral injury may occur. The incidence of ECT induced shoulder injury has been markedly reduced, leaving epileptic seizures as the overwhelmingly dominant cause of bilateral fracture-dislocation of the shoulders [2]. The association of posterior dislocation with a seizure has long been known [3] and the first bilateral dislocation due to epilepsy was reported by Coover in 1932 [4]. The injury may be the only evidence of a seizure [5]. However, it is not widely recognized as a complication of epilepsy and both the fit and resultant injury frequently go undetected for a considerable time.

We believe that our patient suffered his first epileptic fit while asleep, injured both shoulders and awoke from his post-ictal sleep as a result of the pain. The right shoulder injury was just visible on the chest radiograph when it was viewed by a radiologist, but unfortunately this film is again unavailable. Missing this subtle radiographic sign, combined with failure to recognize the association of epilepsy with fracture-dislocation of the shoulder, meant that the correct diagnosis was not suspected, despite an epileptic fit being witnessed. Cardiac investigations and CT of the brain were normal.

References

1. Samilson RL, Prieto V. Dislocation arthropathy of the shoulder. J Bone Joint Surg 1983;65A:456–60.
2. Shaw JL, Kansas T. Bilateral posterior fracture-dislocation of the shoulder and other trauma caused by convulsive seizures. J Bone Joint Surg 1971;53A:1437–40.
3. Cooper A. On the dislocation of the os humeri upon the dorsum scapulae and upon fractures near the shoulder joint. Guys Hosp Report 1839;4:265.
4. Coover C. Double posterior luxation of the shoulder. Pennsylvania Med J 1932;35:566.
5. Pear BL. Bilateral posterior fracture dislocation of the shoulder—an uncommon complication of a convulsive seizure. New Engl J Med 1970;283:135–6.

The case of the bloated nurse

J E JACKSON and A M K THOMAS

Department of Radiology, Hammersmith Hospital, Du Cane Road, London W12 0HS, UK

A 46-year-old nurse who had been treated at this hospital for several years presented with a history of a severely bloated feeling after meals, with resultant loss of appetite and weight. She had previously suffered from dysphagia secondary to a benign oesophageal stricture which had improved after oesophageal dilatation several months previously. Her abdominal radiograph on admission is shown in Figure 1. She subsequently had a barium meal and follow-through examination (Figure 2).

What features are seen and what is the likely diagnosis?

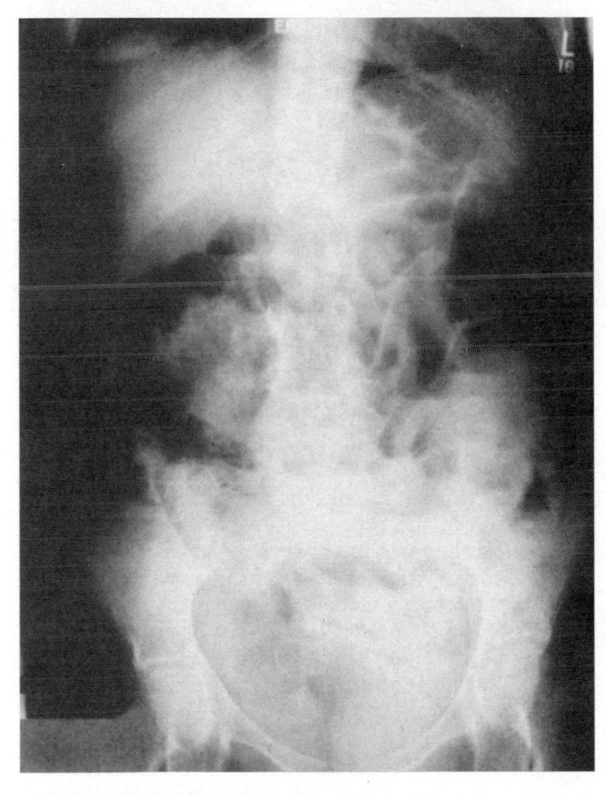

Figure 1. Erect abdominal radiograph.

(a)

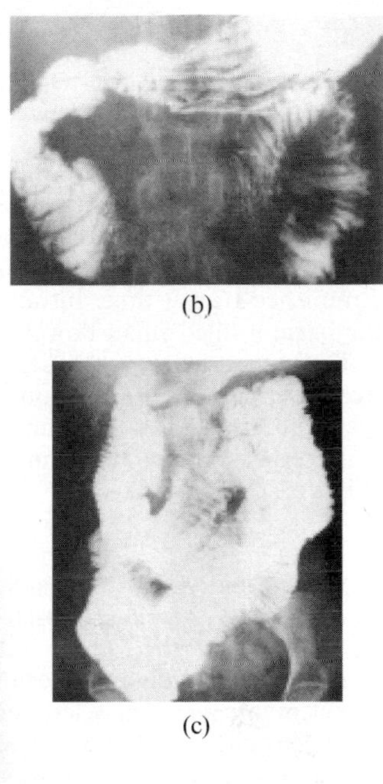

(b)

(c)

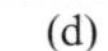

(d)

Figure 2. Series of radiographs from barium meal and follow-through: (a) oesophagogram, (b) duodenal loop, (c) small bowel, and (d) detail from small bowel study.

Based on the case of the month originally published in Br J Radiol 1987;60:721–2.

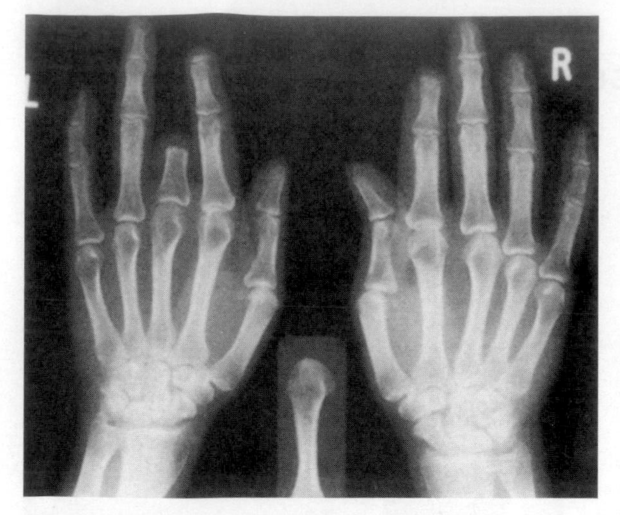

Figure 3. Hands of patient showing acro-osteolysis (the left middle finger had to be amputated).

The plain abdominal radiograph (Figure 1) showed small bowel dilatation and intramural pneumatosis. The barium studies showed oesophageal, duodenal and jejunal dilatation with gastro-oesophageal reflux and a diminished transit time. Intramural air is seen clearly in the barium-filled small bowel.

The patient had severe systemic sclerosis and had been treated for Raynaud's phenomenon. She had atrophy of the soft tissues of the fingers with acro-osteolysis (Figure 3) and basal pulmonary interstitial fibrosis (Figure 4).

Table 1. Causes of linear pneumatosis

Bowel infarction	Carcinoma
Small bowel obstruction	Gastric-outlet obstruction
Collagen vascular disease	Whipple's disease
Peptic ulceration	Perforated jejunal diverticula
Post-endoscopy	Caustic ingestion
Post-bowel anastomosis	Phlegmonous gastritis
Steroid therapy	Intestinal parasites
Necrotizing enterocolitis	Toxic megacolon

Information from Bryk [4], Rice et al [5] and Meyers et al [2].

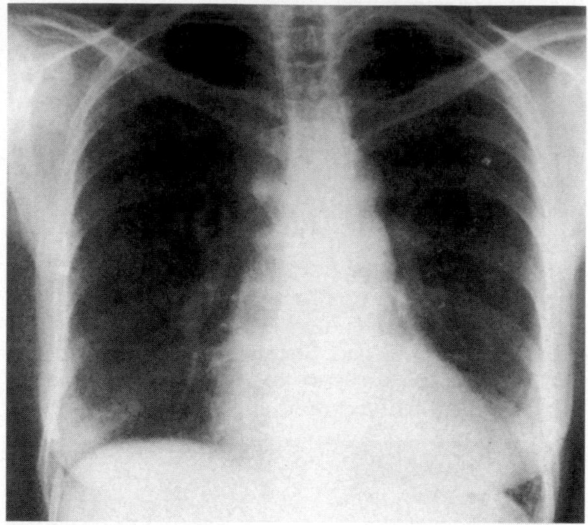

Figure 4. Chest radiograph showing basal interstitial shadowing.

This patient shows the classic features of scleroderma (progressive systemic sclerosis). The oesophagus is usually involved, the small intestine less commonly. Pseudodiverticula may be seen in the large bowel. Small bowel involvement in scleroderma is associated with a worse prognosis. Meihoff et al [1], while recognizing that intestinal pneumatosis was probably a benign complication, saw it as a grave prognostic sign. The intramural gas is probably produced by the raised intraluminal pressure secondary to diminished intestinal motility forcing gas into the submucosa and subserosa; occasionally there may be an associated pneumoperitoneum [2]. It is interesting to note that oesophageal stenosis secondary to caustic (lye) ingestion is a cause of pneumatosis [3] although at the time of presentation the oesophageal stricture was no longer a problem with our patient. Gas in the bowel wall has usually been attributed to primary and secondary causes. In the primary form, called pneumatosis cystoides intestinalis, gas-filled non-communicating cysts are seen in the colon of adults. In a secondary form, linear streaks of gas are seen in the walls of the large or small bowel. In a patient with acute symptoms, the presence of linear gas is usually ominous because it implies the presence of bowel infarction. However, more benign causes of intestinal linear pneumatosis are increasingly being recognized (Table 1). A knowledge of the causes of linear pneumatosis may save the patient an unnecessary laparotomy if the clinical features are appropriate. It may be difficult to exclude vascular ischaemia by clinical features and a plain radiograph alone, and in these cases angiography or a water soluble contrast medium study may be indicated.

References

1. Meihoff WE, Hirschfield JS, Kern F. Small intestinal scleroderma with malabsorbtion and pneumatosis cystoides intestinalis. J Am Med Assoc 1968;204:102–6.
2. Meyers MA, Ghahremani GG, Clements JL, Goodman K. Pneumatosis intestinalis. Gastrointest Radiol 1977;2:91–105.
3. Koss JG. Abdominal gas cysts (pneumatosis cystoides intestinorum hominis). Arch Pathol 1952;53:523–49.
4. Bryk D. Unusual causes of small bowel pneumatosis: perforated duodenal ulcer and perforated jejunal diverticula. Radiology 1973;106:299–302.
5. Rice RP, Thompson WM, Gedgaudas RK. The diagnosis and significance of extraluminal gas in the abdomen. Radiol Clin North Am 1982;20:819–37.

A leaking laparoscopy wound

F REGAN and M E CROFTON

Department of Radiology, The Samaritan Hospital for Women, Marylebone Road, London NW1, UK

A 34-year-old Bahrainian woman presented to the Accident and Emergency Department complaining of fluid leaking from a recent laparoscopy scar. She spoke very little English so no further history was available. Examination of the abdomen was unremarkable. She was referred for an ultrasound examination of the abdomen to exclude an intraabdominal collection or urinoma.

A midline sagittal scan of the pelvis and a parasagittal scan to the left are shown (Figures 1 and 2). What is the diagnosis? What were the likely indications for the laparoscopy?

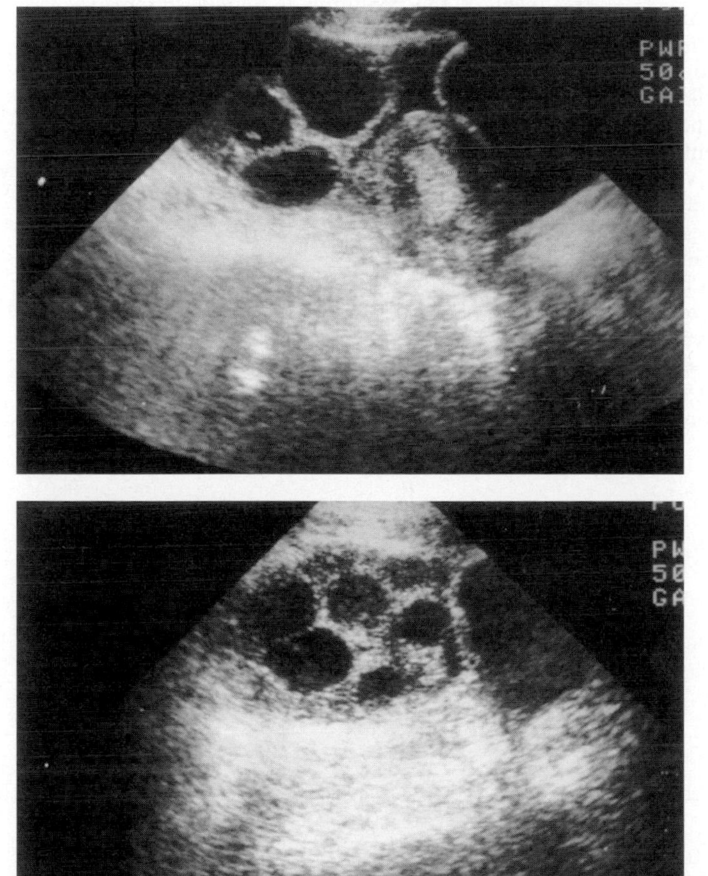

Figure 1. Parasagittal scan of the pelvis.

Figure 2. Parasagittal scan to the left.

Based on the case of the month originally published in Br J Radiol 1991;64:1073–4.

The ultrasound examination showed a moderate amount of ascites, later confirmed to be the source of the leaking fluid. The uterus was normal in size (Figure 1) but had a very thickened endometrial echo (16–18 mm anteroposterior diameter). Both ovaries were enlarged (8 × 4 cm approximately) and contained multiple 1.5–2.0 cm cysts (Figure 2). These appearances are those of ovarian hyperstimulation syndrome (OHSS). It was subsequently learned that she had undergone ovulation induction therapy prior to *in vitro* fertilization. Laparoscopic egg collection had been performed in Belgium 2 days before presentation, but unfortunately none of the retrieved oocytes had fertilized so no embryos had been returned to her uterus. The patient insisted on returning to Bahrain following her diagnosis and as far as we are aware made an uneventful recovery.

The OHSS has frequently been described in the literature since Gemzell first described successful induction of ovulation and pregnancy in humans in 1958. The syndrome is usually of minimal consequence but can be a potentially life threatening condition, characterized by enlarged ovaries containing multiple cysts and extravascular fluid collections, ascites and pleural effusions. Exceptionally, pleural effusions may occur without an increase in ovarian size. There is haemoconcentration and in severe cases circulatory collapse and various coagulation disorders including disseminated intravascular coagulation can occur. Abnormally high levels of oestrogen are found in the patient's serum, urine and follicular fluid and there are raised plasma levels of progesterone, 17-hydroxyprogesterone and testosterone. It is usually seen in association with various ovulation induction regimes (to treat ovarian dysfunction in infertility or to induce superovulation prior to *in vitro* fertilization), but has been reported in association with hydatidiform moles and multiple pregnancies occurring without the aid of ovulation inducing agents.

The severe form of the disease is rare with a reported incidence of 0.4–4% of patients on ovulation induction therapy. The milder form is much commoner (reported rates vary from 3 to 80%) and many cases undoubtedly go unrecognized.

The pathogenesis and aetiology of the syndrome are unclear. There is thought to be a sudden increase in the permeability of the ovarian vessels and the fact that the extravascular fluid collections are transudates supports this. Crooke et al [1] found that high follicle stimulating hormone (FSH)/luteinizing hormone (LH) ratios resulted in a lower incidence of OHSS, but subsequently this could not be confirmed. Schenker and Weinstein [2] showed the dose of gonadotrophins was significant but that the critical dose varied enormously between individuals.

Histamine release blocking agents and prostaglandin inhibitors have been tried with variable success, but treatment of the condition is mainly supportive with correction of any fluid and electrolyte imbalance. It usually resolves spontaneously in 7–10 days. Primarily, effort should be directed at preventing development of the syndrome by careful monitoring of all ovulation induction regimes and removal of the stimulating agent should the condition arise.

[*See also Kim and Lee [3] for a description of imaging appearances, ED*]

References

1. Crooke AC, Butt WR, Palmer RF, Morris R. Clinical trial of human gonadotrophins. J Obstet Gynaecol 1963;70:604.
2. Schenker JG, Weinstein G. Ovarian hyperstimulation syndrome—a current survey. Fertility Sterility 1978;30:255–68.
3. Kim IY, Lee BH. Ovarian hyperstimulation syndrome: US and CT appearances. Clin Imaging 1997;21:284–8.

The forgotten incident

T L TRAN and M MCCARTY

Department of Radiology, St Mary's Hospital, Praed Street, London W2 1NY, UK

A 47-year-old man was referred by his general practitioner to the medical outpatient clinic with a 4-week history of colicky pain in the epigastrium and periumbilical region, anorexia and weight loss. He also complained of flatulence and abdominal distension after meals. The only relevant past medical history was bilateral inguinal hernia repairs 12 months previously.

Abdominal examination in the outpatient clinic did not show any abnormality. His complaints were thought to be related to gall bladder or peptic ulcer disease. Initial investigations included an upper abdominal ultrasound which was normal. 2 weeks later, the patient attended for a barium meal. The oesophagus, stomach and duodenum were normal. A barium follow-through examination was then carried out. The findings are illustrated in Figures 1 and 2.

What is your provisional diagnosis?

What further clinical history should be sought?

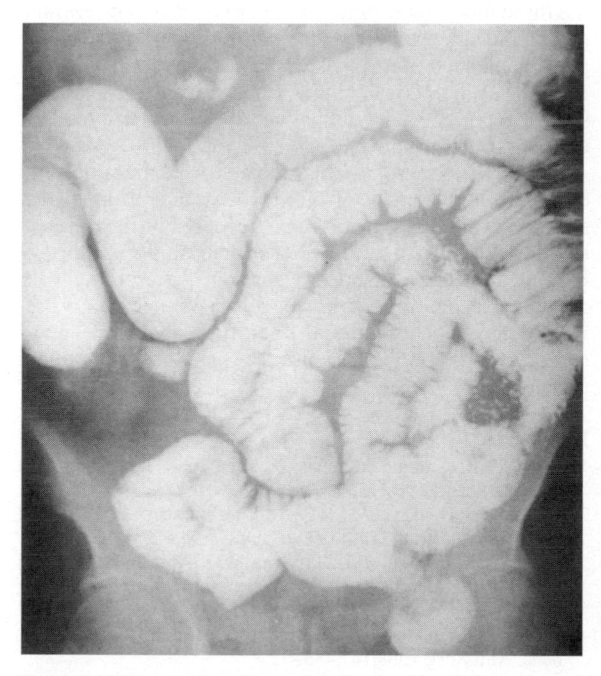

Figure 1. Abdominal radiograph of a barium follow-through study.

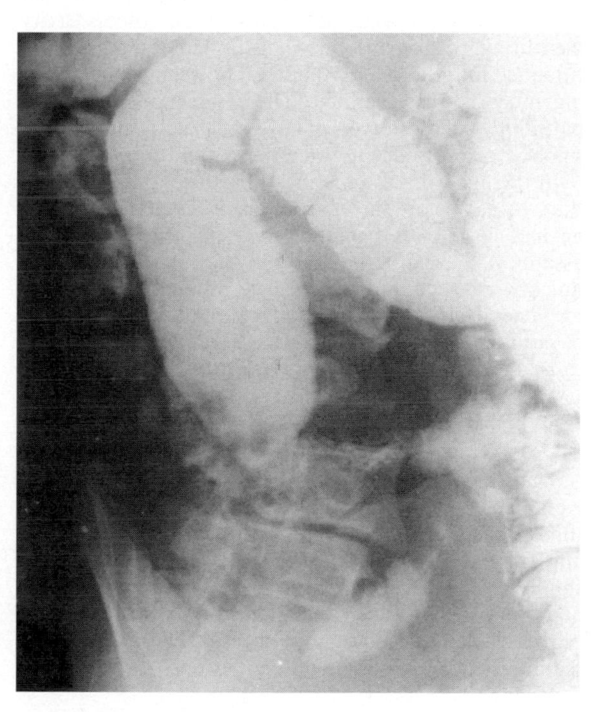

Figure 2. Further delayed film.

Based on the case of the month originally published in Br J Radiol 1990;63:659–60.

The barium follow-through study demonstrated a short segment of narrowing in the distal ileum with gross dilatation of the small bowel proximal to it. The stricture showed abrupt tapering with mucosal irregularity, and there appeared to be an associated mass in the right iliac fossa. There was incidentally a recurrent left inguinal hernia. In view of the small bowel obstruction, the patient was referred directly from the radiology department to the surgical team for further management. Examination of the abdomen this time demonstrated a mass in the right iliac fossa and obstructive bowel sounds. The provisional differential diagnosis was carcinoid tumour of the small bowel, carcinoma, Crohn's disease or adhesions due to previous hernia repairs.

A laparotomy followed. In the right iliac fossa, the ileal stricture was encased in a fibrous mass to which the sigmoid colon was also adherent. The mass together with 10 cm of the sigmoid colon and the encased loop of ileum were excised. On histology, the small bowel was tethered to the sigmoid colon and sharply bent on itself. At the point where it was tethered, there was a 2 cm perforation in the sigmoid colon with an abscess cavity, measuring 1.5 cm × 1 cm × 1 cm. The abscess had extended into the wall of the small bowel and the overlying mucosa was ulcerated. There was no other bowel pathology such as diverticular disease or tumour in the sigmoid colon to account for the perforation.

In the light of these findings, specific enquiry revealed that, 1 week before the onset of his presenting symptoms, he had been kicked in the lower abdomen during an assault. Although he had pain in that region initially, it quickly subsided and the incident was not disclosed to his general practitioner. As the site of injury and the site of pathology were well correlated, trauma was assumed to be the cause of the bowel perforation.

The differential diagnosis of a small bowel stricture would include adhesions, Crohn's disease, carcinoid tumour, carcinoma, lymphoma, metastasis, ischaemia and trauma. Adhesions are the most common cause of small bowel obstruction, even in patients who have not had an operation. The latent small bowel obstruction in our case is due to colonic perforation with subsequent sealing by adjacent tissue and adhesions.

Delayed intestinal obstruction due to bowel strictures is an infrequent sequel of blunt abdominal trauma and may manifest at variable time after the initial injury. Raf [1] reviewed a series of 95 benign bowel strictures reported over a period of 12 years and found only one report of post-traumatic stricture. The underlying pathophysiological mechanisms of delayed bowel obstruction include bowel ischaemia, contusion of the bowel wall, intramural hemorrhage and/or bowel perforation with fibroblastic reaction. These factors, alone or in combination, result in cicatricial narrowing of the bowel wall and/or adhesions with resultant mechanical obstruction. Other mechanisms are mesenteric or diaphragmatic disruption with subsequent internal hernia and serosal contusion resulting in adhesions.

The mechanism of blunt trauma to the bowel is compression with shearing between two surfaces such as the spine and the abdominal wall [2]. Bowel rupture occurs when intestinal wall tension exceeds its bursting potential because of rapidly displaced intestinal content. The most frequently damaged bowel and associated mesentery are the duodeno-jejunal junction, the proximal and terminal ileum, and the transverse and sigmoid colon because the peritoneal fixed points place these segments of bowel over the spine [3]. A similar mechanism may account for the types of injury associated with the lap-type seat belt, sustained in automobile collision [4].

Finally, in patients with complete or partial intestinal obstruction, a history of blunt abdominal trauma may remain occult and is not often considered in the differential diagnosis. As a result of the increasing incidence of blunt trauma in our society, patients, presenting with complete or incomplete bowel obstruction with no previous history of abdominal operation, should be questioned about previous episodes of blunt abdominal trauma.

References

1. Raf LE. Ischaemic stenosis of the small intestine. Acta Chirurg Scand 1969;135:253–9.
2. Williams RD, Sargent, FT. The mechanism of intestinal injury in trauma. J Trauma 1963;3:288–94.
3. Martin JD, Perdue GD, Harrison WH. Abdominal visceral injury due to non-penetrating trauma. Arch Surg 1960; 80:192–7.
4. Witte CL. Mesentery and bowel injury from automotive seat belts. Ann Surg 1968;167:486–92.

Pseudo-tumour of the posterosuperior mediastinum

J F M MEANEY, D E ROBERTS and H CARTY

Department of Radiology, Alder Hey Children's Hospital, Liverpool, UK

A 6-month-old male child with known cystic fibrosis and a previously normal chest radiograph had a routine chest radiograph. What does it show? An ultrasound examination and enhanced CT were also performed. Do these help?

What is the most likely diagnosis and what would you do next?

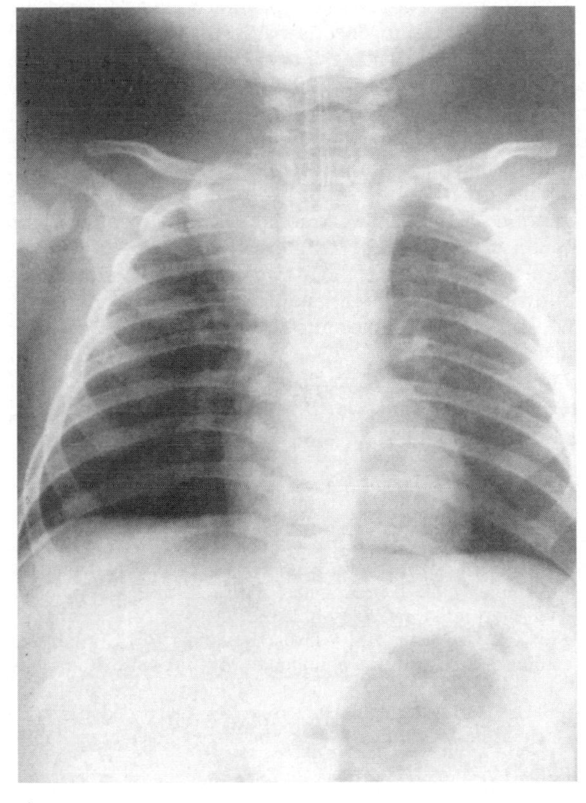

Figure 1. AP chest radiograph.

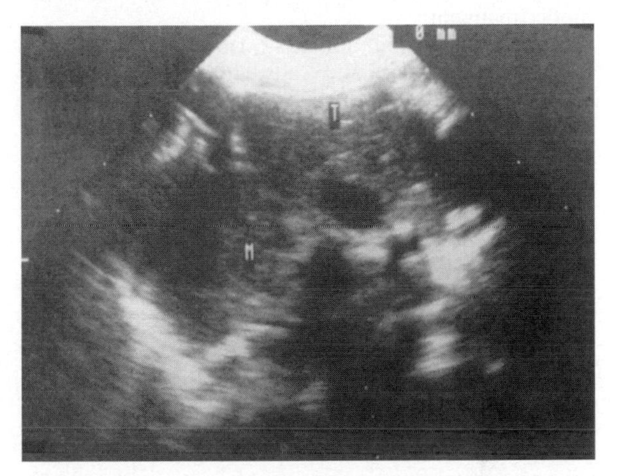

Figure 2. Ultrasound examination. M, mass; T, thymus.

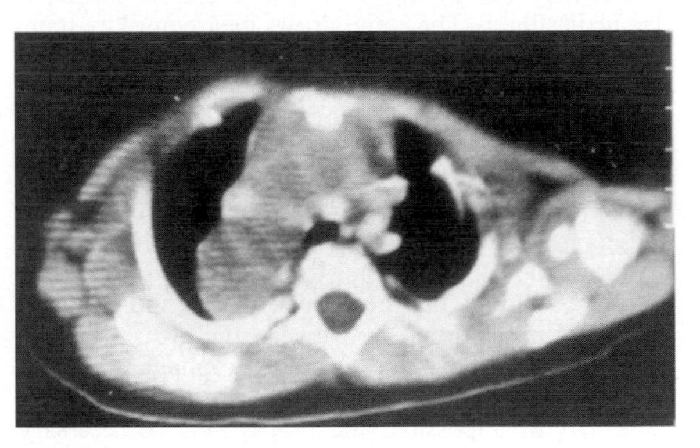

Figure 3. Contrast enhanced CT at the level of the mass.

Based on the case of the month originally published in Br J Radiol 1993;66:741–2.

The chest radiograph showed an opacity in the right upper mediastinum extending from the right hilum to the apex of the lung (Figure 1). There was no calcification or rib erosion. In view of a recent normal chest radiograph a malignant neurogenic tumour was considered the most likely diagnosis. Serum and urinary catecholamines were normal. Atelectasis of the right upper lobe was considered unlikely on both clinical and radiological grounds and, furthermore, there was no change in the mass following physiotherapy and antibiotic treatment.

Ultrasound examination was performed via the second left intercostal space and showed a hypoechoic mass lesion isoechoic with normal thymus (Figure 2). The mass could not be clearly delineated from the thymus anteriorly. Contrast enhanced CT (Figure 3) confirmed the ultrasound findings and showed a homogeneously enhancing mass extending into the right costovertebral sulcus. There was no evidence of calcification or rib destruction. The mass had an attenuation value identical to that of normal thymus and there was no discernible plane of cleavage between the mass and thymus. The possibility of an aberrantly positioned thymus was considered but, because a mediastinal neoplasm could not definitely be excluded, a percutaneous CT-guided biopsy was performed using a posterior approach. A good core of tissue was obtained and pathological examination showed normal thymic tissue.

The thymus is a normal bilobed structure lying in front of the great vessels in the anterior mediastinum. It is most prominent radiologically in infancy, at which time it may occupy up to 50% of the cross-section of the mediastinum. The gland grows in size until it attains its greatest absolute size at puberty, after which fatty involution occurs.

The thymus is derived embryologically from the third pharyngeal pouches by paired primordial buds. By the end of the seventh week of gestation the primordia have lost connection with their parent pouches, fused medially and migrated into the anterior mediastinum. Ectopic thymic tissue can thus persist anywhere along this line of migration and has been reported in the posterior mediastinum, in the neck, between the great vessels in the thorax and above the left brachiocephalic vein. Even when normally sited, differentiation from a mediastinal mass may be impossible and biopsy may be necessary. Aberrant location of the thymus poses an even greater problem and is an uncommon event [1–4]. The presence of thymic tissue at such sites can result in great confusion, especially in the context of a known clinical problem such as the follow-up of a patient with known malignancy or, as in our case, cystic fibrosis, where lobar atelectasis may be mimicked.

Extension of the thymus into the posterior mediastinum is rarely seen with conventional imaging modalities, but may be more frequently seen with MRI [3] where posterior extension was seen in four out of 47 cases. When it occurs it is almost invariably on the right, as in our case. CT demonstrates an attenuation coefficient identical to that of normal thymus, similar enhancement with intravenous contrast medium, and absence of a discernible plane of cleavage between the normally situated anterior thymus and the posterior extension [2]. MRI shows a homogeneous signal intensity identical to normal thymus on all pulse sequences and absence of a plane of cleavage between the posterior limb and the more normally sited anterior thymus [3, 4]. The sonographic features of a posterior thymus corroborate the CT and MRI appearances and demonstrate a hypoechoic homogeneous mass with evenly distributed echoes isoechoic with thymus, once again without an evident plane of cleavage. Ultrasound is cheap, readily available and easy to perform, and, despite the fact that it has been shown to be of use in demonstrating a prominent mediastinal outline to be thymic in origin [5], remains greatly under-utilized. We believe that the combination of these newer modalities will in many cases result in the correct diagnosis being made without recourse to surgery and, furthermore, if doubt exists following multiplanar imaging, percutaneous biopsy is the procedure of choice and should obviate the need for open thoracotomy.

[*There is an excellent review of imaging of mediastinal masses, which includes the thymus, by Meza et al [6], ED*]

References

1. Saade M, Whitten DM, Necheles TF, et al. Posterior mediastinal accessory thymus. J Pediatr 1976;88:71–2.
2. Cohen MD, Weber TR, Sequeira FW, et al. The diagnostic dilemma of the posterior mediastinal thymus: CT manifestations. Radiology 1983;146:691–2.
3. Siegel MJ, Glazer HS, Wiener JJ, Molina PL. Normal and abnormal thymus in childhood: MR imaging. Radiology 1989;172:367–71.
4. Bach AM, Hilfer CL, Holgersen LO. Left sided posterior mediastinal thymus—MRI findings. Paediatr Radiol 1991:440–1.
5. Carty H. Ultrasound of the normal thymus in the infant: a simple method of resolving a clinical dilemma. Br J Radiol 1990;63:737–8.
6. Meza MP, Benson M, Slovis TL. Imaging of mediastinal masses in children. Radiol Clin North Am 1993;31:583–604.

A lump in the throat

[1]P GUEST and [2]J HUSBAND

[1]Department of Radiology, Queen Elizabeth Hospital, Edgbaston, Birmingham B15 2TH, and [2]Department of Diagnostic Radiology, Royal Marsden Hospital, Downs Road, Sutton, Surrey SM2 5PT, UK

A 46-year-old man previously treated for spinal cord compression complained of a painless swelling in his neck. He had no difficulty in breathing or swallowing.

A plain radiograph of his neck and a chest radiograph are shown (Figures 1 and 2).

What is the abnormal structure in the neck and what diagnosis can you reach from the films?

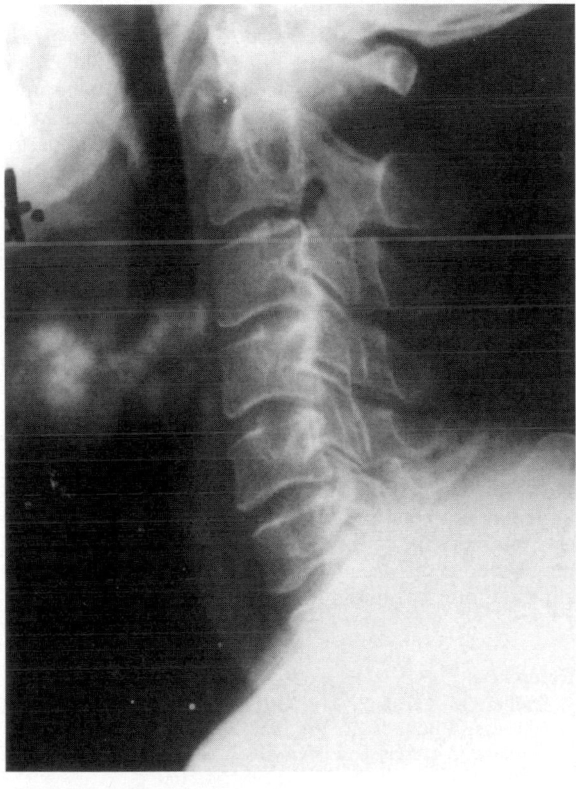

Figure 1. Lateral radiograph of the neck.

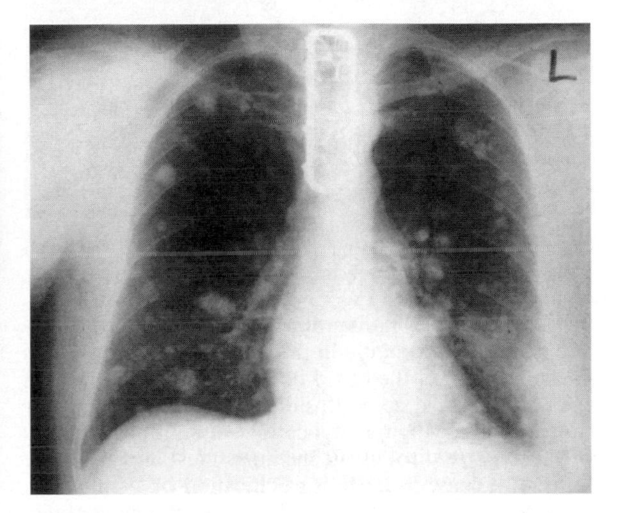

Figure 2. Frontal chest radiograph.

Based on the case of the month originally published in Br J Radiol 1994;67:1279–80.

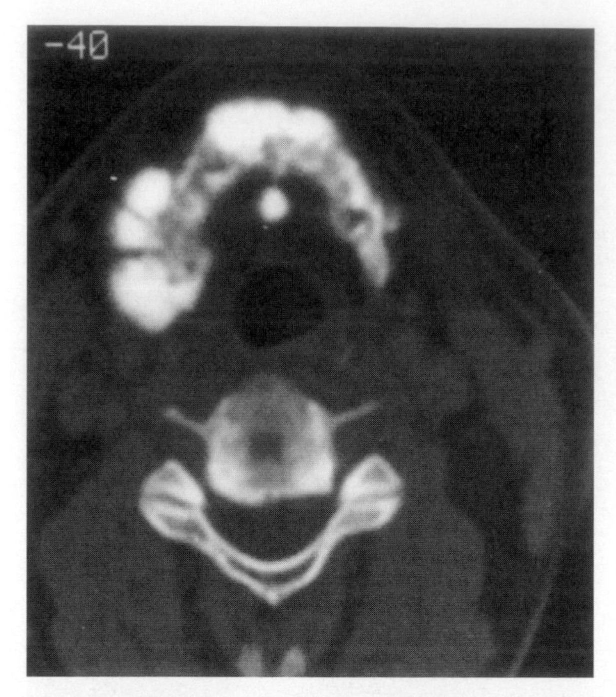

Figure 3. CT section through the neck at the level of the hyoid bone which is demonstrably expanded by bone forming tumour.

The plain lateral radiograph of the neck showed cloud-like new bone formation in the pre-epiglottic soft tissues in the position of the hyoid bone (Figure 1). The film of the chest showed spinal fusion apparatus in the upper thoracic spine (Figure 2). There were multiple opacities of varying size throughout the lungs most of which were unusually dense indicating calcification or ossification. Expansile and exophytic bone lesions were demonstrated in the left lower ribs and right clavicle. The head of the right humerus was inhomogeneously sclerotic and expanded up to the articular surface.

The findings in the lungs together with the multiple lesions in the bones indicated metastatic disease from an osteogenic sarcoma. The lesion in the neck was a metastasis to the hyoid bone. This was exquisitely shown on a CT section of the neck on bone windows. There was marked expansion of the hyoid bone by amorphous new bone with some exophytic elements but with preservation of the overall shape of the hyoid (Figure 3).

At the time of presentation 3 years earlier this patient already had multiple bone lesions throughout the skeleton including the spine and pelvis. Although not symptomatic a bone scan had demonstrated increased uptake in the hyoid bone (not shown) consistent with metastasis. The dominant lesion appeared to be in the right humeral head. The diagnosis of osteosarcoma was confirmed on surgical decompression of the spinal cord from thoracic spine disease.

Osteosarcoma is a tumour occurring most often in the second decade, although 50% will be found outside this age group. Usually no predisposing cause is apparent, but irradiation, Paget's disease or osteochondromata may be associated, particularly in older age groups [1]. Of those who die of their disease 90% have pulmonary metastases and 80% have bone metastases. Although extrapulmonary involvement is usually a late manifestation this has been increasingly recognized in recent years due to the success of adjuvant chemotherapy [2]. Hence it is relatively unusual, as in this case, to find multiple lesions at the time of presentation. When this does occur it may be termed osteosarcomatosis *i.e.* synchronous involvement of multiple sites [3, 4]. However, this term is a matter of some dispute because it is usually possible to identify a single dominant tumour. The disease is therefore best considered as unifocal with multiple early synchronous metastases, rather than multifocal osteosarcomatosis [4]. The presence of osteoblastic metastases occurring in an organ such as the lung which does not normally form bone, further indicates that a unifocal origin is a more likely mechanism as osteoblastic pulmonary metastases were found in the majority of the 29 cases of "osteosarcomatosis" identified by Hopper et al [4]. Thus, unifocal disease with early widespread metastases is the most likely explanation for the findings demonstrated in this report.

Osteosarcoma may metastasize to almost any structure including the thyroid gland and cervical nodes [5]. However, to our knowledge, a metastasis to the hyoid bone has not been previously reported. This case serves as a reminder that even the most innocuous of structures may harbour disease and present with striking and puzzling radiological findings.

References

1. Dahlin DC, Coventry MB. Osteogenic sarcoma. A study of 600 cases. J Bone Joint Surg 1967;49A:101–11.
2. Giuliano AE, Feig S, Eilber FR. Changing metastatic patterns of osteosarcoma. Cancer 1984;54:2160–6.
3. Edeiken-Monroe B, Edeiken J, Jacobsen HG. Osteosarcoma. Semin Roentgenol 1989;24:153–73.
4. Hopper KD, Moser RP, Haseman DB, et al. Osteosarcomatosis. Radiology 1990;175:233–9.
5. Jeffree GM, Price CHG, Sisson HA. The metastatic patterns of osteosarcoma. Br J Cancer 1975;32:87–107.

A child at heart?

M L ERRINGTON and J H REID

Department of Radiology, Royal Infirmary, 1 Lauriston Place, Edinburgh EH3 9YW, UK

An 80-year-old woman presented with a 2 month history of progressive fatigue and ankle swelling. She had a past history of polymyalgia rheumatica but had never smoked and denied chest pain.

On examination she had signs of right heart failure with an elevated jugular venous pressure (JVP) and pitting oedema. There were systolic and early diastolic murmurs in the left parasternal region with an accompanying systolic thrill. She was not cyanosed. Her chest radiograph is shown in Figure 1.

What is the differential diagnosis of the radiographic findings? What question would you ask the patient and what further investigation would you undertake?

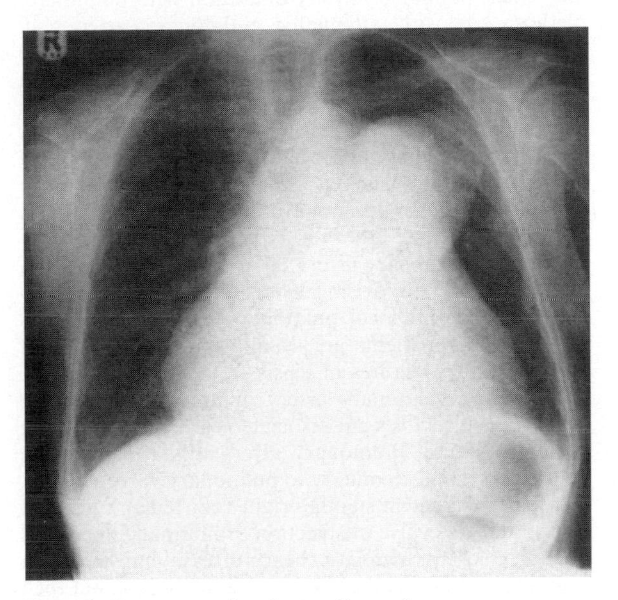

Figure 1. Posteroanterior chest radiograph.

Based on the case of the month originally published in Br J Radiol 1996;69:195–6.

The chest radiograph showed marked cardiac enlargement with dilatation of the main pulmonary artery. The peripheral pulomonary vascularity and lung fields were normal.

Pulmonary artery dilatation in an adult is usually caused by pulmonary hypertension, either idiopathic or secondary to embolic or respiratory disease. However, the striking degree of cardiomegaly in our patient would be unusual with these conditions. Left to right shunts may cause pulmonary artery dilatation with pulmonary plethora, or with attenuated pulmonary arteries in Eisenmenger's syndrome, and may result in cardiac enlargement due to volume overload. Shunts associated with murmurs sufficiently intense to cause a thrill include ventricular septal defect (VSD), patent ductus arteriosus (PDA), aortopulmonary window and coronary artery fistulas. However, such a shunt was unlikely in our patient because she was not cyanosed and the lung fields were not plethoric.

Marked pulmonary artery dilatation may represent a mycotic aneurysm, arising from either septic embolization or adjacent local pulmonary parenchymal infection, but such patients are usually unwell with clinical and laboratory features of sepsis.

Idiopathic pulmonary artery dilatation results from cystic medial necrosis but associated cardiac enlargement is not a feature. Pulmonary artery dilatation may be post-stenotic and secondary to pulmonary valve stenosis. Cardiac enlargement signifies right ventricular and atrial response to the valve obstruction. Pulmonary stenosis is documented in rheumatic heart disease but rarely in isolation and may complicate carcinoid disease, but then a clinical history of flushing, wheeze and weight loss might be expected. Congenital pulmonary stenosis would cause such radiographic appearances if severe although it would be unusual at the age of our patient.

One would ask the patient whether she has ever been known to have a heart murmur. Cardiac ultrasound would then be the investigation of choice. This patient had a heart murmur diagnosed in childhood and was refused entry to theological college at the age of 20 because of a "narrow valve". Despite this she lived a full life until her recent illness. Ultrasound showed massive dilatation of the main and both right and left pulmonary arteries (Figure 2—compare with the normal aortic root dimension). The pulmonary valve was thickened, calcified and severely stenotic. Its immobility also caused detectable regurgitation.

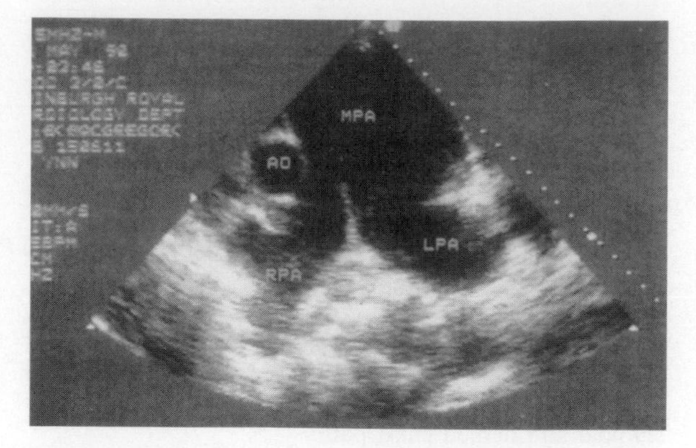

Figure 2. Cardiac ultrasound transversely through the pulmonary arteries. MPA, LPA and RPA, main, left and right pulmonary arteries; Ao, aorta.

Pulmonary stenosis is one of the commonest congenital heart lesions, but few patients are described with symptoms developing in late adulthood [1]. Presentation at the age of 80 years has never been described. Many young adults show no deterioration when followed for up to 24 years [2], but symptoms may supervene in later life when right ventricular failure results from the sustained struggle against stenosis, possibly compounded by further degenerative calcific stiffening of the valve [1]. Patients then present with breathlessness, fatigue and sometimes oedema as in this case.

Accurate diagnosis is important for correct management. The chest radiograph of pulmonary stenosis in adulthood, as in childhood, may show a normal or near-normal cardiac silhouette if the lesion is mild or moderate. Severe stenosis is manifested by enlargement of the cardiac silhouette, secondary to right heart chamber enlargement, with post-stenotic dilatation of the main and predominantly left pulmonary arteries. Ultrasound findings are characteristic and permit Doppler grading of stenosis severity [1].

Management may be either medical therapy for heart failure and arrhythmias or intervention. Recently, balloon valvuloplasty has largely obviated the need for cardiac surgery in pulmonary stenosis. There has been long-term success in children and young adults with pliable valves [3], but the long-term outcome in elderly patients with calcified valves is not yet known [4].

Radiological suspicion of congenital heart disease should not be discounted because of the patient's age, especially as new techniques may facilitate correction in all age groups.

References

1. Perloff JK. The clinical recognition of congenital heart disease. Philadelphia; WB Saunders, 1987.
2. Johnson LW, Grossman W, Dalen JE, Dexter L. Pulmonic stenosis in the adult. New Engl J Med 1972;287:1159–63.
3. Stanger P, Cassidy SC, Girod DA, et al. Balloon pulmonary valvuloplasty: results of the valvuloplasty and angioplasty of congenital anomalies registry. Am J Cardiol 1990;65:775–83.
4. Goudvenos J, Wren C, Adams PC. Balloon valvotomy of calcified pulmonary valve stenosis. Cardiology 1990;77:55–7.

A rare cause of a common symptom

[1]P J CLOSE and [2]P L MONKS

Departments of [1]Radiology and [2]Gynaecology, Princess Alexandra Hospital, Woolloongabba, Brisbane, Queensland 4102, Australia

A 34-year-old woman presented with a short history of painless vaginal bleeding. Her last menstrual period had been approximately 8 weeks previously and a recent pregnancy test had been positive. She had a history of two previous lower segment Caesarean sections. On general examination she was mildly shocked. Vaginal examination showed an enlarged dumb-bell shaped 8–10 week uterus. The cervix was enlarged, invaginating the bladder. The external os was closed.

An initial diagnosis of incomplete abortion was made and pelvic ultrasound was requested. A midline sagittal transabdominal ultrasound image is shown (Figure 1).

What does the image demonstrate? What diagnoses should be considered? How might management be influenced?

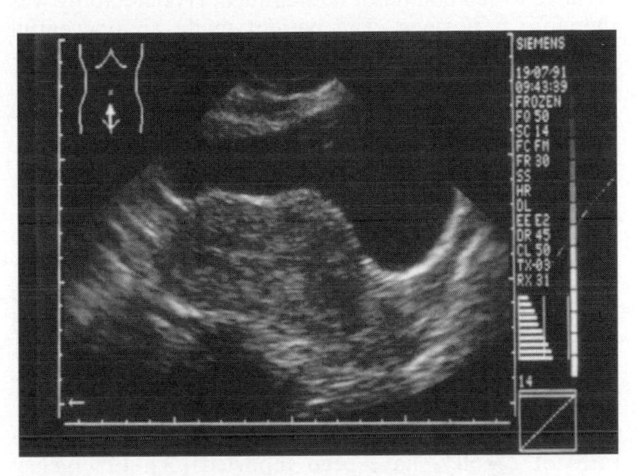

Figure 1. A midline sagittal transabdominal image.

Based on the case of the month originally published in Br J Radiol 1992;65:729–30.

Ultrasound demonstrated a normal midline cavity echo in the body of the uterus. Inferiorly products of conception occupied the lower uterine segment and cervix. The mass bulged into the bladder. No fetal parts were seen and the external os appeared closed. No free blood was seen in the pouch of Douglas. The diagnoses to consider were cervical pregnancy or cervical abortion. The former was considered more likely.

At operation products of conception were located in the cervical canal. Gentle removal resulted in brisk haemorrhage which could not be stemmed. Hysterectomy was therefore performed. The patient made an uneventful recovery. Histological examination of the resected specimen confirmed a cervical ectopic pregnancy.

Cervical ectopic pregnancy is a rare occurrence with a reported incidence of between one per 1000 to one per 24 000 pregnancies [1, 2]. Predisposing factors include previous gynaecological surgery and multiparity [1], so as the incidence of Caesarean section and other uterine procedures increase, so might the incidence of cervical implantation. Without pre-operative diagnosis, dilatation and curettage for misdiagnosed spontaneous abortion is likely to cause life threatening haemorrhage or rupture the weakened uterine wall. Maternal morbidity rates of 20–50% have been reported [3]. Emergency hysterectomy is usually required to achieve haemostasis with obvious consequences for future fertility. Clinically, patients present as a miscarriage. A clue to the diagnosis is if pelvic examination reveals a disproportionately enlarged cervix compared with the body of the uterus. Ultrasonic findings include a minimally enlarged uterine fundus with a swollen and bulging cervical canal containing an inhomogenous mass and decidual reaction. Sometimes a poorly defined gestation sac is visible [3]. Fetal parts may be detected and, if visible, the internal os should appear closed.

Cervical pregnancy is mimicked very closely by cervical abortion, both clinically and ultrasonically. The latter is defined as spontaneous abortion of an intra-uterine pregnancy into the cervix where the abortus is retained by a resistant external os. Vas et al [3] reported four cases of cervical abortion in which the endometrial cavity appeared more prominent than with cervical pregnancies. Blood clots and products of conception rather than a decidual cast were seen. The uterine fundus was larger for the state of gestation, giving less of an "hourglass" appearance, and the internal os was open.

MRI has been used to aid diagnosis of cervical pregnancy, complementing ultrasound, and confirming the suspicion that implantation had occurred at the site of a previous Caesarean section scar [4]. Endovaginal sonography (EVS) should be expected to provide further information in cases of cervical pregnancy due to excellent visualization of the cervix. EVS was not available at this institution.

If diagnosed early and accurately, management strategies are available to reduce maternal morbidity and preserve the uterus. Lobel et al [2] reported two cases of cervical pregnancy detected by ultrasound. Before termination of pregnancy the uterine arteries were successfully embolized using angiographic techniques. As a result, surgical evacuation was performed with minimal haemorrhage. Hysterectomy was not required and the patient's potential fertility was retained. Other reported management strategies to achieve the same aim include use of feticidal agents [5], ligation of internal iliac and uterine arteries, circumsuture and intracervical obturator and intracervical balloon tamponade [2].

In this case the patient was in shock and it was not prudent to delay surgery any longer than necessary. As this 34-year-old patient had three previous children, hysterectomy was not as devastating as for a young nulliparous woman.

[*See also Frates et al [6], ED*]

References

1. Werber J, Prasadarao PR, Harris VJ. Cervical pregnancy diagnosed by ultrasound. Radiology 1983;149:279–80.
2. Lobel SM, Meyerovitz MF, Benson CC, Goff B, Bengtson JM. Pre-operative angiographic uterine artery embolization in the management of cervical pregnancy. Obstet Gynecol 1990;76:938–41.
3. Vas W, Suresh PL, Tang-Barton P, Salimi Z, Carlin B. Ultrasonic differentiation of cervical abortion from cervical pregnancy. J Clin Ultrasound 1984;12:553–7.
4. Bader-Armstrong B, Shah Y, Rubens D. Use of ultrasound and magnetic resonance imaging in the diagnosis of cervical pregnancy. J Clin Ultrasound 1989;17:283–6.
5. Segna RA, Mitchell DR, Misas JE. Successful treatment of cervical pregnancy with oral etoposide. Obstet Gynecol 1990;76:945–7.
6. Frates MC, Benson CB, Doubilet PM, et al. Cervical ectopic pregnancy: results of conservative treatment. Radiology 1994;191:773–5.

Inside a thin man—an engrossing problem

J P HUGHES and E WYN JONES

Department of Radiology, Morriston Hospital, Morriston, Swansea, West Glamorgan, UK

A 21-year-old male presented with a 12 month history of progressive symptoms in his right leg, consisting of weakness and numbness, with a limp which was initially fluctuant, but becoming more persistent. He also complained of lower dorsal back pain which seemed to be posture-related, and over the past 2–3 months he had developed some frequency of micturition. He had been seen 10 years previously on account of clumsiness, but no clear diagnosis had been reached. His general health was normally good and he was on no medication.

On examination he appeared a fit young man. There was no scoliosis and no spinal tenderness. The cranial nerves and upper limbs were normal. In the lower limbs, there was mild spasticity with global weakness of the right leg, and hypoasthesia to light touch and pin-prick on the right side from T12/L1 through to S4 inclusive. The knee and ankle jerks were brisk bilaterally, particularly on the right. Both plantar responses were flexor. Biochemical tests, including a fasting cortisol level were all normal.

What does MRI (Figures 1 and 2) show, and what is the diagnosis?

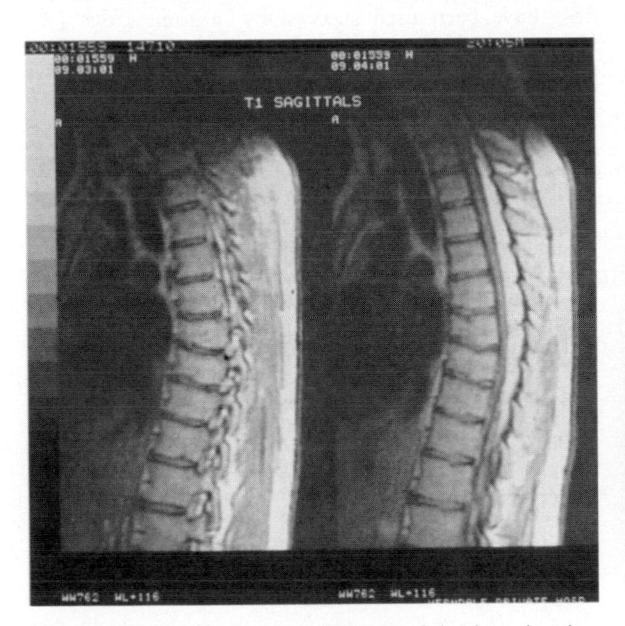

Figure 1. Sagittal T_1 weighted MRI scan of the thoracic spine.

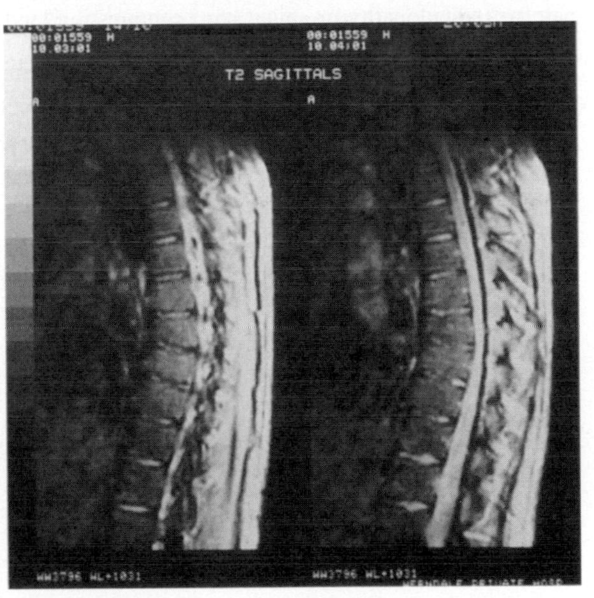

Figure 2. The corresponding T_2 weighted sagittal MRI scan of the thoracic spine.

Based on the case of the month originally published in Br J Radiol 1995;68:213–4.

MRI demonstrated an extensive extradural soft tissue mass of hyperintense signal on both T_1 and T_2 sequences. The lesion was situated posterolaterally within the spinal canal and extended over several segments of the mid-lower dorsal spine; significant anterior displacement and compression of the spinal cord was demonstrated on axial scans (Figure 3). A diagnosis of epidural lipomatosis was made and confirmed at operation. An extensive laminectomy was undertaken from T3–T10 and a 1.0–1.5 cm thick adipose mass was found, causing marked dural compression. The lesion was readily dissectable from the dura, which appeared satisfactorily decompressed. Post-operatively there was immediate and complete resolution of all neurological signs.

Epidural lipomatosis is pathological overgrowth of adipose tissue within the epidural space. This may lead to dural or cauda-equina compression.

The condition has most often been reported in patients either with elevated endogenous steroids, or those receiving long-term steroid therapy for a variety of medical conditions [1, 2]. However, a small number of cases have been reported in which symptomatic epidural lipomatosis occurred in otherwise normal, healthy patients [3, 4]. Presentation may vary from non-specific back pain to radiculopathy or spinal cord compression, and is typically progressive.

The distribution of excess adipose tissue may be circumferential, but tends to be predominantly posterior and posterolateral, usually within the thoracic region, although the lumbosacral region can also be affected [5].

Diagnosis is usually made from a combination of imaging, surgical and histological findings. Although myelography may be useful in demonstrating dural compression, and sometimes complete extradural block, appearances are non-specific, and in some cases the myelogram has been normal [5].

CT readily demonstrates the excess epidural fat (tissue density −80 to −120 Hounsfield units) and compression of the dura, which may become distorted, typically into a triangular shape.

MRI has the advantage of allowing multiplanar imaging, so that the extent of the lesion can be demonstrated on sagittal images. The fatty nature of the tissue can be readily appreciated from the hyperintense signal obtained on both T_1 and T_2 weighted images. In the thoracic region, the T_2 weighted scan will ensure that the

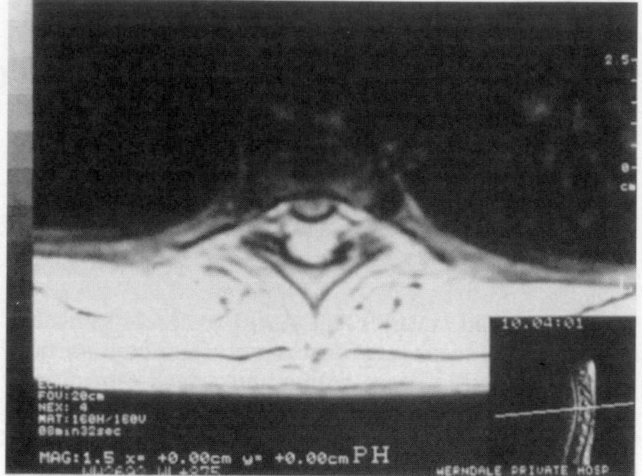

Figure 3. Axial fast T_1 weighted MRI scan at the level of T10, demonstrating anterior displacement and compression of the cord.

high signal dorsal to the cord does in fact represent fat, rather than the haemorrhagic component of an epidural abscess or haematoma.

Treatment depends on the clinical findings. Weight reduction in the obese, and slow tapering of the steroid dose have been used successfully in some cases [2]. However, in patients with acute progressive symptoms, and where conservative management fails, decompressive laminectomy is indicated.

Although it is rare, awareness of this condition is necessary in view of the potentially reversible neurological effects.

References

1. Roy-Camille R, Mazel CH, Husson JL, Saillant G. Symptomatic spinal epidural lipomatosis induced by a long term steroid treatment. Review of the literature and report of two additional cases. Spine 1991;16:1365–71.
2. Fessler RG, Johnson DL, Brown FD, et al. Epidural lipomatosis in steroid treated patients. Spine 1992;17:183–8.
3. Bednar DA, Esses SI, Kucharczyk W. Symptomatic lumbar epidural lipomatosis in a normal male. A unique case report. Spine, 1990;15:52–3.
4. Haddad SF, Hitchon PW, Godersky JC. Idiopathic and glucocorticoid-induced spinal epidural lipomatosis. J Neurosurg 1991;74:38–42.
5. Quint DJ, Boulos RS, Sanders WP, et al. Epidural lipomatosis. Radiology 1988;169:485–90.

Calcified leg

J FLINN and I BEGGS

Department of Radiology, Princess Margaret Rose Orthopaedic Hospital, Fairmilehead, Edinburgh, EH10 7ED, UK

A 74-year-old man presented with a feeling of heaviness in his right leg on walking. He had fractured his right tibia 50 years previously, sustaining severe neurovascular damage. Subsequently, he had required sympathectomy for trophic ulcer, tenotomies and toe fusion. He needed an orthopaedic boot to compensate for his shortened leg. There was no other relevant history and the patient was otherwise well.

On examination, he had thin skin on his right shin and foot and had varicose eczema, diminished sensation on the sole of the foot and absent posterior tibial and dorsalis pedis pulses.

Plain radiographs and a CT scan were performed (Figures 1 and 2). What is the diagnosis?

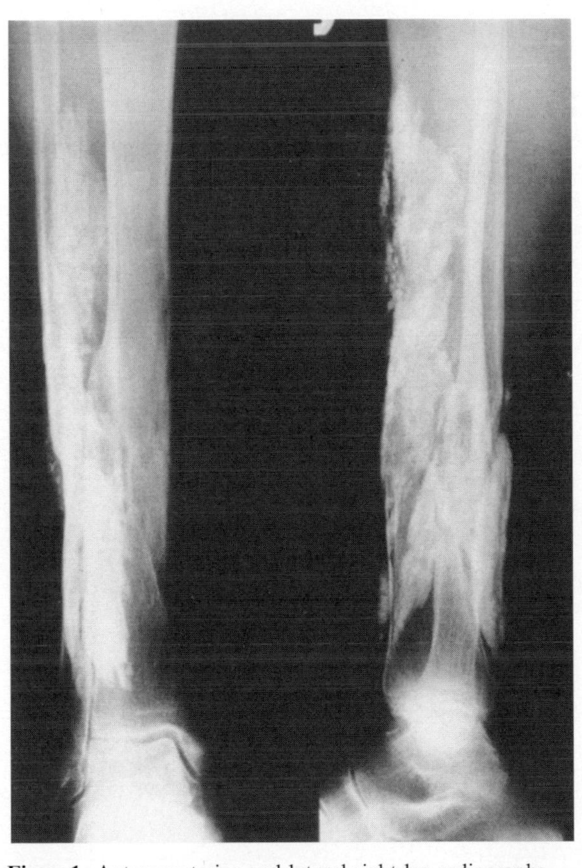

Figure 1. Anteroposterior and lateral right leg radiographs.

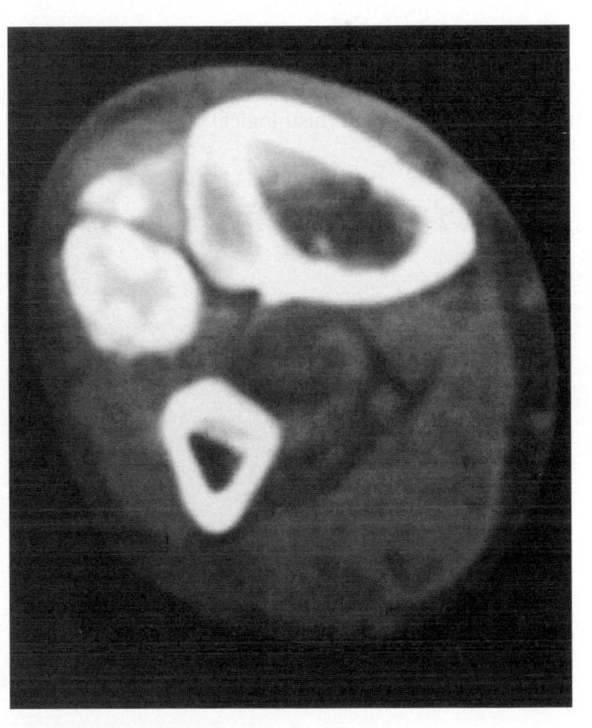

Figure 2. CT of the right calf.

Based on the case of the month originally published in Br J Radiol 1996;69:371–2.

Plain radiographs showed healed fractures of the tibia and fibula which were partly obscured by an extensive sheet of calcification. CT confirmed that the calcification was in the anterior compartment, predominantly in tibialis anterior.

The appearance of a sheet of calcification which corresponds to an individual muscle or compartment in the arm or leg is characteristic of an old severe compartment syndrome, although an old calcified tuberculous abscess could cause a similar appearance.

Acute compartment syndromes usually result from trauma. Haemorrhage, oedema and muscle swelling occur within a compartment surrounded by inelastic fascia [1]. The pressure within the compartment is elevated and exceeds the tissue capillary perfusion pressure. Decompression by fasciotomy is required within hours to prevent irreversible necrosis of the muscles and nerves which traverse the compartment. The anterior compartment of the leg is the most frequently involved site.

Long-term complications of compartment syndrome include contractures and motor and sensory deficits. Calcification of the involved muscles is a rare but recognized complication [2–4] which usually presents with local swelling at the site of the calcification, 20–60 years after the original injury. Incision of the calcified masses produces large amounts of sterile, creamy or gelatinous material. This is not recommended as chronic infection with discharging sinuses may result. Our patient had no swelling and only minor symptoms and was happy to be reassured and have no other treatment.

References

1. Hargens AR, Mubarak SJ (editors). Definition and terminology. In: Compartment syndromes and Volkman's ischaemic contracture. Philadelphia: WB Saunders, 1981:1–5.
2. Janzen DL, Connell DG, Vaisler BJ. Calcific myonecrosis of the calf manifesting as an enlarging soft-tissue mass: imaging features. AJR 1993;160:1072–4.
3. Malisano LP, Hunter GA. Liquefaction and calcification of a chronic compartment syndrome of the lower limb. J Orthop Trauma 1992;6:245–7.
4. Viau MR, Pederson HE, Salcicioli GG, Manoli A. Ectopic calcification as a late sequela of compartment syndrome. Clin Orthop 1983;176:178–80.

Jekyll and Hyde chest radiographs

M COBBY, A DUNCAN and G HARTNELL

Department of Radiology, Bristol Royal Hospital for Sick Children, St Michael's Hill, Bristol BS2 8BJ, UK

A full-term, male infant was admitted to the Special Care Baby Unit immediately following birth with cyanosis and respiratory distress. The pregnancy had been uneventful and the mother had three other children who were all well. The baby was intubated and ventilated but remained persistently hypoxic with a respiratory acidosis. The chest radiograph on admission is shown in Figure 1.

Treatment for a presumed streptococcal pneumonia was instituted but the baby remained unwell.

What abnormalities are shown on the three chest radiographs (Figures 1–3)? What is your differential diagnosis and what further investigations would you perform?

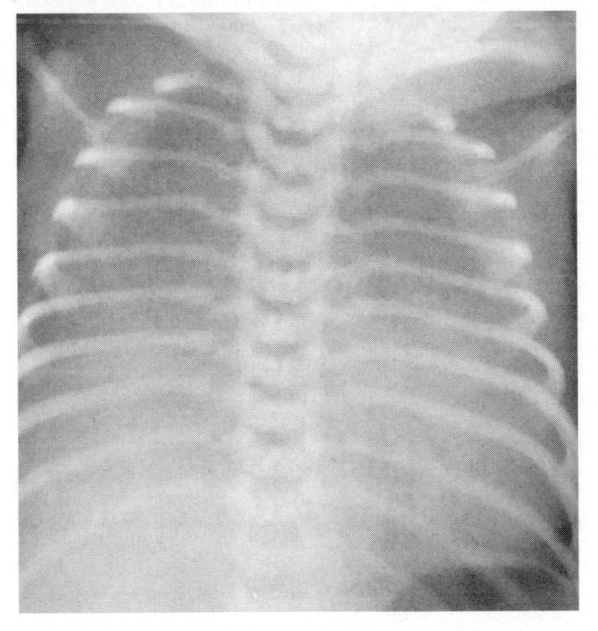

Figure 1. Chest radiograph on admission to the Special Care Baby Unit.

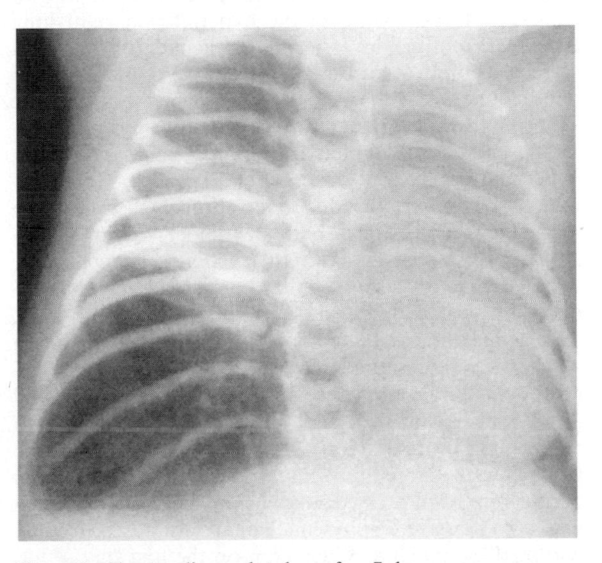

Figure 2. Chest radiograph taken after 7 days.

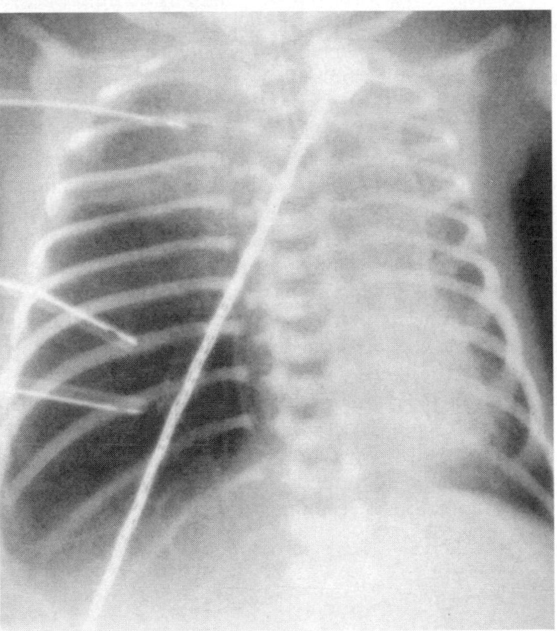

Figure 3. Chest radiograph taken on the 10th day.

Based on the case of the month originally published in Br J Radiol 1989;62:561–2.

On the initial chest radiograph (Figure 1) the cardiac apex was shifted to the left as was the upper mediastinum, shown by the position of the endotracheal tube. There was diffuse shadowing throughout both lungs, compatible with retained fetal fluid, and more dense opacification of the right lower zone. The second radiograph (Figure 2) showed marked overexpansion of the right lung, with emphysematous changes of the lower and middle lobes, and mediastinal shift to the left. This was even more severe on the third radiograph (Figure 3) with considerable herniation of the hyperinflated right lung across the midline, inversion of the hemidiaphragm and increased emphysematous changes in the right lower and middle lobes. The chest drain tubes were inserted on the assumption that a pneumothorax was present.

The chest radiographic appearances could be due to hyperinflation from obstruction of a bronchus. In a neonate [1, 2], this may be due to intrabronchial obstruction by a mucus plug, foreign body or tumour, extrinsic compression by a mediastinal mass (such as a bronchogenic cyst), or a vascular ring. Similar appearances can be produced by bronchial stenosis, congenital lobar emphysema, a congenital lung cyst or cystic adenomatoid malformation when the cystic component predominates. A tension pneumothorax should not cause confusion if a lung edge and absent vessels are observed, and in cases of difficulty a horizontal beam lateral view should be obtained. Congenital lobar emphysema presents in the neonatal period with respiratory distress due to air trapping, which results in massive emphysema, collapse of adjacent lobes and mediastinal shift. When seen on the first day of life, the affected, distended lobe may initially be fluid filled, as shown in Figure 1. However, the upper lobes, most commonly the left, and sometimes the middle lobe, are usually involved, and only rarely the lower lobes [3].

The most important differential diagnosis was considered to be compression of the right main bronchus by a vascular ring. Contrast-enhanced CT of the mediastinum was initially performed but, due to artefacts from the endotracheal tube, failed to provide any diagnostic information. An anomalous left pulmonary artery, which arose from the right pulmonary artery and crossed to the left behind the trachea, was confirmed by cine angiography, which also showed a small patent ductus arteriosus (Figure 4). Division of the pulmonary sling and re-implantation of the left pulmonary artery into the main pulmonary artery was performed 13 days after the child was born and at the same time the patent ductus was divided.

An anomalous left pulmonary artery usually arises from the first part of the right pulmonary artery, passes over the right main bronchus and crosses the midline between the trachea and oesophagus. This presents with obstructive symptoms and signs due to compression of any of the airways with which the anomalous artery is intimately related, usually the right main bronchus, as in our patient. It can be simply differentiated from the variety of other aberrant vessels and vascular rings on a lateral barium swallow [4] as it is the only vascular anomaly to pass between the trachea and oesophagus, resulting in anterior oesophageal indentation. Although this is an unusual cause of unilateral emphysema in the neonate it is important to consider it in the differential diagnosis as the surgical management is quite different from that required for congenital lobar emphysema or other causes of this appearance.

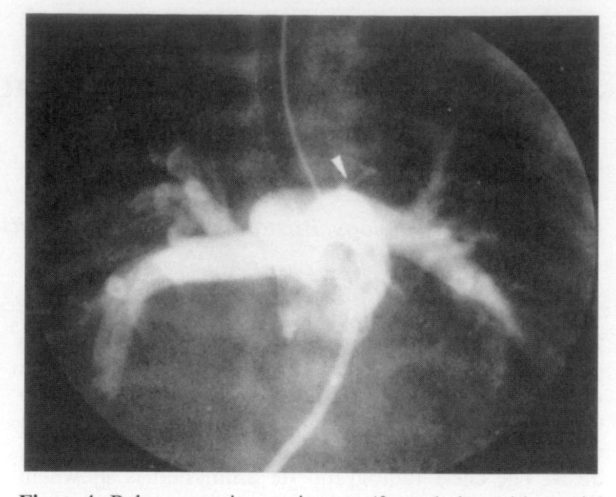

Figure 4. Pulmonary cine angiogram (frontal view with cranial tilt). The tip of the catheter lies in the main pulmonary artery. The anomalous origin of the left pulmonary artery passes over the right main bronchus and behind the trachea to reach the left hilum. The arrowhead points to the patent ductus arteriosus. The endotracheal tube is in the left main bronchus.

References

1. Caffey J. Pediatric X-ray diagnosis. Chicago: Year Book Publishers, 1978:1682–9.
2. Alford BA, Armstrong P. In: Grainger RG, Allison DJ. Diagnostic radiology. Edinburgh: Churchill Livingstone, 1986:364–5.
3. Cremin BJ, Movsowitz H. Lobar emphysema in infants. Br J Radiol 1971;44:692–6.
4. Berdon WB, Baker WE. Vascular anomalies and the infant lung: rings, slings, and other things. Semin Roentgenol 1972;7:39–64.

Hypokalaemic hypertension: a real con!

L S HUNTLEY and N R MOORE

Oxford Magnetic Resonance Imaging Centre, John Radcliffe Hospital, Oxford OX3 9DU, UK

A 40-year-old baker was referred for investigation of increasingly frequent episodic fast irregular palpitations with slight chest discomfort and dizziness. There was no dyspnoea. He was hypertensive at 150/105 mmHg. His general practitioner had commenced atenolol 50 mg daily for the hypertension and potassium supplements as a low serum potassium concentration had been discovered during initial investigation. Further assessment showed mild asymmetric left ventricular hypertrophy and confirmed a low serum potassium concentration of 3.2 mmol l^{-1} with normal renal function. 24 h urinary catecholamine assessment and supine/standing serum assays of renin and aldosterone were normal. After control of his hypertension he was discharged to the care of his general practitioner.

2 years later he presented as an emergency with similar symptoms. His treatment had been changed to verapamil 160 mg twice daily with potassium supplementation. His blood pressure was 150/100 mmHg and serum potassium concentration was 3.0 mmol l^{-1}. Supine and standing serum samples now showed suppressed renin levels with elevated aldosterone, confirming primary hyperaldosteronism. A CT examination of the adrenals was performed (Figure 1a, b). What does this show?

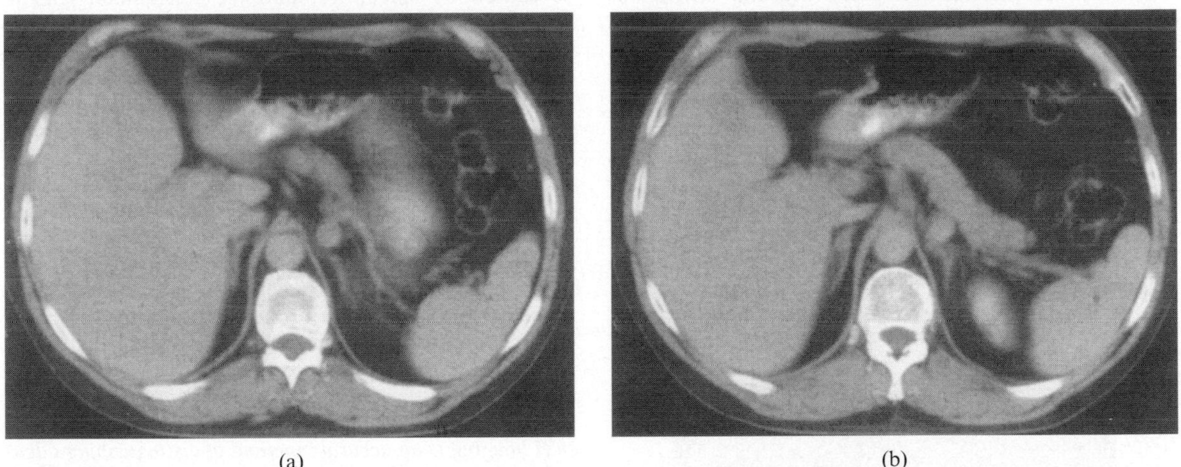

(a) (b)

Figure 1. Two contiguous 10 mm thick images from a CT study. Intravenous contrast medium had been given.

Based on the case of the month originally published in Br J Radiol 1993;66:1197–8.

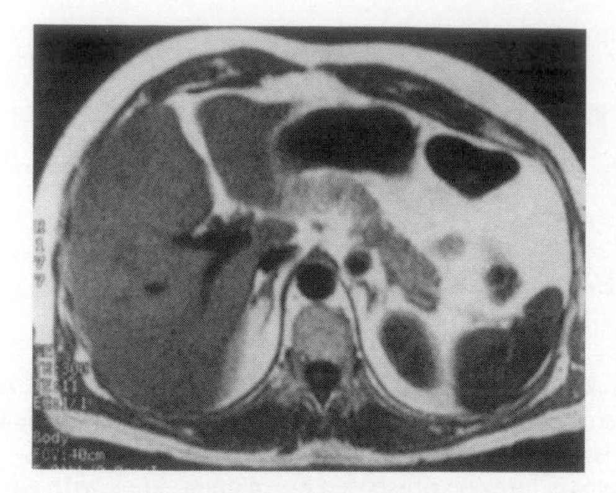

Figure 2. T_1 weighted spin echo image (TR 300 ms, TE 11 ms, 256 × 192 matrix, 4 excitations) showing a 1.5 cm mass adjacent to the body of the left adrenal gland. Note the central signal void.

There was a 1.5 cm diameter mass related to the body of the left adrenal gland. A left adrenal aldosterone secreting tumour was diagnosed initially. At review it was appreciated that the CT had not been performed with meticulous technique. Contiguous 10 mm rather than 5 mm sections had been performed, and intravenous contrast medium had been given as a bolus at the start of the study rather than as a dynamic enhancement technique. Instead of recalling the patient for a repeat CT examination, an MRI study was performed. The T_1 weighted spin echo image (Figure 2) showed the left adrenal lesion to have a central signal void which was of high signal intensity on a breathhold gradient recalled acquisition in the steady state (GRASS) image (Figure 3). These features indicated that the abnormality was vascular with flowing blood centrally [1]. A coronal image (Figure 4) and adjacent transverse sections showed a dilated tortuous splenic artery masquerading as an adrenal tumour. In the absence of any other adrenal mass a diagnosis of adrenal hyperplasia was made. This has not been confirmed by adrenal vein sampling.

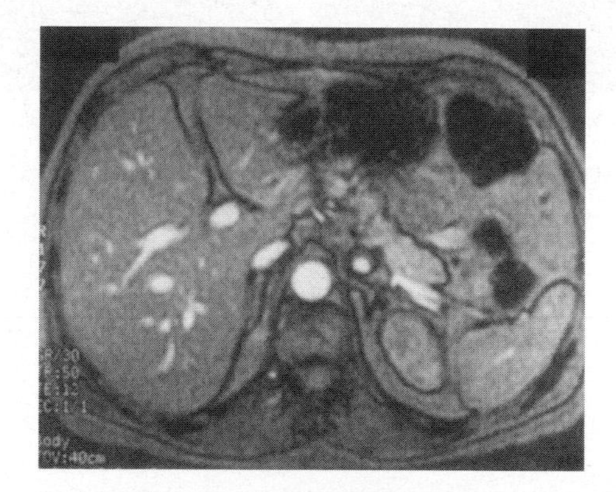

Figure 3. A gradient recalled acquisition in the steady state (GRASS) image obtained in a breath hold (TR 50 ms, TE 12 ms, 30° flip angle, 256 × 128 matrix, 2 excitations, scan time 13 s). This flow sensitive image shows high signal owing to flowing blood within the lesion.

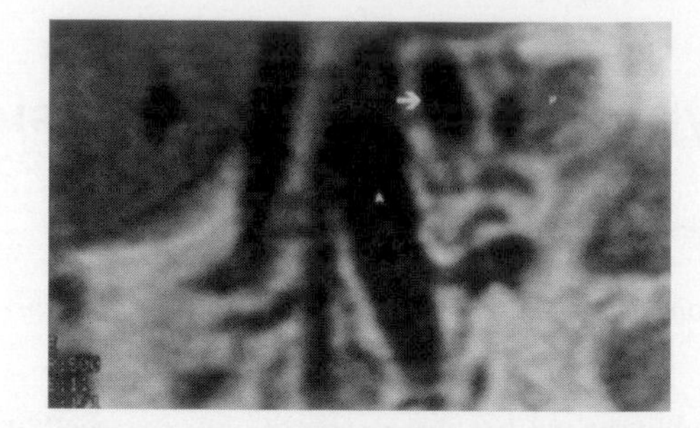

Figure 4. A coronal T_1 weighted spin echo image (TR 500 ms, TE 11 ms, 256 × 128 matrix, 2 excitations) shows the dilated splenic artery (arrow) between the aorta (A) and body of the pancreas (P).

The adrenal pseudotumour is a recognized pitfall in the search for aldosterone secreting adenomas. Pseudotumours are more common on the left and may be caused by splenic lobulations, splenunculi, gastric fundus, gastric or jejunal diverticula, renal or pancreatic masses and adjacent vessels [2–4]. A tortuous splenic artery or a dilated inferior phrenic vein (a porto-systemic shunt in portal hypertension) are the usual vascular mimics [4]. Careful attention to technique (contiguous thin sections, good bowel opacification, dynamic intravenous contrast enhancement) usually resolves most pseudotumours [3]. Berliner et al indicated that occasionally other imaging techniques such as ultrasound and angiography are needed [3].

This case reiterates the potential for a tortuous dilated splenic artery to simulate an adrenal tumour. MRI was valuable because it identified with confidence the vascular nature of this pseudotumour. MRI can be used as a non-invasive alternative if CT is indeterminate.

[*On the subject of MRI in adrenal masses, chemical shift imaging is an accurate method of distinguishing adenomas from metastases [5], ED*]

References

1. Atlas SW, Mark AS, Fram EK, Grossmann RI. Vascular intracranial lesions: applications of gradient-echo MR imaging. Radiology 1988;169:455–61.
2. Sample WF, Sarti DA. Computed tomography and gray scale ultrasonography of the adrenal gland: a comparative study. Radiology 1978;128:377–83.
3. Berliner L, Bosniak MA, Megibow A. Adrenal pseudotumors on computed tomography. JCAT 1982;6:281–5.
4. Brady TM, Gross BH, Glazer GM, Williams DM. Adrenal pseudomasses due to varices: angiographic–CT–MRI–pathologic correlations. AJR 1985;145:301–4.
5. Outwater EK, Siegelman ES, Radecki PD, et al. Distinction between benign and malignant adrenal masses: value of T_1-weighted chemical-shift MR imaging. AJR 1995;165:579–83.

"... or plat du jour"

J BHATTACHARYA, C FRASER and L M MACDONALD

Department of Radiology, St Thomas' Hospital, Lambeth Palace Road, London SE1 7EH, UK

A 37-year-old man with psoriasis complained of mild neck and back stiffness at a regular visit to a dermatology outpatient clinic. His skin involvement had been widespread for the last 4 years, although he had never suffered from psoriatic arthropathy.

Several common therapeutic regimens had failed to procure significant improvement and 2 years prior to this visit his treatment had again been changed.

What do the radiographs show and what is the aetiology?

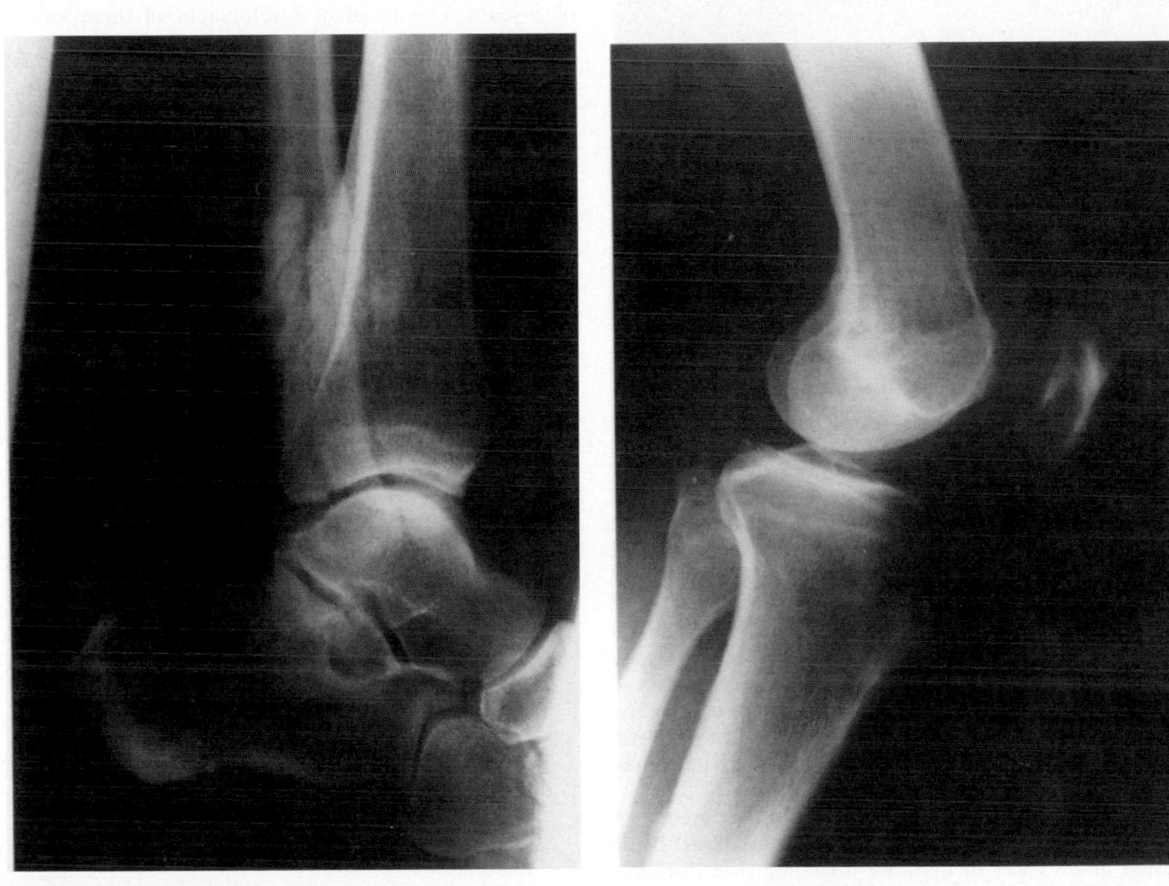

Figure 1. Ankle radiograph.

Figure 2. Knee radiograph.

Based on the case of the month originally published in Br J Radiol 1995;68:545–6.

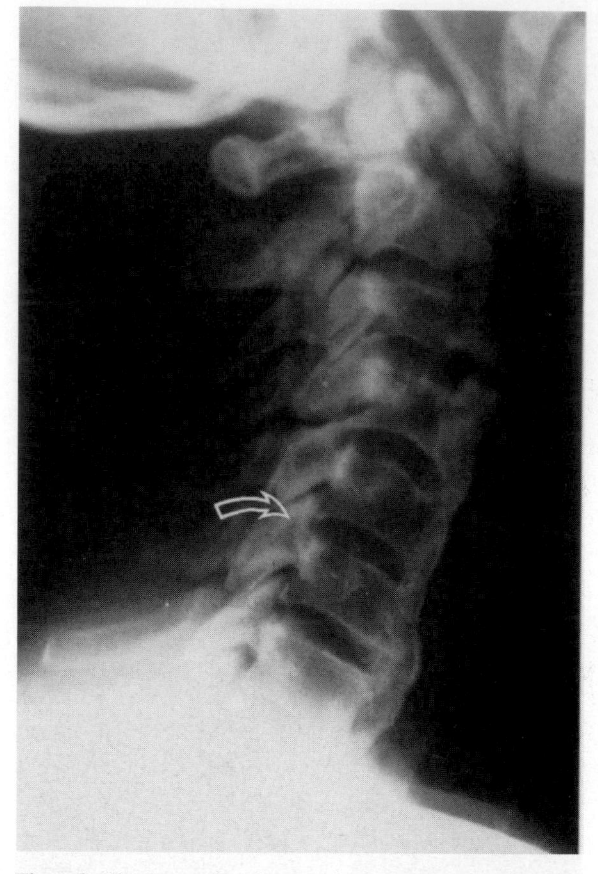

Figure 3. Flowing ossification and hyperostosis of the anterior longitudinal ligament with localized ossification of the posterior longitudinal ligament at the C5/6 level (arrow). The disc spaces are preserved.

Ossification and hyperostosis of the interosseous ligament above the ankle joint and calcaneal spurs are present (Figure 1). There was sub-periosteal new bone formation on the distal femur and proximal tibia (Figure 2).

The cervical spine (Figure 3) demonstrated flowing ossification of the anterior longitudinal ligament and cortical hyperostosis to produce an appearance suggestive of diffuse idiopathic skeletal hyperostosis (DISH). There was also ossification of the posterior longitudinal ligament at the C5/6 level, which may potentially cause spinal stenosis.

Our patient had commenced oral retinoid therapy with etretinate 2 years previously. Widespread skeletal hyperostoses are an increasingly common complication.

Synthetic derivatives of vitamin A (retinoids) are being tested in a variety of diseases, including skin disorders (psoriasis, cystic acne and keratinization disorders), joint diseases (rheumatoid and psoriatic arthropathy) and cancers (bladder, breasts and skin). They are already widely used in dermatology.

Skeletal toxicity, resulting from chronic vitamin A (retinoid) poisoning, was first described nearly 50 years ago, causing bone demineralization, thinning of long bones, cortical hyperostosis, periostitis and premature epiphyseal closure.

More recently an ossifying diathesis resembling DISH was found in patients taking high doses of 13-cis-retinoic acid for refractory ichthyosis. These changes are the result of accelerated bone and cartilage resorption and new bone formation. Indeed, given the similarity of retinoid associated hyperostosis to DISH, it has been suggested that the latter may be metabolic in origin [1].

The DISH-like syndrome associated with etretinate has been the subject of several reports [2, 3]. The former authors described a prospective study of 38 patients with keratinization disorders on etretinate. These patients developed features resembling principally the extraspinal manifestations of DISH with widespread tendon and ligament calcification after a mean duration of 5 years. The speed of development of these lesions has been variously reported, however, and a more recent report described hip and spine hyperostoses after 18 months continuous etretinate therapy [4]. Patients on 13-cis-retinoic acid have developed this complication in as little as 6 months [1, 5].

The potential rapidity in the evolution of this syndrome together with the increasing therapeutic use of retinoids mean that this complication is likely to be encountered with increasing frequency in the future.

References

1. Pennes D, Ellis C, Martel W. Early skeletal hyperstoses secondary to 13-cis-retinoid acid. AJR, 1984;141:979–83.
2. Digiovanna MD, Roberta K, Peck G. Extraspinal tendon and ligament calcification associated with etretinate. N Engl J Med 1986;315:1177–82.
3. Burge S, Ryan T. Diffuse hyperostosis associated with etretinate. Lancet 1985;2:397–8.
4. Cerio R, Wells R, McDonald DM. Calcifying artropathy of the hips and diffuse hyperostosis associated with etretinate. Clin Exp Dermatol 1987;12:129–31.
5. Pennes D, Martel W, Voorhees J. Evolution of skeletal hyperstosis caused by 13-cis-retinoic acid therapy. AJR 1988; 151:967–73.

A real headache!

[1]J E JACKSON and [2]C J O'DONNELL

[1]*Department of Diagnostic Radiology, Hammersmith Hospital, Du Cane Road, London W12 0HS, UK and*
[2]*Department of Radiology, Royal Melbourne Hospital, Parkville 3050, Victoria, Australia*

This 31-year-old female patient had recently undergone a uterine myomectomy. Histology of the resected surgical specimen had demonstrated borderline sarcomatous change in a fibroid and, in view of a complaint of headaches, the patient was referred for further radiological investigation to exclude cerebral metastatic disease. There had been no previous history of trauma. Neurological examination was unremarkable. A plain frontal skull radiograph (Figure 1) and contrast enhanced CT at the level of the lateral ventricles (Figure 2), are shown. What abnormalities are present and what are the likely causes of these appearances?

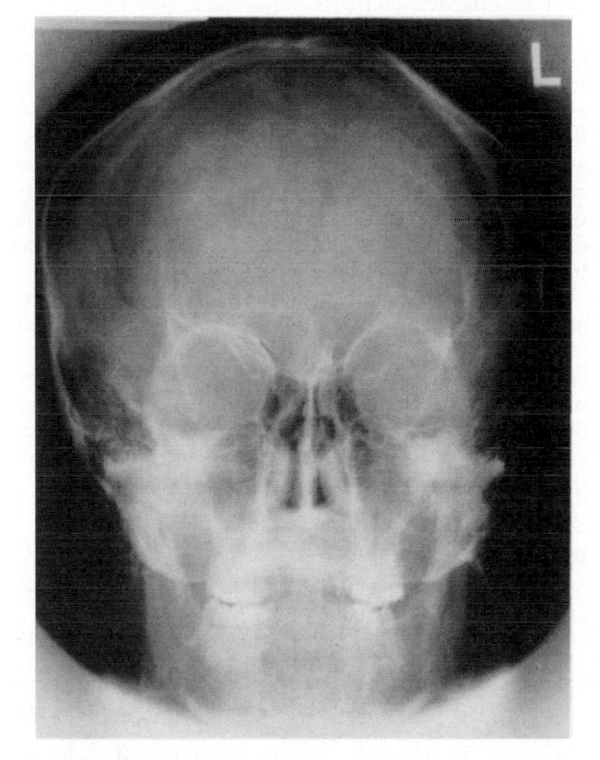

Figure 1. Plain frontal skull radiograph.

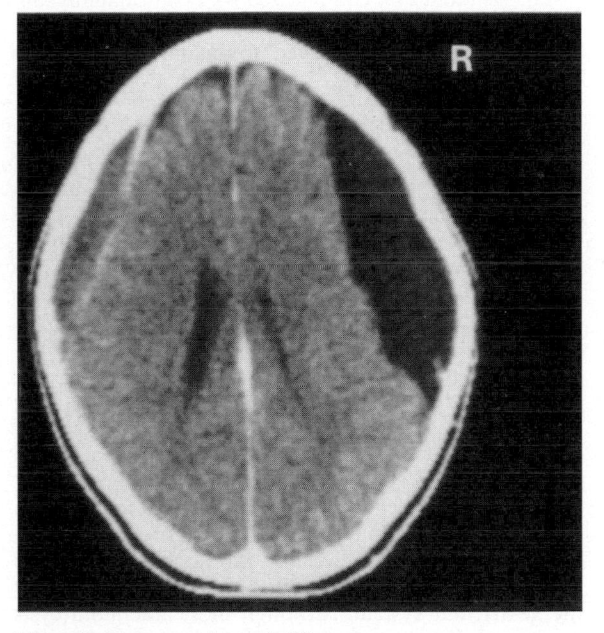

Figure 2. Contrast enhanced CT scan.

Based on the case of the month originally published in Br J Radiol 1989;62:867–8.

The plain frontal skull radiograph (Figure 1) demonstrated elevation of the right lesser wing of sphenoid. CT (Figure 2) showed a water density extracerebral mass over the right cerebral convexity and a higher density extracerebral collection over the left frontoparietal convexity, which showed enhancement of its wall. The combination of the elevation of the lesser wing of sphenoid on the plain radiograph, which suggests long-standing mass effect, and a water density extracerebral mass on the same side was highly suggestive of an arachnoid cyst of the middle cranial fossa. CT at the level of the middle cranial fossa showed forward displacement and thickening of the greater wing of sphenoid and confirmed that the water density mass arose from the floor of the middle cranial fossa. The features on the left side, of a crescentic low density extracerebral collection with linear enhancement medially, were those of a chronic subdural haematoma. The diagnosis was therefore a right middle cranial fossa arachnoid cyst complicated by a contralateral subdural haematoma. Because of the lack of significant symptoms the patient received no treatment and is to be followed-up in clinic.

Arachnoid cysts are believed to represent a congenital anomaly of the developing subarachnoid cistern in early intrauterine life. They are relatively uncommon, comprising approximately 1% of all intracranial space-occupying lesions, and occur in a variety of different sites including the middle cranial fossa, the supracollicular area, the cerebellopontine angle, the vermian area, the clival zone, the sellar and parasellar areas, the interhemispheric fissure and over the cerebral convexity.

The aetiology of intracranial arachnoid cysts has been discussed by several authors [1–3]. Robinson [2] initially postulated agenesis of the temporal lobe with overlying cerebrospinal fluid loculation. It is now generally believed, however, that arachnoid cysts occur as a consequence of anomalous development of the subarachnoid cisterns, and are actually intraarachnoid with no communication with either the subarachnoid space or the ventricular system. Although most arachnoid cysts are regarded as being congenital, and unrelated to previous trauma, haemorrhage or inflammation, it is impossible to dissociate completely such factors from cases described in the literature. Many affected patients are reported as having a history of old and relatively minor head trauma, such as a minor birth injury, which may initiate cyst formation. [*An interesting theory on the aetiology of arachnoid cysts is described by Garcia Santos et al [6], ED*].

Of the various intracranial arachnoid cysts, those that occur in the middle cranial fossa are the most common, accounting for nearly 50% of cases [3]. They are usually asymptomatic and, since the advent of CT, are frequently found incidently during investigation for unrelated disease. When symptomatic, their most usual presentation is with headache, which is generally not severe, or with asymmetric bulging of the head. Less commonly, but more importantly, they can present with symptoms and signs of raised intracranial pressure usually secondary to an associated subdural or intracystic bleed. This complication is more likely to occur in children or adolescents and is uncommon over the age of 21 years [2]. The majority of haemorrhagic complications have occurred in males.

The association between arachnoid cysts, especially of the middle cranial fossa, and subdural haematomata is well recognized but unexplained. An ipsilateral haematoma may result from tearing of unsupported blood vessels around the periphery of the cyst, either spontaneously or following relatively minor trauma. Operative findings in five patients of abnormal small veins running on the surface of the membranous capsule of the arachnoid cyst and bridging the Sylvian fissure support this view [4].

The occasional occurrence of a contralateral subdural haematoma may be explained by intermittent changes in intracranial pressure, due to either expansion of the cyst or blockage, by the cyst, of the lateral cerebrospinal fluid (CSF) route to its site of absorption. Alternatively, a redistribution of the CSF by the cyst may disturb the mechanical buffer for the brain [5]. Any of these may cause abnormal traction and compression of brain tissue and subsequently increase the likelihood of a subdural bleed.

Although well demonstrated in this case, it is important to remember that a subdural haematoma will not always be as well defined on CT because it may be isodense with brain tissue. As middle cranial fossa arachnoid cysts usually produce no mass effect, if signs of brain compression are present, an associated subdural collection must be suspected. This is more commonly on the same side but may be contralateral.

References

1. Starkman SP, Brown TC, Linell EA. Cerebral arachnoid cysts. J Neuropathol Exp Neurol 1958;17:484–500.
2. Robinson RG. The temporal lobe agenesis syndrome. Brain 1964;87:87–106.
3. Rengachary SS, Watanabe I. Ultrastructure and pathogenesis of intracranial arachnoid cysts. J Neuropathol Exp Neurol 1981;40:61–83.
4. Kushida Y, Terao H, Shibata I, Shisido M, Seiki Y, Tsutsumi S. Chronic subdural haematoma associated with middle fossa arachnoid cyst. No-Shinkei-Geka 1983; 11:1211–7.
5. van der Meche FGA, Braakman R. Arachnoid cysts in the middle cranial fossa: cause and treatment of progressive and non-progressive symptoms. J Neurol Neurosurg Psychiatr 1983;46:1102–7.
6. Garcia Santos JM, Martinez-Lage J, Ubeda AG, et al. Arachnoid cysts of the middle cranial fossa: a consideration of their origins based on imaging. Neuroradiology 1993; 35:355–8.

"But fell like autumn fruit that mellowed long" (John Dryden)

[1]W T YANG, [1]R M EVANS and [2]S C CHUNG

Departments of [1]Diagnostic Radiology and Organ Imaging, and [2]Surgery, Prince of Wales Hospital, Chinese University of Hong Kong, Shatin, Hong Kong

An 89-year-old lady presented in the month of October with vomiting, colicky abdominal pain and abdominal distention. 3 years prior to presentation she underwent a Bilroth I partial gastrectomy for a gastric carcinoid tumour. Physical examination revealed that she was dehydrated and there was a positive succession splash.

A clinical diagnosis of high intestinal or gastric outlet obstruction was made and a contrast study of the upper gastrointestinal tract was performed (Figure 1). What abnormalities are shown and what is your diagnosis?

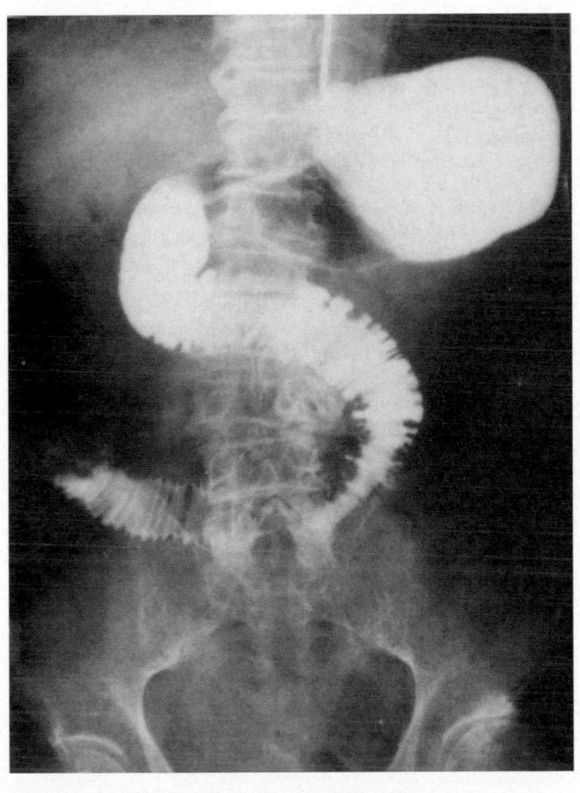

Figure 1. Contrast study via nasogastric tube.

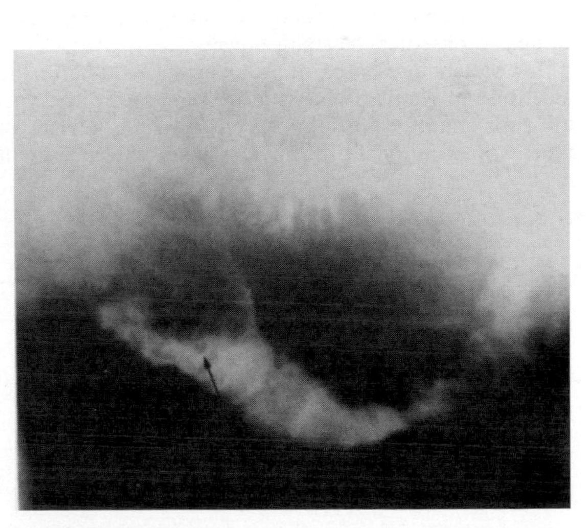

Figure 2. Spot view.

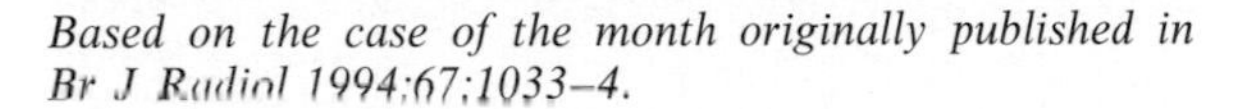

Based on the case of the month originally published in Br J Radiol 1994;67;1033–4.

A large intraluminal filling defect was seen in the proximal jejunum causing obstruction. Mild thickening of the valvulae conniventes was seen proximally. The mass had a stippled appearance (Figure 2, arrow).

A diagnosis of either recurrent carcinoid tumour or phytobezoar impaction was made. At laparotomy a 5 cm diameter phytobezoar was found impacted in the proximal jejunum which was removed via an enterostomy. The patient has been well since discharge.

A phytobezoar is a concretion composed of vegetable matter such as skins, seeds and the fibres of fruit and vegetables. The word "bezoar" derives from either the Arabic term "badzehr" or the Persian word "padzahr" both of which translate as counter poison or antidote. This word was applied to a greenish, hard concretion found in the fourth stomach of the Syrian goat. The stone was thought to prevent poisoning and came to Europe as the bezoar-stone which was highly prized for its medical properties [1].

Small bowel phytobezoars are a rare cause of small bowel obstruction (2.9%) [2]. The commonest phytobezoar encountered worldwide is related to the ingestion of the persimmon fruit [3]. It has been proposed that the formation of persimmon bezoars is due to a soluble tannin termed "shibuol" which forms a coagulum when the astringent unripe fruit comes into contact with dilute hydrochloric acid in the stomach. This probably explains why most phytobezoars encountered nowadays are in patients who have recently undergone peptic ulcer surgery. Vagotomy decreases gastric motility, allowing prolonged contact of the ingested persimmon fruit with gastric acid, which increases the coagulation of shibuol. A pyloroplasty or gastroenterostomy results in an enlarged gastric outlet that allows large fragments of bezoar to enter the small bowel. Normally the intact pylorus prevents the passage of food particles large enough to obstruct the small bowel.

Our patient presented in October at the time of the mid-Autumn festival when the persimmon fruit is traditionally eaten. Chisholm et al [4] in a review of patients presenting with phytobezoars causing small bowel obstruction in Hong Kong found that 70% of the patients presented in the months of September and October, *i.e.* when the persimmon fruit is in season. On direct questioning our patient did give a history of eating persimmon fruit.

Obstruction caused by small bowel phytobezoars frequently occurs in the jejunum or proximal ileum. Barium studies are useful in differentiating obstruction due to post-operative adhesions from obstruction caused by bezoars [5]. The classic appearance of bezoars on barium studies is of an intraluminal filling defect of variable size with no constant site of attachment to the bowel wall. Barium may fill the interstices giving a mottled appearance mimicking a villous tumour of the small bowel, *e.g.* carcinoid, leiomyoma, lymphangioma, lipoma and lymphoma. Because of the high incidence of synchronous gastric bezoars (17.5% [1]; 21% [3]) the stomach should always be assessed for the presence of a residual bezoar.

Small bowel obstruction due to a phytobezoar is uncommon and often overlooked. Any patient having undergone previous gastric or ulcer surgery with a suggestive dietary history presenting with small bowel obstruction should raise the suspicion of this diagnosis. Contrast studies can play a vital role in the management of these patients.

References

1. De Bakey M, Oschner A. Bezoars and concretions. Surgery 1938;5:132–60.
2. Vellar DJ, Veller ID, Puciaus R, Steedman PK. Phytobezoars—an overlooked cause of small bowel obstruction following vagotomy and drainage operations for duodenal ulcer. Austral NZ J Surg 1986;56:635–8.
3. Krausz MM, Moriel EZ, Ayalon A, et al. Surgical aspects of gastrointestinal persimmon phytobezoar treatment. Am J Surg 1986;152:526–30.
4. Chisolm EM, Leung HT, Chung SCS, Li AKC. Phytobezoar—an uncommon cause of small bowel obstruction. Ann R Coll Surg Engl 1992;74:342–4.
5. Verstandig AG, Klin B, Bloom RA, et al. Small bowel phytobezoars: detection with radiography. Radiology 1989; 172:705–7.

Inflammatory back pain

S A RENOWDEN and M W J HAYWARD

Department of Radiology, University of Wales College of Medicine, Heath Park, Cardiff, UK

A 57-year-old male was admitted as an emergency with a 3 day history of thirst, frequency and severe low back pain radiating to his right flank for 24 h. He was apyrexial and examination was normal. An elevated plasma glucose confirmed late onset diabetes. Urinalysis did not show any evidence of infection.

He developed a temperature of 39 °C 24 h later and his erythrocyte sedimentation rate (ESR) was raised at 133. Blood cultures demonstrated Gram negative (G – ve) bacilli, later confirmed as *Salmonella enteritidis*. Appropriate intravenous antibiotics were commenced, stool cultures, ultrasound of his renal tract, gallbladder and plain films of the lumbar spine were normal.

In view of his severe back pain, a three phase bone scan was performed (Figures 1 and 2). What does it demonstrate and, given the clinical history, what is the most likely diagnosis?

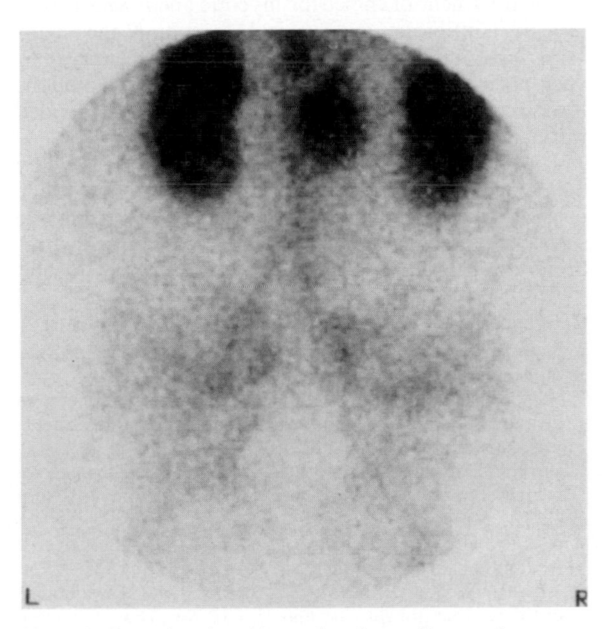

Figure 1. Posterior view of vascular phase of isotope bone scan.

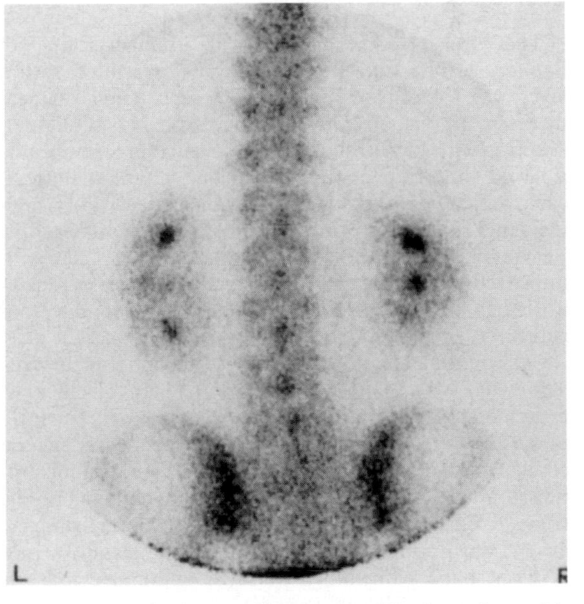

Figure 2. Posterior image of bone scan of lumbar spine at 3 h.

Based on the case of the month originally published in Br J Radiol 1991;64:969–70.

The vascular phase of the bone scan demonstrated abnormal vascularity just below the level of the renal arteries. The 3 h scan was normal. The most likely diagnosis, in view of the clinical history, was a mycotic aortic aneurysm, as a result of Salmonella septicaemia.

CT (Figure 3) demonstrated a 6 cm right sided aortic aneurysm, with a narrow neck at the level of the renal arteries. There was marked compression of the inferior vena cava and an associated soft tissue mass extending caudally adjacent to the psoas muscle representing either a haematoma or an abscess. A technetium labelled white cell study showed increased activity in the right upper abdomen confirming an infective process. Angiography demonstrated a huge aneurysm arising just below the level of the renal arteries. Embolization was considered hazardous and he underwent resection of the false aneurysm with oversewing of the aorta and an axillobifemoral graft. At surgery, the extensively friable and indurated aneurysm had perforated on the right, producing a false aneurysm. Histology showed some atheromatous degeneration with acute inflammation and *Salmonella enteritidis* was demonstrated in the pathological specimen.

Post-operatively the patient made a good recovery and continued oral antibiotic therapy for a further 6 weeks.

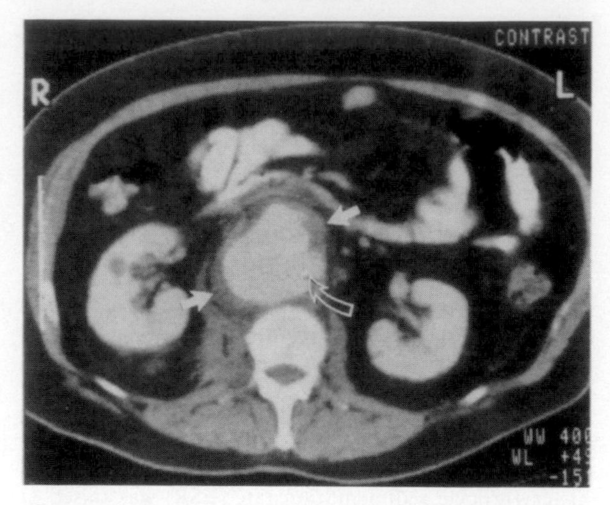

Figure 3. CT, just below the level of the renal arteries, demonstrating the aneurysm (closed straight arrows) and its neck (open curved arrows).

The most common clinical manifestation of Salmonella infection is gastroenteritis associated with a fever, but 7% of cases present with septicaemia or focal disease [1], usually in the appendix or gallbladder. Arteritis with or without mycotic aneurysm formation is a severe but rare complication and, if not diagnosed early and treated aggressively, is associated with a high incidence of either aortic rupture or overwhelming sepsis. Before 1969, only one survivor was reported [2]. With improved treatment and more rapid diagnosis the prognosis has improved. Even so, 40% of patients die from rupture or sepsis prior to surgery.

Salmonella accounts for 35% of mycotic aneurysms associated with G−ve septicaemia [3]. Involvement is more common in men [4] and occurs most frequently in the fourth to sixth decade. Predisposing factors include clinical sepsis, pre-existing medical illness, immunosuppression and congenital and traumatic vascular lesions. Clinical features are usually non-specific, fever being by far the most common symptom [4]. The classical triad of fever, back pain and a pulsatile abdominal mass is present only in 50% of cases [4].

Characteristically, CT demonstrates a well localized aortic dilatation, with a paucity of calcification and an encasing mass which may contain gas. There may be neighbouring osteomyelitis and a juxtaaortic retroperitoneal abscess [5]. Angiography typically demonstrates a saccular, eccentric aneurysm [6].

The treatment of choice for mycotic aneurysms is bacteriocidal antibiotics and surgical resection of the aneurysm. No one has survived without surgery. Interpositional grafts are inadequate; the aorta should be ligated and vascularization to the lower limbs provided through clean tissue planes.

The prognosis of mycotic aneurysms caused by Salmonella remains bleak. If diagnosis is not to be delayed, with potentially fatal consequences, it must be suspected and aggressively investigated in the appropriate clinical setting.

References

1. Saphra I, Winter JW. Clinical manifestations of Salmonellosis in man. N Engl J Med 1957;256:1129–34.
2. Meade RH, Moran JM. Salmonella arteritis—a preoperative diagnosis and cure of salmonella typhimurium aortic aneurysm. N Engl J Med 1969;281:310–2.
3. Jarret F, Darling RC, Mundth ED, Ansten WG. The management of infected arterial aneurysms. J Cardiovasc Surg 1977;18:361–6.
4. Mendelowitz DS, Ramstedt R, Yao JST, Bergan JJ. Abdominal aortic Salmonellosis. Surgery 1979;85:514–9.
5. Weschler RJ, Kurtz AB, Wang Y, Steiner RM. CT evaluation of the retroperitoneal vasculature. Crit Rev Diagn Imaging 1985;24:237–91.
6. Kaufman SL, White RI, Harrington DP, Barth KH, Stegelman SS. Protean manifestations of mycotic aneurysms. AJR 1978;131:1019–25.

A case of post-operative paresis

J F C OLLIFF, S J GWYTHER and G HART

Royal Marsden Hospital, Downs Road, Sutton, Surrey SM2 5PT and Atkinson Morley Hospital, Copse Hill, Wimbledon SW20 0NE, UK

An 82-year-old man was admitted for biopsy of an anal mass lesion. Histology showed a moderately well differentiated squamous cell carcinoma originating at the anal margin. Post-operative pyrexia resolved with intravenous antibiotics. 5 days after this he developed neck stiffness, urinary retention and left-sided weakness with a sensory level at C4. Radiographs of the cervical spine were obtained and a cervical myelogram performed (Figures 1 and 2).

What features are seen on the two examinations and what are the likely causes?

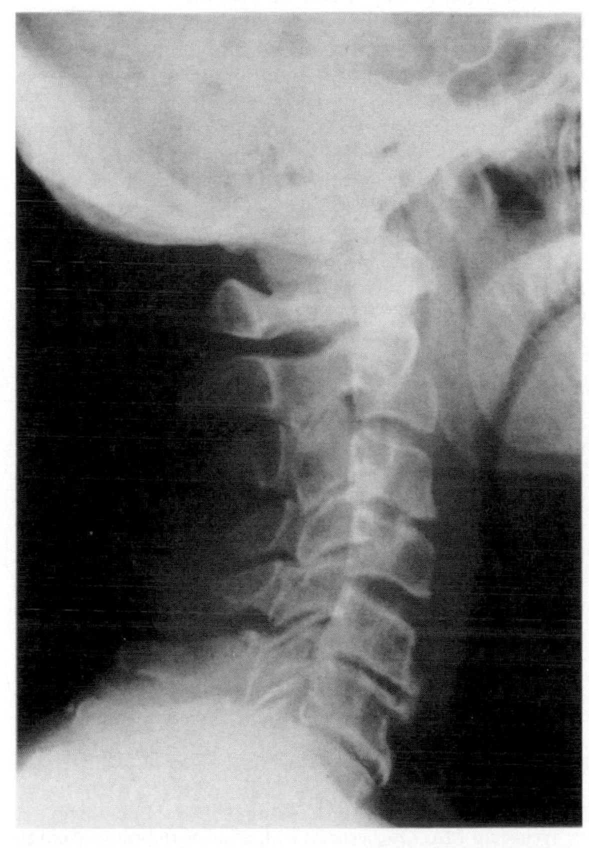

Figure 1. Lateral plain radiograph of the cervical spine.

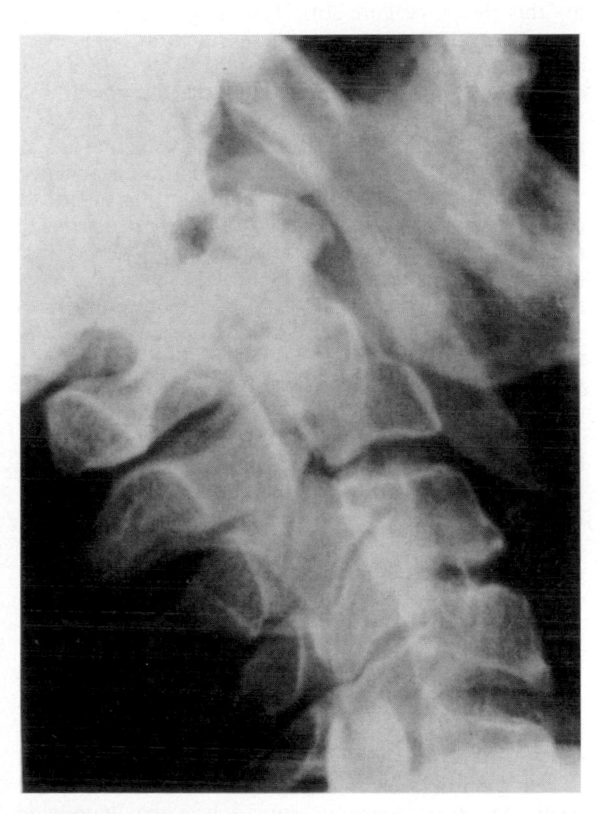

Figure 2. Prone lateral view of the cervical spine from a myelographic series.

Based on the case of the month originally published in Br J Radiol 1990;63:819–20.

The cervical spine radiograph (Figure 1) showed degenerative changes with reduced height of the disc joint and osteophyte formation at C5/6 and C6/7. The height of the disc joint was also reduced at C3/4 with grade 1 backward slip of C3 on C4. The marginal hypertrophic changes were relatively slight. Subtle prevertebral soft tissue swelling could be recognized anteriorly at this level. The myelogram showed almost complete obstruction to flow of contrast medium at the level of the C4/5 disc joint. The theca was displaced posteriorly at this level and the appearances were in keeping with an extradural obstruction: only a small amount of contrast medium being visible superiorly at C2.

On MRI of the neck, the sagittal T_1 weighted (repeat time (TR) 500 ms, echo time (TE) 17 ms) image demonstrated abnormal low signal in the vertebral bodies of C3 and C4 with thickening of the pre-vertebral, retropharyngeal soft tissues anteriorly (Figure 3a). Abnormal soft tissue also extended in a linear fashion posterior to these vertebral bodies within the spinal canal, anterior to the spinal cord. On the T_2 weighted (TR 2.1 s, TE 90 ms) image, abnormal high signal was seen in the vertebral bodies of C3 and C4 adjacent to the intervening intervertebral disc which also showed high signal only at this level (Figure 3b). The soft tissue swelling anteriorly and posterior to these vertebral bodies was also confirmed by abnormal high signal. This T_2 weighting gave a "myelographic effect" and the extradural soft tissue mass anterior to the cord at C3/4 was better appreciated on this image than on the T_1 weighted image.

These are the features of a discitis and associated vertebral osteomyelitis. On the plain film the slight loss of disc joint height at C3/4 could be interpreted as being a result of degenerative disease, although there was little marginal hypertrophy and subtle soft tissue swelling was seen anteriorly. At this level the pre-vertebral soft tissues should not measure greater than one-third of the sagittal diameter of the vertebral body or more than 4 mm, provided conventional examination can be made without magnification [1]. The myelogram showed the pattern of extradural obstruction to flow of contrast from the level of C4/5. The differential diagnosis of an extradural block includes extradural malignancy, degenerative hypertrophy, infection and haematoma.

Squamous cell carcinomas of the anal margin very rarely metastasize to bone and with the recent history of pyrexia, infection seemed the most likely cause.

The three major pathogenetic mechanisms of acute osteomyelitis are haematogenous spread, direct inoculation secondary to trauma or surgery and contiguous spread from adjacent or soft tissue infection [2]. In this patient with no history of the last two causes it would seem that haematogenous spread was the underlying mechanism. Acute haematogenous osteomyelitis predominantly affects the long tubular bones. In adults the vertebral bodies are also often affected. In a post-surgical patient, one risk factor is the use of indwelling catheters for vascular access; another factor is a distant focus of infection such as an abscess or cellulitis.

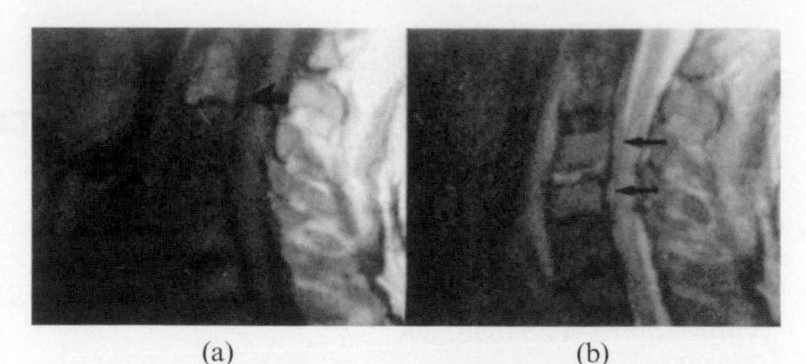

Figure 3. (a) Sagittal T_1 weighted (TR 50 ms TE 17 ms) view of the neck demonstrates abnormal low signal in the vertebral bodies of C3 and C4. Subtle soft tissue swelling is noted anterior to these vertebral bodies. Abnormal signal is also seen extending in a linear fashion posterior to the vertebral bodies of C3 and C4 (arrow). (b) Sagittal T_2 weighted (TR 2.1 s TE 90 ms) view of the neck which demonstrates abnormal high signal within the vertebral bodies of C3 and C4 with high signal in the intervening disc joint. Abnormal high signal is also seen in the soft tissues anteriorly and extending posterior to these vertebral bodies within the spinal canal (arrows).

MRI elegantly demonstrates the features of an infective process centred on the C3/4 disc joint with adjacent vertebral osteomyelitis. Inflammation causes prolongation of the T_1 and T_2 relaxation times of the vertebral marrow and adjacent soft tissue. On T_1 weighted images there is reduction of signal from the marrow of the infected vertebral bodies. On T_2 weighted images the infected vertebral bodies, disc and inflamed tissue have a higher signal intensity than adjacent normal structures. The multi-planar imaging ability of MRI allows accurate assessment of the superior and inferior limits of the extradural mass. This is not always possible on myelography which is less precise.

MRI is more sensitive and specific for vertebral osteomyelitis than either plain radiography or radioisotope bone scans. [*See [4], ED*] Changes of vertebral osteomyelitis on MRI are apparent sooner than on plain radiographs, but appear at about the same stage in evolution as can be detected by increased isotope concentration on radionuclide scan. In follow-up of treated patients, the resolution of disc joint infection with appropriate therapy is accompanied by a return to normal of the signal intensity changes on both T_1 and T_2 weighted images [3].

References

1. Weir DC. Roentgenographic signs of cervical injury. Clin Orthopaed 1975;109:9–17.
2. Wald RW. Risk factors for osteomyelitis. Am J Med 1985;78:206–212.
3. Modic MT, Feiglin DH, Piraino DW, Boumphrey F, Weinstein MA, Duchesneau PM, et al. Vertebral osteomyelitis assessment using MR. Radiology 1985;157:157–66.
4. Gillams AR, Chaddha B, Carter AP. MR appearances of the temporal evolution and resolution of infectious spondylitis. AJR 1996;166:903–7.

Painful ankle swelling—diagnosis by MRI

[1]W C G PEH and [2]K M C CHEUNG

Departments of [1]Diagnostic Radiology and [2]Orthopaedic Surgery, University of Hong Kong, Queen Mary Hospital, Hong Kong

A 39-year-old man presented with recurrent left ankle swelling. The patient had had a similar mass excised from the same ankle 10 years previously but did not know the nature of the lesion. The mass recurred after 3 years, producing progressive swelling of the left ankle. The patient developed increasing left ankle pain in the 3 years prior to the current presentation. He had no other joint involvement or systemic symptoms. On examination, there was nodular swelling around the ankle joint with a consistency which varied from soft to hard on palpation. The overlying skin was normal except for scars from previous surgery. The range of left ankle movement was reduced. All blood investigations, including erythrocyte sedimentation rate, were normal.

What do the plain radiograph (Figure 1) and MRI scans (Figures 2 and 3) show? What is the diagnosis?

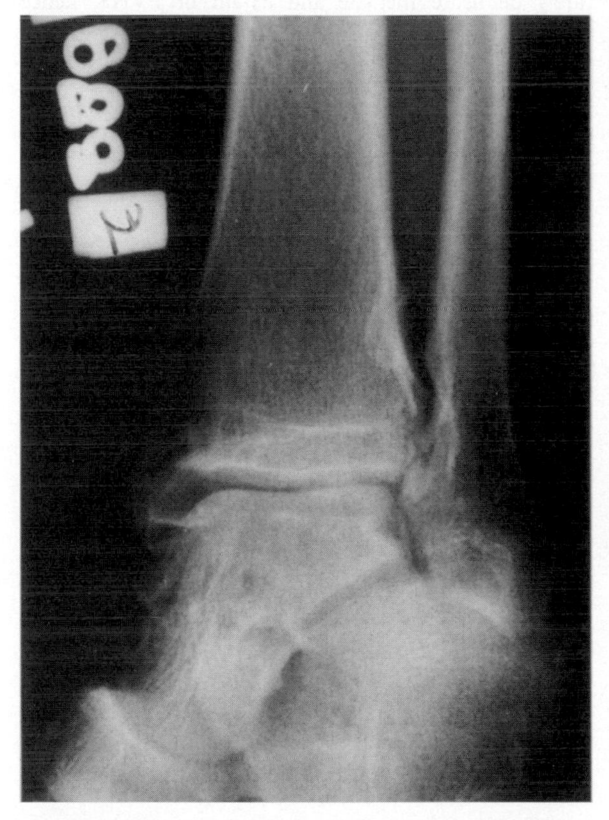

Figure 1. Anteroposterior (AP) radiograph of the left ankle.

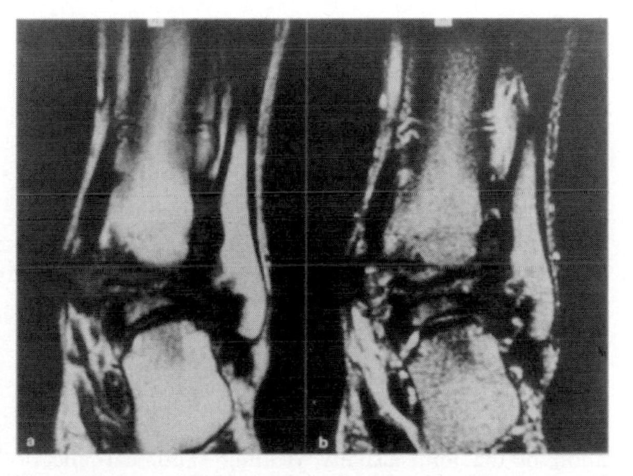

Figure 2. Coronal MRI through the left mid ankle. (a) T_1 and (b) T_2 weighted images.

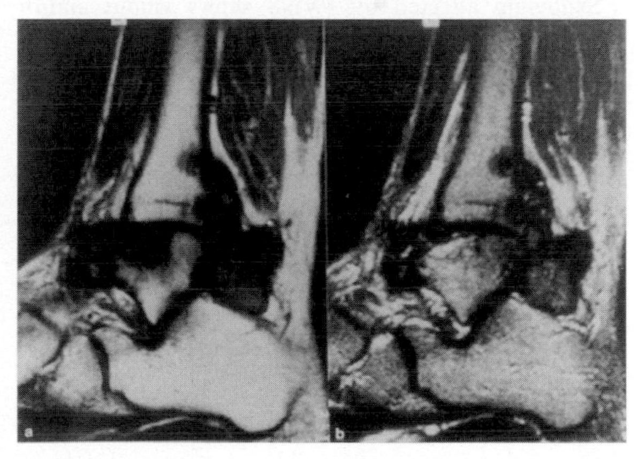

Figure 3. Sagittal MRI through the left mid ankle at the level of the lateral aspect of the tibia. (a) T_1 and (b) T_2 weighted images.

Based on the case of the month originally published in Br J Radiol 1996;69:881–2.

The plain radiograph (Figure 1) showed widening of the inferior tibiofibular joint. There were smooth, concave defects with sclerotic rims in the adjacent subchondral bones. There was no soft tissue calcification. MRI (Figures 2 and 3) showed a large lobulated soft tissue mass in the tibiotalar and tibiofibular joints, with anterior, medial and posterior extraarticular extensions. The mass was of low to intermediate signal intensity on T_1 weighted images (Figures 2a and 3a) and, although it had some areas of intermediate signal intensity, was largely hypointense on T_2 weighted images. A small amount of synovial fluid, seen as high signal intensity with T_2 weighting, was present. Intraarticular masses having low to intermediate T_1 signal and remaining low in signal on T_2 weighted images are characteristic of haemosiderin-laden hyperplastic synovium found in pigmented villonodular synovitis (PVNS). A near total synovectomy was performed and the diagnosis of PVNS was histologically proven.

PVNS is an uncommon benign proliferative disorder of the synovium of joints, bursae or tendon sheaths. The aetiology remains unknown. PVNS can be classified into diffuse or localized forms, depending on the extent of synovial involvement [1].

Diffuse PVNS of joints occurs most frequently in the third to fourth decades of life, with an equal sex distribution. The knee is the most common joint affected, being involved in 80% of cases. Other joints afflicted, in descending order of frequency, are the hip, ankle and shoulder. The process is usually monoarticular. Clinically, patients present with progressive pain, swelling and decreased range of movement of the affected joint. Laboratory investigations are negative, with aspiration of the joint usually yielding xanthochromic or serosanguinous fluid. In the past, the definitive diagnosis depended on synovial biopsy [1].

Synovium affected by PVNS shows villous and/or nodular proliferation, and is often rust-coloured from haemosiderin deposition. Histologically, the lesion consists of masses or strands of hyperplastic synovium, with characteristic multinucleated giant cells loaded with lipid and haemosiderin. Presence of intracellular and extracellular haemosiderin produces the pigmentation typical of PVNS [1–4]. Plain radiographs are not helpful in the diagnosis of PVNS, sometimes showing soft tissue swelling and, in about half of the cases, osteochondral changes such as erosions or subchondral cysts [1]. Arthrography demonstrates multiple nodular filling defects, while CT may show a soft tissue mass with high attenuation due to haemosiderin deposits [1, 2]. Early phase blood flow isotope studies and angiography have been used to assess the vascularity of PVNS [4].

The distinctive MRI appearance of PVNS is due to the presence of hyperplastic synovium, as well as its tendency to bleed, with resultant deposition of haemosiderin. Haemosiderin is paramagnetic and produces lowering of the T_2 relaxation time, especially with increased field strengths, resulting in decreased signal intensity best seen on T_2 weighted images. The unique tissue combination of variable amounts of haemosiderin and fat in PVNS produces a significant effect on tissue signal intensities. On spin echo images, PVNS typically appears inhomogeneous with a mixture of low and intermediate signals on both the T_1 and T_2 weighted images [5].

Lesions which may possibly mimic PVNS on MRI include synovial chondromatosis, haemangioma, rheumatoid arthritis, haemophilia and chronic traumatic synovitis. These conditions can usually be distinguished on the basis of clinical history, laboratory findings, plain radiographic findings, as well as the characteristic intraarticular distribution of PVNS [3, 4].

Besides providing the diagnosis, MRI can also accurately delineate the site and extent of PVNS, hence enabling pre-operative planning and post-treatment follow-up of residual or recurrent disease. The treatment of choice is total synovectomy but there is a high local recurrence rate due to the difficulty of complete excision [3].

[*See also the review by Bravo et al [6], ED*]

References

1. Goldman AB, DiCarlo EF. Pigmented villonodular synovitis. Diagnosis and differential diagnosis. Radiol Clin North Am 1988;26:1327–1347.
2. Kottal RA, Vogler III JB, Matamoros A, et al. Pigmented villonodular synovitis: a report of MR imaging in two cases. Radiology 1987;163:551–3.
3. Steinbach LS, Neumann CH, Stoller DW, et al. MRI of the knee in pigmented villonodular synovitis. Clin Imaging 1989;13:305–16.
4. Jelinek JS, Kransdorf MJ, Utz JA, et al. Imaging of pigmented villonodular synovitis with emphasis on MR imaging. AJR 1989;152:337–42.
5. Wilson AJ. Nonarticular soft tissues. Top Magn Reson Imaging 1989;1:1–16.
6. Bravo SM, Winalski CS, Weissman BN. Pigmented villonodular synovitis. Radiol Clin N Am 1996;34:311–26.

Painless testicular nodularity in a young man

D C HOWLETT, A J JONES and A J S SAUNDERS

Department of Radiology, 2nd Floor Guy's Tower, Guy's Hospital, Guy's and St Thomas' NHS Trust, St Thomas' Street, London SE1 9RT, UK

A 25-year-old Caucasian male presented with a 6 month history of painless, non-enlarging testicular lumps. He was otherwise well. At 3 weeks of age, congenital adrenal hyperplasia had been diagnosed. He had been on maintenance replacement therapy since that time, currently hydrocortisone 35 mg and fludrocortisone 200 mg daily. There was no family history of the condition.

On examination the patient looked well, with no Cushingoid or Addisonian features. There was no lymphadenopathy or hepatosplenomegaly. Bilateral, firm testicular nodularity was present, although the testes were of normal size.

Serological results including urea and electrolytes, liver function tests, TSH, LH, FSH, cortisol and testosterone levels were within normal limits. The testicular tumour markers AFP and B-HCG were also within the normal range.

An ultrasound scan of the testes was performed using an Acuson 128 XP/7.5 MHz linear array transducer. This showed normal sized testes containing a single 2 cm intratesticular mass on the right and a pair of similar sized lesions on the left, with only a narrow rim of normal testicular tissue at the periphery (see Figures 1 and 2). These masses were well defined, hypoechoic and did not contain flow on colour Doppler examination.

What is the diagnosis?

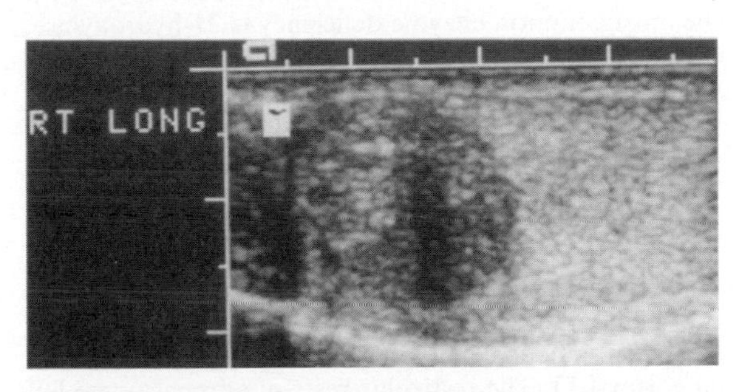

Figure 1. Longitudinal ultrasound scan through the right testis showing a well circumscribed hypoechoic lesion in the mid-testis.

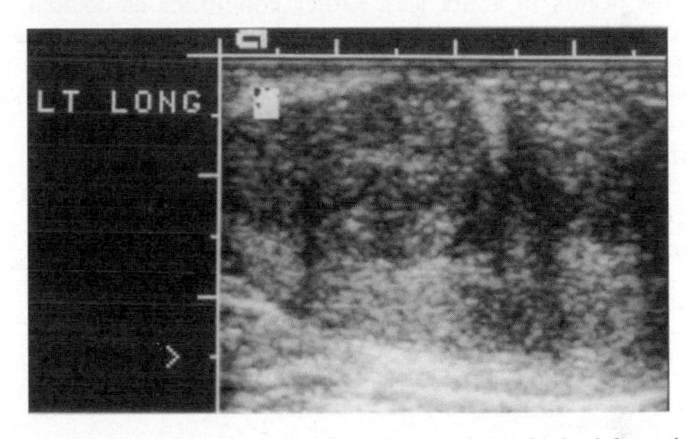

Figure 2. Longitudinal ultrasound scan through the left testis showing two lesions within the left testis of a similar nature to that seen in Figure 1. A narrow rim of normal surrounding testicular tissue is identified.

Based on the case of the month originally published in Br J Radiol 1997;70:1195–6.

The hypoechoic testicular masses represent ectopic rests of adrenal tissue which occur in patients with congenital adrenal hyperplasia. Follow-up ultrasound scans at 6 months and a year have shown no change in the lesions.

Congenital adrenal hyperplasia (CAH) is due to an autosomal recessive adrenocortical enzyme defect which may become clinically apparent in the neonatal period or in early adulthood. Affected males may become hyperandrogenic, hypoadrenal and hypercorticotrophic [1]. The most common enzyme deficiency is 21-hydroxylase, as in this patient, which occurs in 90% of cases. It may present with pre-natal virilization, with or without salt-wasting, as a late-onset form or as an asymptomatic form [2]. Deficiencies of 11-hydroxylase and 17-hydroxylase cause a minority of cases of CAH [2].

The exact origin of testicular adrenal rests is unclear, although they are thought to arise from aberrant adrenal cortical cells which migrate with the gonadal tissues in fetal life. They are not pre-malignant. The testicular masses are biochemically identical to hyperplastic adrenal cortex [3]. The testicular rests of adrenal tissue fail to involute in the presence of a chronically raised ACTH, which is due to the defective glucocorticoid synthesis that occurs in CAH [1]. Other conditions associated with elevated ACTH levels, such as Addison's disease and Cushing's syndrome, can also develop such testicular rests [4].

This ectopic adrenal tissue may hypertrophy when there is inadequate glucocorticoid replacement and may atrophy with high dose glucocorticoid replacement. Growth of the testicular lesions whilst on treatment may indicate poor patient compliance or inadequate control [5]. The ectopic adrenal rests may rarely occur in an extratesticular site, such as the epididymis [6].

The ultrasound features of testicular adrenal rest tumours are well described [3, 6]. Adrenal rests detected on ultrasound are common in CAH with an incidence of 24% in one series [3]. The tumours are usually bilateral and multiple. They tend to be hypoechoic, cause minimal disruption of surrounding testicular tissue and are most often seen near the mediastinum testis. Sound attenuation is frequent, may be patchy or uniform and is due to the adrenal rest cells. Patterns of colour flow are variable, but if vessels traverse the mass they are not deviated by it [3].

The detection of multiple, bilateral testicular lesions should raise the possibility of undiagnosed CAH. It is important to recognize the association of intratesticular adrenal rests and CAH, in order to prevent unnecessary surgery if a testicular mass is identified.

References

1. Seidenwurm D, Smathers RL, Kan P, Hoffman A. Intratesticular adrenal rests diagnosed by ultrasound. Radiology 1985;155:479–81.
2. Miller WL, Levine L. Molecular and clinical advances in CAH. J Pediatr 1987;11:1–17.
3. Avila A, Premkumar A, Shawher TH, et al. Testicular adrenal rest tissue in congenital adrenal hyperplasia: findings at grayscale and colour Doppler ultrasound. Radiology 1996; 198:99–104.
4. Hamwi GJ, Gwinup G, Mostow JH, Besch PK. Activation of testicular adrenal rest tissue by prolonged excessive ACTH production. J Clin Endocrinol Metab 1963;23:861–9.
5. Rutgers JL, Young RH, Scully RE. The testicular tumour of the adrenogenital syndrome: a report of six cases and review of the literature on testicular masses in patients with adrenocortical disorders. Am J Surg Pathol 1988;12:503.
6. Vanzulli A, Delmaschio A, Paesano P, et al. Testicular masses in association with adrenogenital syndrome: ultrasound findings. Radiology 1992;183:425–9.

An unusual case of pneumonia

R CHAUDHURI

Queen Mary's Hospital, Roehampton, London SW15, UK

A 41-year-old European man presented with a 4-week history of increasing dyspnoea, left pleuritic chest pain, productive cough and 7 kg weight loss. He had smoked 60–70 cigarettes per day for many years, and he drank 3 pints of beer daily. He had had a myocardial infarction 5 years before, and had paranoid schizophrenia, well controlled on monthly flupenthixol injections.

On examination, he was pyrexial with signs of consolidation at the left lung base. There was no adenopathy. His fingers were heavily nicotine stained and his dental hygiene very poor. Investigations showed a mild anaemia, elevated white blood cell count and ESR 100 mm h^{-1}.

An initial chest radiograph showed a left basal effusion loculated posteriorly (Figure 1). What is the differential diagnosis at this stage?

He was discharged on trimethoprim, with some weight gain, erythrocyte sedimentation rate (ESR) 32 mm h^{-1}, but little resolution on chest radiography. 2 months later he had developed a woody indurated mass over the left anterior ribs, with a central discharging sinus. He had again lost 3 kg, and the ESR had risen. Sputums were negative for acid fast bacilli and malignant cells. Bronchoscopy was normal and bronchial biopsy and washings were unhelpful. No pleural fluid could be aspirated.

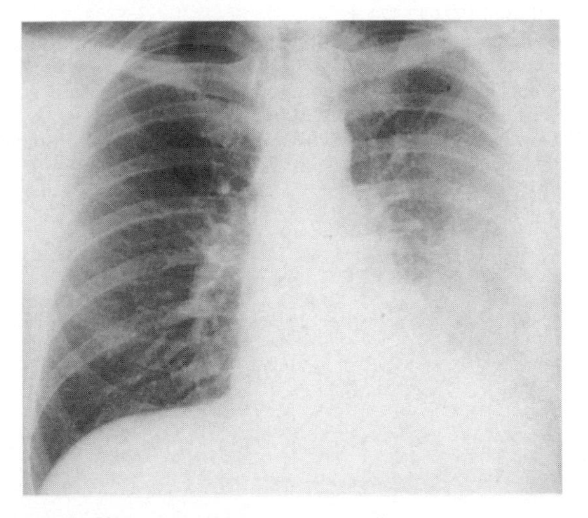

Figure 1. Chest radiograph on presentation.

Based on the case of the month originally published in Br J Radiol 1991;64:175–6.

The chest radiograph at this stage is shown (Figure 2). How would you modify the differential diagnosis and how could the diagnosis be comfirmed?

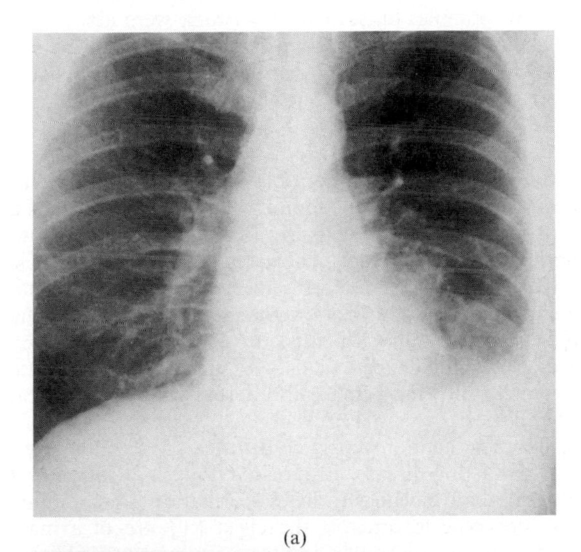

(a)

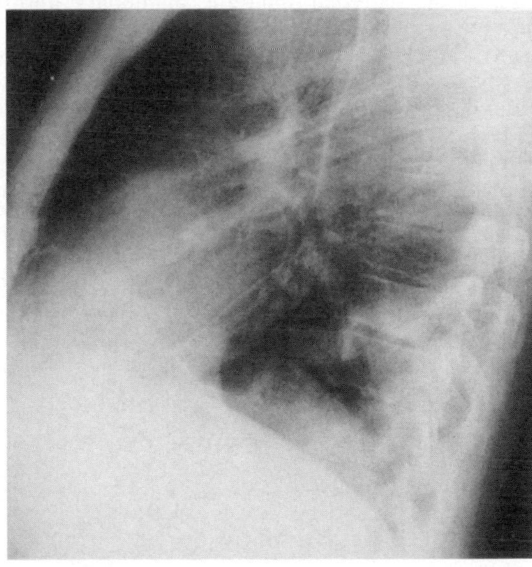

(b)

Figure 2. Chest radiographs after antibiotic treatment.

At presentation the differential diagnosis was of infection, including atypical pneumonias and tuberculosis, carcinoma of the bronchus with metastatic effusion or possibly pulmonary infarction or a collagen disorder. The second chest radiograph showed considerable pleural thickening over the left lower lobe with a solid looking mass posteriorly, but no associated rib involvement. In view of his history, the differential diagnosis was modified to either a neoplastic cause (including bronchial carcinoma with cutaneous metastasis, lymphoma or malignant mesothelioma) or a chronic infective cause (including tuberculosis, actinomycosis and fungal disease).

A diagnosis was made by gram-staining of aspirated sinus fluid and biopsy of the chest wall lesion, which revealed a 5 cm subcutaneous abscess. Pathognomonic sulphur granules of *Actinomyces israeli* were identified.

The patient was treated with high dose tetracycline. 1 year later, the chest radiograph was almost completely clear.

Since the advent of antibiotics, actinomycosis has become increasingly uncommon. *Actinomyces israeli* is a saprophytic anaerobe existing freely in the mouth and upper respiratory tract. The usual source for thoracic disease is from carious teeth, infected gums, periodontal membranes and tonsils. Diagnosis depends on finding the sulphur granule, which is a mycelium surrounded by radiating club-shaped rods. It produces proteolytic enzymes, allowing penetration across usual anatomical boundaries.

Thoracic actinomycosis constitutes 15% of all cases. It is a wasting disease. Progressive lung infiltration and pleural involvement with fistula formation are common. Radiographic features in the chest [1] are of a mass lesion, chronic alveolar infiltrate, pulmonary fibrosis, cavitation, pleural effusion or empyema. Spread is directly through the chest wall with associated wavy periostitis or frank rib destruction, or extension of pulmonary lesions across interlobar fissures. Dermal lesions may be local or peripheral [2]. Sinus tracts on the chest wall may fistulate into the lung, pleural cavity, trachea, oesophagus or abdomen. Mediastinal widening, spinal involvement, pulmonary osteoarthropathy and erosion into blood vessels with haematogeneous dissemination have also been described. Rarely, congestive heart failure, constrictive pericarditis, endocarditis and peripheral effusions occur secondary to direct spread from the pleura.

The radiological features of pulmonary actinomycosis are largely non-specific. Bates and Cruickshank [3] suggested that periostitis of several adjacent ribs in the absence of empyema was the only pathognomonic finding, a view supported by Flynn and Felson [1]. However, only one of a series of six described by Frank and Strickland [4] showed this sign, while none of six in Slade's series [5] or our patient showed periostitis. [*CT and ultrasound may be helpful in showing presence and extent of chest wall involvement [6, 7], ED*]

A misdiagnosis of carcinoma of the bronchus or tuberculosis, with subsequent lobectomy or pneumonectomy has been well documented [3, 5]. These studies have shown both bronchial carcinoma and pulmonary tuberculosis can co-exist with actinomycosis. However, association with a thymoma has not been described.

In summary, inappropriate antibacterial therapy or surgery may be prevented if pulmonary actinomycosis is considered at an early stage in unusually presenting pneumonias. Potentially more serious superadded or causally related complications such as TB or malignancy should be remembered.

References

1. Flynn MW, Felson B. The roentgen manifestations of thoracic actinomycosis. AJR 1970;110:707–16.
2. Webb AK, Howell R, Hickman JA. Thoracic actinomycosis presenting with peripheral skin lesions. Thorax 1978;33:818–9.
3. Bates M, Cruickshank G. Thoracic actinomycosis. Thorax 1957;12:99–124.
4. Frank P, Strickland B. Pulmonary actinomycosis. Br J Radiol 1974;47:373–8.
5. Slade P, Slesser BV, Southgate J. Thoracic actinomycosis. Thorax 1978;28:73–85.
6. Webb R, Sagel SS. Actinomycosis involving the chest wall: CT findings. AJR 1982;139:1007–10.
7. Dershaw DD. Actinomycosis of the chest wall. Ultrasound findings in empyema necessitans. Chest 1984;86:779–84.

An epidemic tumour

[1]R G HENDERSON and [2]T D RAHMATULLA

Departments of [1]Diagnostic Radiology and [2]General Medicine, St Stephen's Hospital, Fulham Road, London SW10 9TH, UK

A 40-year-old homosexual man presented with a history of vague, increasing abdominal pain, weight loss and fatigue, but no fever. He gave a past history of multiple episodes of sexually transmitted infection, including hepatitis B and genital herpes. On examination, he was noted to have a faint purple macular and nodular skin rash and generalized lymphadenopathy. Examination was otherwise unremarkable. Routine blood count and chest radiography were normal, and biochemical analysis showed a low serum albumin level ($31\ g\,l^{-1}$) but no other abnormality. The patient had antibodies to HTLV III virus. A barium meal was requested. Figures 1 and 2 show two radiographs from this examination.

What does the barium meal show, and what is the differential diagnosis?

What should be the next investigation?

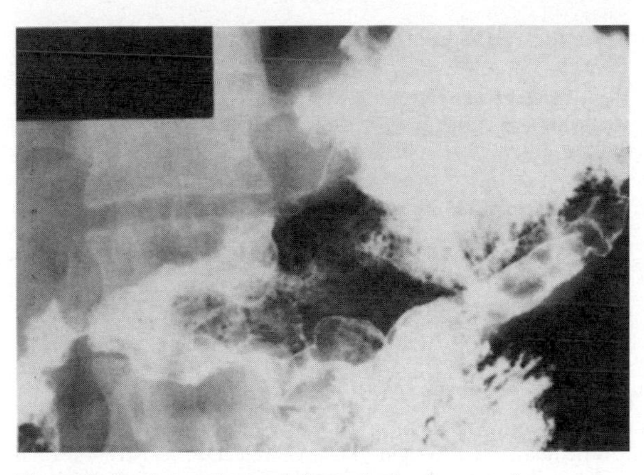

Figure 1. Supine radiograph from the barium meal.

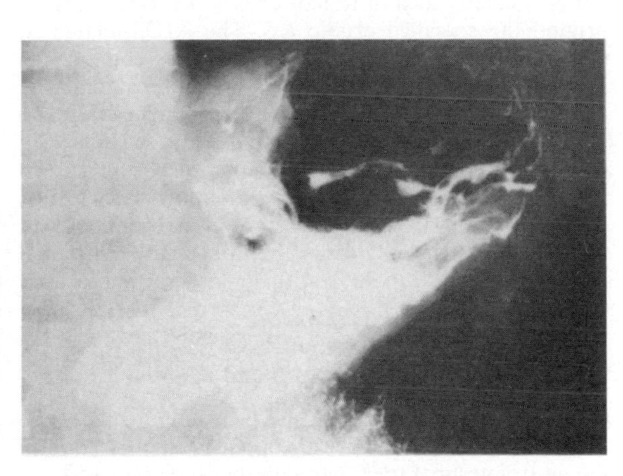

Figure 2. Erect radiograph from the barium meal.

Based on the case of the month originally published in Br J Radiol 1987;60:511–2.

The barium meal showed a rigid stomach with grossly thickened and rather nodular folds. The differential diagnosis included lymphoma, metastases, polyps, carcinoma and Crohn's disease. In a patient with this history, Kaposi's sarcoma should be suspected. An upper gastrointestinal endoscopy (Figure 3) showed the characteristic appearances of Kaposi's sarcoma (KS) involving all the stomach and the first part of the duodenum. This was confirmed by endoscopic biopsy. There was no evidence of opportunistic infection. The skin rash was that of KS, and the diagnosis was acquired immune deficiency syndrome (AIDS).

Kaposi's sarcoma, a multifocal neoplasm of the reticuloendothelial system, is found in about a third of homosexual AIDS cases in the USA. It is, however, rare in heterosexual AIDS patients, for example those who are haemophiliacs, drug abusers or from Haiti [1]. Kaposi's sarcoma is one of the criteria which establish a diagnosis of AIDS [2]. The condition was, however, first described by Kaposi in 1872 occurring predominantly in the lower limbs of elderly men of Italian or East European Jewish origin—the so-called classic KS. The AIDS-related or epidemic KS resembles a variant quite common in Uganda, where it accounts for 3–9% of all malignancies.

Kaposi's sarcoma almost invariably involves the skin, with pink or purple macules, papules and nodules [2]. Gastrointestinal involvement is common, being seen in 77% of cases at post-mortem examination in one series. An antemortem diagnosis of the bowel involvement was, however, made in only 40%; the upper gastrointestinal tract was involved in 32% and the large bowel in 20% of patients [3].

The radiological features of bowel involvement with KS are nodularity and thickening of the mucosal folds, which is seen in 66% of patients. Polypoid lesions are less common, being seen in 18% [4]. The lesions are frequently multifocal and associated with opportunistic infection of the gastrointestinal tract, particularly candidiasis [5].

The diagnosis is more likely to be made by endoscopy than radiology and, indeed, the appearance at endoscopy may be so characteristic that biopsy is unnecessary. Complications described include haemorrhage, obstruction, perforation and malabsorption. These are all unusual and visceral KS rarely produces symptoms. It is, however, associated with a poor prognosis compared with skin KS alone, although the deaths are not directly due to KS but to the associated opportunistic infections [3]. [*See also the useful review by Radin [6], ED*]

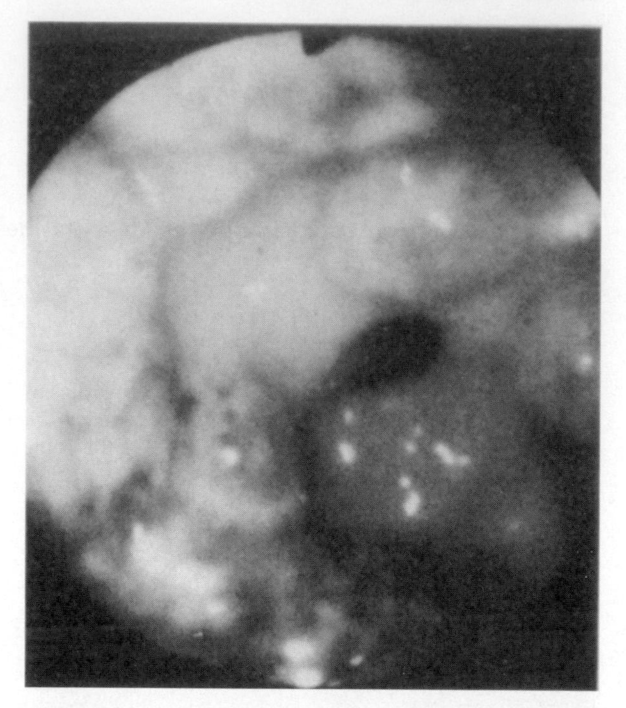

Figure 3. Endoscopic photograph of the pyloric region of the stomach. Note the grossly thickened and oedematous folds. Several polypoid lesions are also seen.

References

1. Rose HS, Balthazar EJ, Megibow AJ, Horowitz L, Laubenstein LJ. Alimentary tract involvement in Kaposi sarcoma: radiographic and endoscopic findings in 25 homosexual men. AJR 1982;139:661–6.
2. Muggia FM, Lonberg M. Kaposi's sarcoma and AIDS. Med Clin North Am 1986;70:139–54.
3. Friedman SL, Wright TL, Altman DF. Gastrointestinal Kaposi's sarcoma in patients with acquired immunodeficiency syndrome. Endoscopic and autopsy findings. Gastroenterology 1985;89:102–8.
4. Wall SD, Friedman SL, Margulis AR. Gastrointestinal Kaposi's sarcoma in AIDS: radiographic manifestations. J Clin Gastroenterol 1984;6:165–71.
5. Wall SD, Ominsky S, Altman DF, Perkins CL, Sollitto R, Goldberg HI, et al. Multifocal abnormalities of the gastrointestinal tract in AIDS. AJR 1986;146:1–5.
6. Radin R. HIV infection in 259 consecutive patients with abnormal abdominal CT findings. Radiology 1995; 197:712–22.

Haemoptysis in a laundry worker

J E JACKSON and D J ALLISON

Department of Diagnostic Radiology, Hammersmith Hospital, Du Cane Road, London W12 0HS, UK

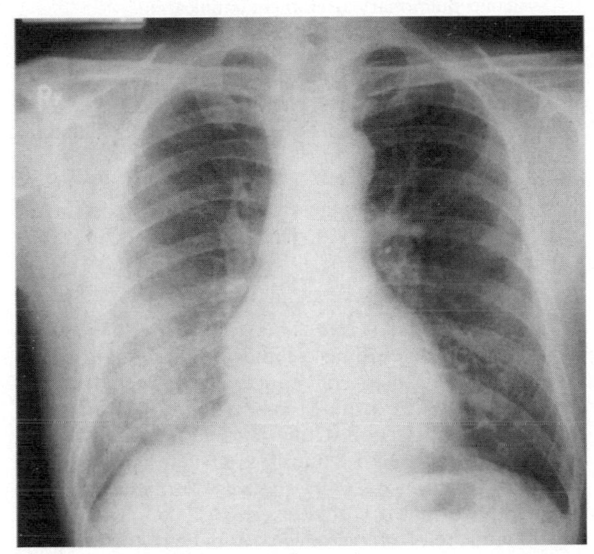

Figure 1. Admission chest radiograph.

A 39-year-old man of Philipino origin, who moved to England in April 1986, presented in January 1987 to his local hospital as an emergency following a massive haemoptysis. He had suffered four smaller haemoptyses during the preceding 4 months. The patient denied any history of cough, sputum, chest pain or wheezing although he had noted mild dyspnoea on exertion and had smoked until about 1 year previously. Bronchoscopy on admission demonstrated friable mucosa but no actual bleeding. He was subsequently referred to this hospital for further investigation.

Physical examination was unremarkable. Baseline laboratory investigations revealed only a mild microcytic anaemia and his arterial blood gases were normal. The chest radiograph on admission (Figure 1) and a ventilation/perfusion lung scan (Figure 2) are shown. What abnormalities are present and what are the possible diagnoses? How would you further investigate this patient?

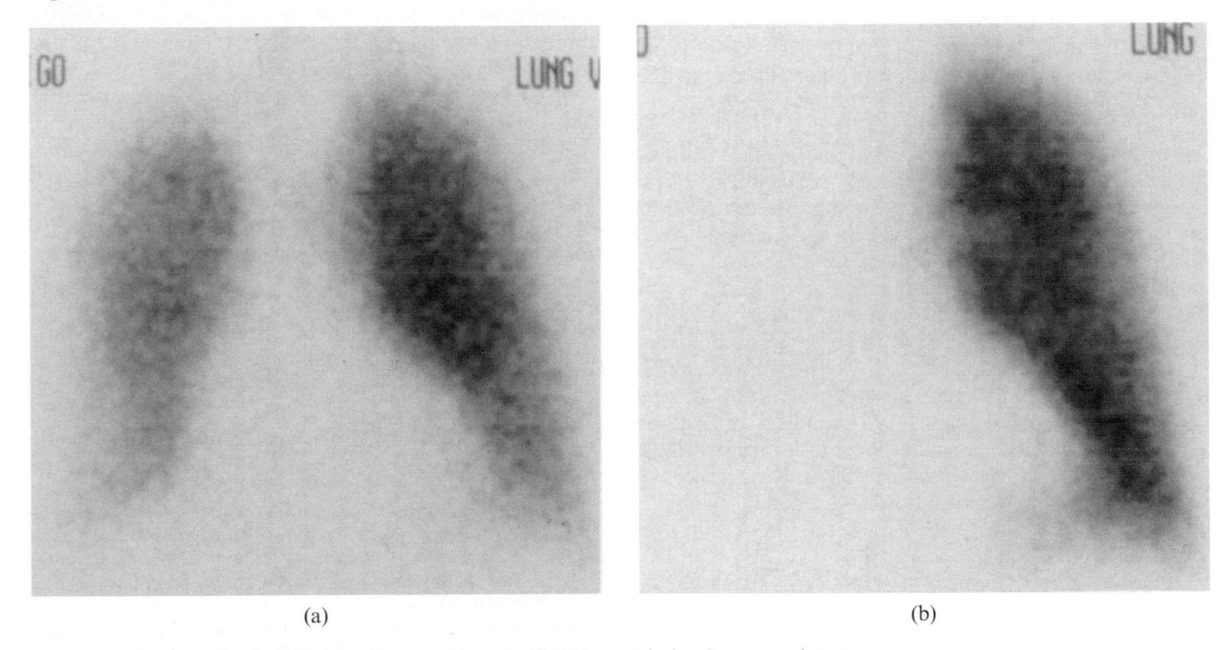

(a) (b)

Figure 2. (a) Anterior ventilation lung scan image. (b) Anterior perfusion lung scan image.

Based on the case of the month originally published in Br J Radiol 1989;62:379–80.

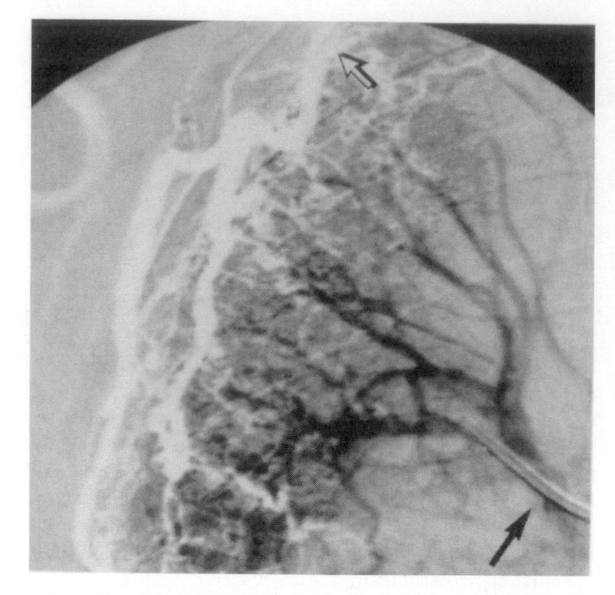

Figure 3. Digital subtraction angiogram showing both the feeding lateral thoracic artery (in white) and the draining pulmonary arterial branches (in black). The contrast medium has been injected through a selectively positioned catheter in the thoracic feeding artery (white arrow); a second catheter (black arrow) has been placed in the pulmonary artery for pressure measurements and blood gas analysis.

The chest radiograph showed a widespread, ill defined area of increased opacity in the right lung field affecting principally the middle and lower zones. The proximal pulmonary arteries appear normal. The radionuclide lung scan shows an almost normal distribution of ventilation with minimal diminution to the right lower zone, but no evidence of any perfusion of the right lung.

The differential diagnosis of unilateral lung non-perfusion includes both congenital and acquired causes, which are listed in Table 1. The relative wellbeing of the patient and the normal gases exclude the diagnosis of massive pulmonary embolism. Chronic granulomatous mediastinitis can uncommonly cause pulmonary artery occlusion and a prominent reticular pattern in the involved lung; however, the mediastinal contour is usually asymmetrically widened [1]. Severe pulmonary artery stenosis is associated with well recognized radiographic findings. Pulmonary artery agenesis may present with recurrent haemoptyses but the chest radiograph usually demonstrates a small, poorly vascularized lung, which is often associated with ipsilateral tracheal deviation, diaphragmatic elevation and a small hilum. A reticular pattern from the collateral circulation can occasionally be seen [2].

A systemic-to-pulmonary arterio-arterial fistula causes reversal of blood flow in the affected pulmonary artery but would have to be very extensive to involve the entire lung.

Coronary arteriography showed an atrial vessel supplying pulmonary anastomotic vessels to the right hilum. A main pulmonary artery arteriogram showed non-

Table 1. Causes of unilateral lung non-perfusion

Congenital
1. Severe pulmonary artery stenosis.
2. Pulmonary artery agenesis.
3. Systemic–pulmonary arterial communication.

Acquired
1. Massive thromboembolism.
2. Chronic granulomatous mediastinitis (usually because of either histoplasmosis or tuberculosis).
3. Extrinsic compression, *e.g.* tumour, lymph node.
4. Systemic–pulmonary arterial communication.

opacification of the right pulmonary artery. The right pulmonary artery was selectively catheterized and showed reversal of flow. Subsequently, aortic, internal mammary and lateral thoracic arteriograms (Figure 3) were performed revealing numerous systemic-to-pulmonary arterial fistulae with reversal of flow in the entire right pulmonary arterial tree. Bronchography was normal.

Fistulous communications between the systemic arteries (excluding the coronaries) and the pulmonary artery are rare. The aetiology of reported cases includes: congenital abnormality; trauma, for example following intercostal catheter insertion, artificial pneumothorax therapy or thoracotomy [3]; inflammation, such as may occur following tuberculosis [4], or severe bronchiectasis; or as a complication of Hodgkin's disease [5]. The lack of any previous relevant history in our patient, the extensive nature of his malformation and the presence of a coronary-pulmonary arterial anastomosis (a known congenital anomaly) all suggest a congenital aetiology for his arterio-arterial communications.

Most patients with such fistulae are asymptomatic, and the anomalies are detected because of the presence of a continuous murmur or an abnormal chest radiograph. Rib notching may be present if the intercostal arteries are involved in the afferent supply of the anomaly. The right lung has been reported as being affected twice as often as the left. Selective arteriography is the diagnostic investigation of choice as it identifies the feeding vessels and the extent of the anomaly. The disorder may be treated by either surgery or therapeutic embolization.

References

1. Kinard RE, Orrison WW, Williams JE. Absent right pulmonary artery flow in a young man. Invest Radiol 1985;20:785–9.
2. Mehta AC, Livingston DR, Kawalek W, Golish JA, O'Donnell JK. Pulmonary artery agenesis presenting as massive hemoptysis: a case report. J Vasc Dis 1987;Jan:67–71.
3. Syme J. Systemic to pulmonary arterial fistula of the chest wall and lung following lobectomy. Australas Radiol 1975;19:326–33.
4. Earl GM, Mohr JA, White RH, Stein PD. Subclavian arterial-pulmonary arterial fistula associated with healed cavitary tuberculosis. Am Rev Respir Dis 1972;106:898–903.
5. Poh SC, Wang YT, Tan LKA. Systemic to pulmonary artery fistulas in Hodgkin's disease. Am Rev Respir Dis 1986;134:1324–6.

Interesting ileus

A J SACKS and R P GOLDSCHMIDT

Department of Radiology, Hillbrow Hospital, University of the Witwatersrand, Johannesburg, South Africa

A 50-year-old black female with well controlled hypertension presented with a neck swelling and a right hypochondrial mass. She had no evidence of neurofibromatosis or mucosal neuromata and no significant family history. A chest radiograph was normal. Serum electrolytes, glucose and full blood count were normal. Urinary vanillylmandelic acid (VMA) levels were elevated, 50.6 $\mu mol\,l^{-1}$ (5–35 $\mu mol\,l^{-1}$) and serum catecholamine levels were markedly elevated, noradrenaline 5530 $pg\,ml^{-1}$ (100/600 $pg\,ml^{-1}$) and adrenaline 831 $pg\,ml^{-1}$ (10–80 $pg\,ml^{-1}$), while dopamine levels were normal 30 $pg\,ml^{-1}$ (10–150 $pg\,ml^{-1}$). Non-contrast CT of the abdomen showed a mixed density 10 × 6 × 5 cm mass in the region of the right adrenal gland (Figure 1). A saggital T_1 weighted MR scan showed a 5 × 4 cm vascular mass in the left neck, anterior to the carotid bifurcation (Figure 2).

In preparation for surgery an alpha-blocking drug was administered orally (Phenoxybenzamine 20 mg 12 hourly). However, on the second day following this, the patient's abdomen became generally distended and tender to palpation, with absent bowel sounds. A plain abdominal radiograph was obtained (Figure 3).

What is the more likely diagnosis of the abdominal mass and how could this be related to the neck mass and the abdominal distention?

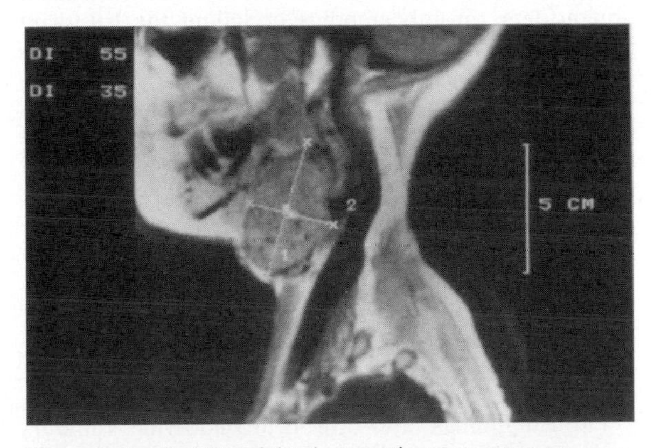

Figure 2. Saggital T_1 weighted magnetic resonance scan.

Figure 1. Non-contrast CT of the abdomen.

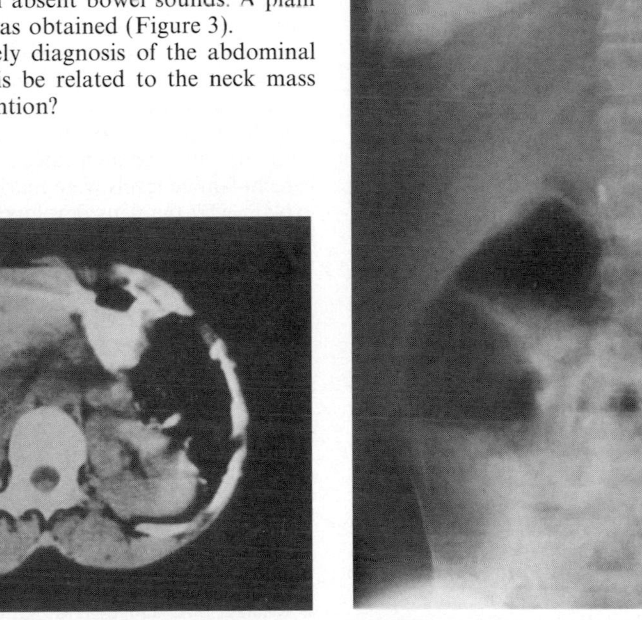

Figure 3. Abdominal radiograph (day 2).

Based on the case of the month originally published in Br J Radiol 1993;66:949–50.

The plain radiographic appearances are in keeping with paralytic ileus. Alpha-blockade was changed to the intravenous route and by day 7 a repeat abdominal radiograph had confirmed resolution of the ileus.

Imaging with meta-iodobenzyl guanidine (MIBG) (Figure 4) showed intense uptake in both the adrenal mass and the neck mass. The adrenal mass was surgically resected and confirmed as a phaeochromocytoma.

On day 4 post-operatively, the patient died following a cardiac arrest. Postmortem examination demonstrated antemortem thromboembolus occluding the left main pulmonary artery associated with deep vein thrombosis bilaterally.

An ovoid tumour measuring 5 × 4 × 2.5 cm was confirmed anterior to the bifurcation of the left common carotid artery. On histology this tumour was diagnosed as a benign paraganglioma, with its location in keeping with a chemodectoma.

The development of paralytic ileus in this patient, with subsequent prompt response to alpha-blocking agents, is in keeping with intestinal pseudo-obstruction associated with phaeochromocytoma.

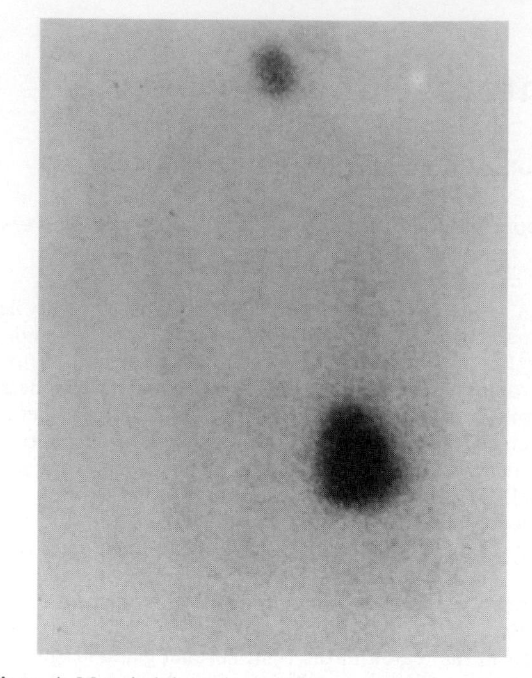

Figure 4. Meta-iodobenzyl guandidine (MIBG) scan (posterior view).

Paragangliomas are rare neuroendocrine tumours arising from paraganglionic tissue that may be distributed from the base of the skull to the floor of the pelvis. The classification of the World Health Organization [1] divides these tumours into four groups *viz* phaeochromocytomas, aorticosympathetic, parasympathetic and paragangliomas not further specified. These tumours may either secrete catecholamines or be non-functional [2]. Phaeochromocytomas secrete a combination of adrenaline and noradrenaline, whereas extraadrenal paragangliomas only secrete noradrenaline. Paragangliomas occasionally produce predominantly dopamine. It is the secretion of these vasopressor amines which produces paroxysmal or permanent hypertension, associated with headaches, palpitations and sweating.

Solitary extraadrenal functioning paragangliomas account for 10–20% of catecholamine producing paragangliomas [3]. Of these up to 85% are located within the abdomen. The remaining 15% can be found in the thorax, head and neck area. In the neck, extraadrenal paragangliomas mainly consist of functioning chemodectomas, which are of parasympathetic origin. The association of phaechromocytomas with extraadrenal paragangliomas (as in this case where a phaechromocytoma and a chemodectoma were demonstrated) has been described in familial and non-familial cases but is thought to be rare.

Intestinal pseudo-obstruction is a rare complication of phaeochromocytomas [4]. Its recognition, however, is important since further diagnostic and therapeutic procedures may be dangerous. Catecholamines relax intestinal smooth muscle largely by activating alpha-adrenergic receptors which inhibit the release of acetylcholine from post-ganglionic nerve terminals. This blocks excitatory post-synaptic potentials in myenteric neurones which allows continued activity of the intrinsic inhibitory neurones. The nett effect of alpha-adrenergic stimulation is to depress peristalsis and constrict the sphincters, producing ileus. The dramatic response to alpha-blockade experienced in this case is in keeping with this mechanism. This clinical picture of pseudo-obstruction in phaechromocytomas may also be produced by catecholamine-induced vasoconstriction of mesenteric vessels. In a review of eight cases of this complication [5] a relationship was demonstrated with large tumours and high catecholamine levels. In this case catecholamine levels were markedly raised and this may explain why the ileus developed on day 2 following the initiation of alpha-blockade orally. This is the first case, to the best of our knowledge, of phaeochromocytoma complicated by intestinal pseudo-obstruction occurring together with an extraadrenal paraganglioma.

References

1. Williams ED, Siebenmann RE, Sobin LH. Histological typing of endocrine tumours. In: WHO International Histological Classifications of Tumours. Geneva: WHO, 1980:33–9.
2. Van Gils APG, Falke THM, Van Erkel AR, et al. RadioGraphics 1991;11:37–57.
3. Goldfarb DA, Novick AC, Bravo EL, et al. Experience with extra-adrenal phaeochromocytoma. J Urol 1989;142:931–6.
4. Khafagi FA, Lloyd HM, Gough IR. Intestinal pseudo-obstruction in phaeochromocytoma. Austral NZ J Med 1987;17:246–8.
5. Cruz SR, Colwell SA. Phaeochromocytoma and ileus. J Am Med Assoc 1972;219:1050–1.

Not all gas and gaiters?

I J McCAFFERTY, K A BRADSHAW and M S MOSS

Department of Radiology, City Hospital NHS Trust, Dudley Road, Birmingham B18 7QH, UK

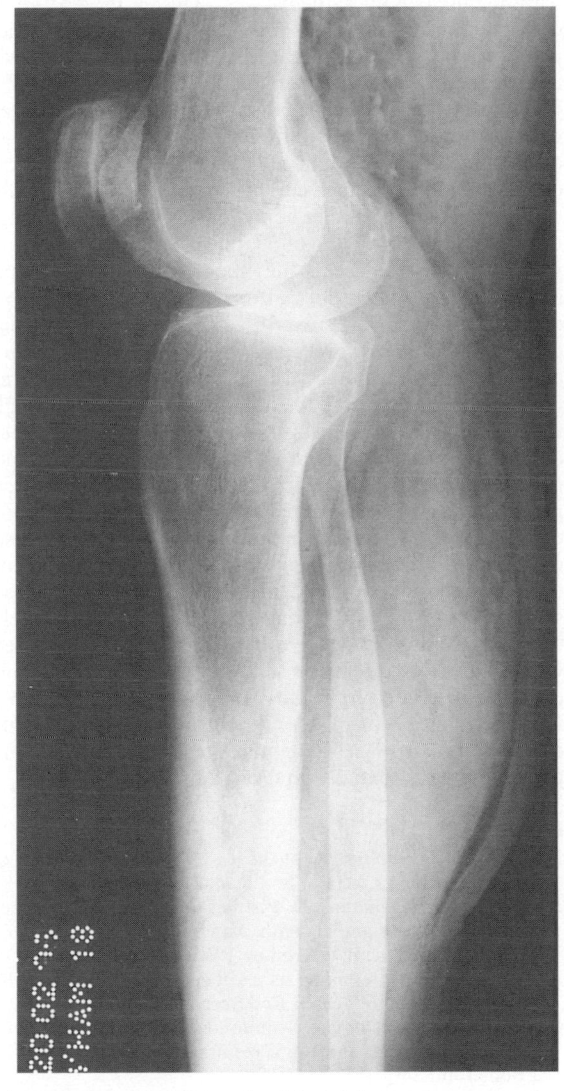

Figure 1. Lateral radiograph of the left leg.

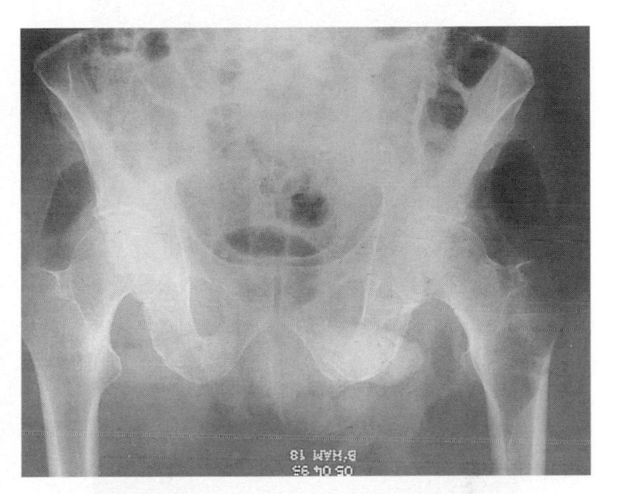

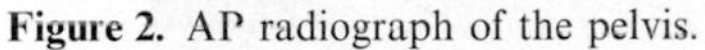

Figure 2. AP radiograph of the pelvis.

A 77-year-old male presented with a 6 week history of anorexia, weight loss and malaise. In the 5 days prior to admission his left leg had become increasingly painful and swollen. His medical history was unremarkable apart from an episode of colonic diverticulitis 2 years previously. On examination he was pyrexial. His entire left leg was swollen, red and tender. Subcutaneous emphysema was palpable along the length of the limb. A clinical diagnosis of gas gangrene was made and the patient treated with multiple excision fasciotomies and intravenous antibiotics. Cultures from the leg showed a mixed growth of coliforms. He made a slow recovery and was eventually discharged. 6 weeks later he presented again, this time with severe pain in the left gluteal region and a palpable abscess over the left greater trochanter. This was treated by surgical incision and drainage. Post-operatively there was persistent leakage of brown fluid from the wound which grew a mixed growth of mainly coliforms. Figure 1 is a radiograph of the lower leg at initial presentation. Figure 2 is a radiograph of the pelvis at the second presentation. What is the diagnosis, and what radiological investigation might confirm it?

Based on the case of the month originally published in Br J Radiol 1997;70:865–6.

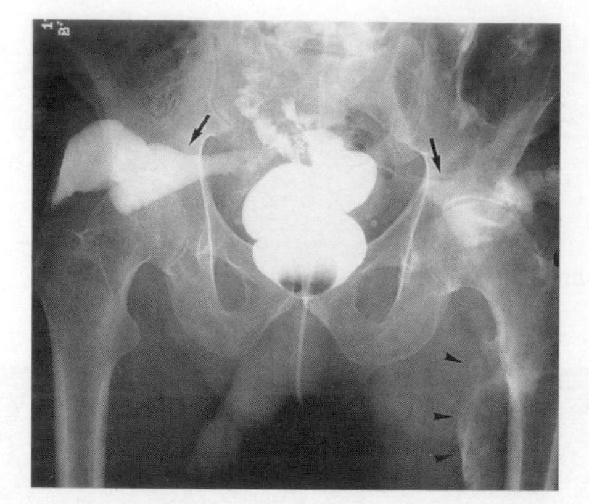

Figure 3. Water soluble contrast enema showing large fistulae from the sigmoid colon passing out through the greater sciatic foramina (arrows). The left one communicates with the proximal thigh (arrowheads).

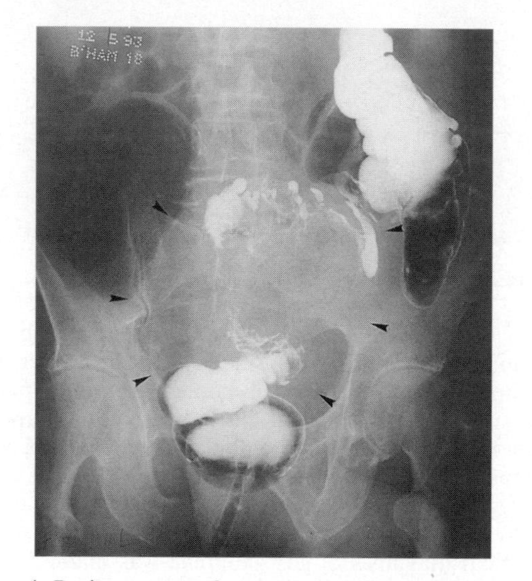

Figure 4. Barium enema 2 years prior to current admission showing a narrowed distorted sigmoid colon with diverticula and the impression of a large associated inflammatory mass (arrows).

The diagnosis is emphysematous cellulitis of the leg secondary to colonic diverticular disease. Figure 1 shows gas throughout the soft tissues and beneath the thickened skin of the lower thigh and calf. Figure 2 shows large locules of gas in the intermuscular planes around the hip joints, particularly on the left where it extends down into the thigh. A water soluble contrast enema examination was performed (Figure 3). This demonstrated the presence of bilateral large fistulous tracks from the sigmoid colon, which passed through the greater sciatic foramina into both gluteal regions. The fistula on the left continued into the proximal thigh and then out onto the skin over the greater trochanter through the surgical incision. Figure 4 demonstrates the severity of the "diverticulitis" 2 years previously. This had been managed non-surgically

The clues to the diagnosis in this case are the previous history of diverticulitis, the nature of the cultured material, and the fact that the gas is in tissue planes rather than within muscle bodies themselves. This latter feature is claimed to distinguish gas simply tracking between fascial planes from gas which might arise *de novo* within tissues as a consequence of gas gangrene [1]. Approximately 20% of patients with diverticular disease who undergo surgery develop fistulae, but spontaneous colocutaneous fistulae are extremely rare [2]. Internal fistulae, such as colovesical and coloenteric, are much commoner and can occasionally communicate with a ureter or any part of the female genital tract [2]. Only 2.6–7.8% of neoplasms of the large bowel perforate, but even then the majority of these remain localized with abscess formation [3]. Although free gas associated with diverticular disease is likely to be from perforation of the bowel, gas-producing organisms are another potential source [1]. Gas may reach the lower limb by tracking beneath the inguinal ligament or through the greater sciatic or obturator foramina [3]. Other abdominal causes of gas in the lower limb include traumatic perforation of the pelvic colon, appendicitis or caecal perforation and Crohn's disease, as well as emphysematous cystitis and pyelonephritis in diabetics [4, 5]. Gas can also extend subcutaneously through the abdominal wall, or develop in the limb as part of an overwhelming generalized septicaemia [3]. Emphysematous cellulitis is more likely to occur in an older age group and is always associated with pre-existing disease. It follows that there is a significant disease-related morbidity and mortality [1, 3, 4, 5]. Early recognition of this condition, and in particular its differentiation from gas gangrene, are important factors in preventing its potentially fatal outcome.

References

1. Ainsworth J. Emphysema of the leg following perforation of the pelvic colon or rectum. Br J Radiol 1959;32:54–5.
2. Colcock BP, Stahmann FD. Fistulas complicating diverticular disease of the sigmoid colon. Ann Surg 1972;175:838–46.
3. Mair WSJ, McAdam WAF, Lee PWR, et al. Carcinoma of the large bowel presenting as a subcutaneous abcess of the thigh: a report of four cases. Br J Surg 1977;64:205–9.
4. Linscheid RL, Kelly PJ, Symmonds RE. Emphysematous cellulitis of the hip and thigh resulting from enteric fistula. J Bone Joint Surg 1963;45A:1691–7.
5. Nicell P, Tabrisky J, Lindstrom R, Peter M. Thigh emphysema and hip pain secondary to gastrointestinal perforation. Surgery 1975;78:555–9.

Communication makes all the difference

K P GILL and A L HINE

Central Middlesex Hospital, Acton Lane, Park Royal, London NW10 7NS, UK

A 64-year-old man was admitted for excision of a mass in the right groin. The mass had been present for 6 months and had recently enlarged. The patient had noticed aching at the end of the day. His past history was non-contributory.

On clinical examination a fixed hard mass was palpated in the right groin. A similar mass was present in the left groin. CT of the pelvis was arranged (Figure 1).

What is the diagnosis?

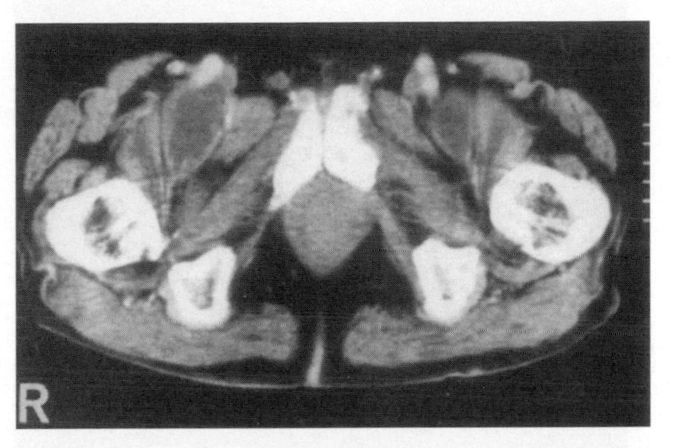

Figure 1. Contrast enhanced CT of pelvis at the level of the symphysis pubis.

Based on the case of the month originally published in Br J Radiol 1994;67:313–4.

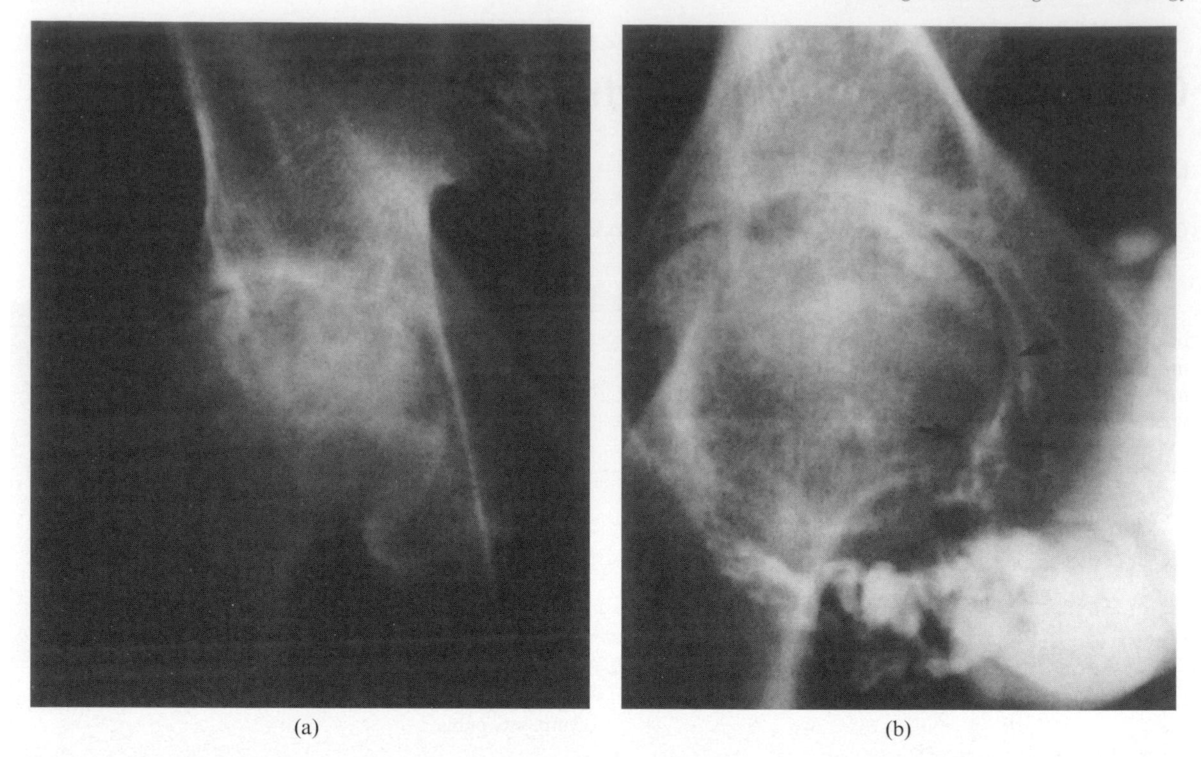

(a) (b)

Figure 2. Degenerative right hip (a) with intraarticular contrast (arrows) following contrast opacification of the iliopsoas bursa (b).

The CT study revealed bilateral bilobulated fluid-containing structures adjacent to the hip joints which were degenerative. The differential diagnosis was of bilateral enlarged iliopsoas bursae or enlarged inguinal nodes with central necrosis.

Under fluoroscopic control the right fluid collection was aspirated and contrast medium instilled into the cavity. The adjacent hip joint capsule was opacified, confirming communication between the bursa and the joint (Figure 2). Cytology of the aspirated fluid revealed scanty lymphocytes. The fluid was sterile on culture. The findings were consistent with iliopsoas bursa enlargement.

The iliopsoas bursa is situated beneath the tendon of the iliopsoas muscle as it crosses the hip joint. It may be found in 98% of subjects and can communicate with the hip joint in up to 15%. Enlargement of the iliopsoas bursa may present as a mass in the groin and is associated with pain and limitation of movement [1].

An enlarged bursa may be associated with pre-existing arthritis, as in our patient. Other associated conditions include synovial chrondromatosis, pigmented villonodular synovitis and septic arthritis. The differential diagnosis includes lymphadenopathy, femoral artery aneurysm, psoas abscess, undescended testis and femoral and inguinal hernia [2].

In our case, opacification of the hip joint following contrast introduction into the bursa confirmed the diagnosis. The use of contrast media in the diagnosis of a distended iliopsoas bursa is, however, surprisingly uncommon [1].

Previous reports have described unilateral distended bursae [1, 3, 4]. Sequential development of bilateral iliopsoas bursae in a 14-year-old female has been described [5]. We believe that this is one of the first cases of simultaneous bilateral iliopsoas bursal enlargement in an adult.

In the assessment of groin masses a distended iliopsoas bursa should be considered; if doubt persists demonstration of communication with the hip joint will confirm the diagnosis.

References

1. Armstrong P, Saxton H. Ilio-psoas bursa. Br J Radiol 1972;45:493–5.
2. Binek R, Levinsohn EM. Enlarged iliopsoas bursa. An unusual case of thigh mass and hip pain. Clin Orthop 1987;224:158–63.
3. O'Connor DS. Early recognition of iliopectineal bursitis. Surg Gynecol Obst 1933;57:674–84.
4. Pritchard RS, Shah HR, Nelson CL, Fitzrandolph RL. MR and CT appearance of iliopsoas bursal distention secondary to diseased hips. JCAT 1990;14:797–800.
5. Dyon JF, Ben Salah S, Baudain P, et al. An abdominal tumor of unusual nature. Synovial cyst in the iliopsoas bursa. Chir Pediatr 1987;28:115–9.

The sheep in wolf's clothing

J F GRIFFITH and P J GUEST

Department of Clinical Radiology, Queen Elizabeth Hospital, Edgbaston, Birmingham B15 2TH, UK

A 57-year-old female was referred for investigation following the discovery of asymptomatic microscopic haematuria during a routine check-up by her general practitioner. She had a 10 year history of hypertension which was well controlled on medication. Her brother had died from disseminated renal carcinoma when aged 40 years. An intravenous urogram (Figure 1) and contrast enhanced renal CT (Figure 2) were performed. What diagnoses would you consider?

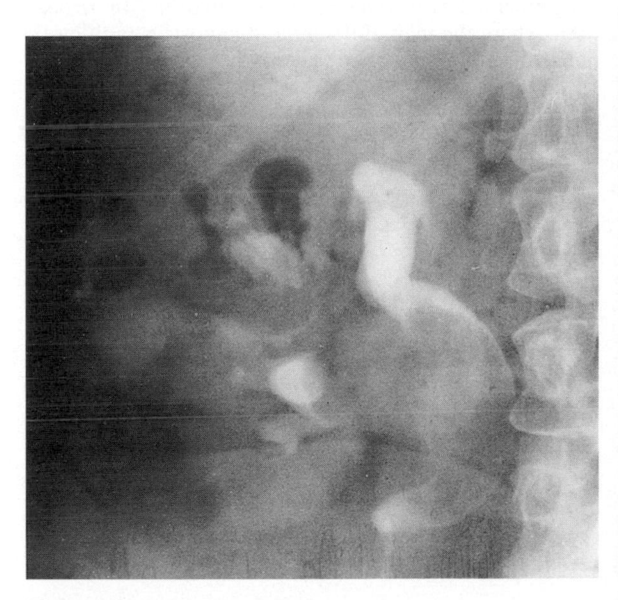

Figure 1. Intravenous urogram.

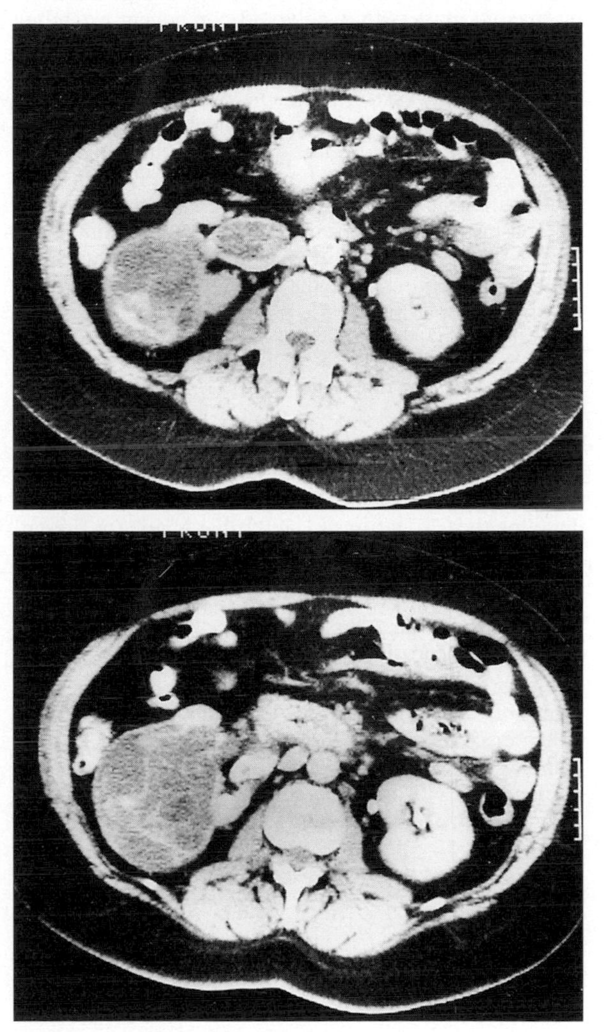

Figure 2. Contrast enhanced CT.

Based on the case of the month originally published in Br J Radiol 1997;70:543–4.

Intravenous urography showed a large renal mass invading the renal pelvis (Figure 1). Ultrasound (not shown) demonstrated a mass with mixed echogenicity arising from the lower pole of the right kidney, extending into the renal pelvis and proximal ureter. Contrast enhanced CT showed a large renal mass of mixed attenuation with evidence of internal septation (Figure 2) and confirmed the extension into the renal pelvis and proximal ureter. A right nephrectomy was performed. Macroscopically, the kidney contained a large multicystic myxoid mass with a polypoid component extending into the renal pelvis. Microscopically, the tumour had a thick fibrous capsule and consisted of many non-communicating cysts varying in size from a few millimetres to a few centimetres and lined by cuboidal epithelium with areas of "hob-nail" epithelium (*i.e.* focal mounds of cuboidal cells). Small foci of calcification were present in some of the cyst walls. These are the radiological and histological appearances of a benign multiloculated cystic nephroma. Both cystic and solid subtypes of renal cell carcinoma are the principal differential diagnoses. Post-operatively, the patient made an uneventful recovery.

Multiloculated cystic nephroma (MLCN) is a rare renal tumour accounting for about 1% of all upper tract renal tumours. Over 100 cases have been reported since it was first described, with only the more recent reports detailing the CT features [1–4]. It has a biphasic presentation [2, 3] in young males aged from 3 months to 4 years when it usually presents as an abdominal mass [2–4] or in adult females with haematuria, hypertension or pain [2, 4]. Herniation into the renal pelvis occurs in approximately 40% of cases [2] and the surface ulceration may lead to microscopic haematuria. Perinephric extension is unusual [2]. Ultrasound demonstrates either discrete cysts with recognizable septa [3] or a complex echogenic mass [2, 4] due to myriad small cysts interspersed with some larger cysts. CT usually shows the multilocular nature of the lesion with cysts containing clear fluid. Occasionally, as in this case, a large number of small cysts with myxoid contents result in the septation being less obvious. Angiographic appearances are variable, the lesion being most commonly hypovascular, although it can be avascular or hypervascular and associated with a tumour blush [2]. On MRI [5], the tumour is hypointense on T_1 weighted sequences and hyperintense on T_2 weighted sequences with well defined irregular hypointense septa.

If cyst formation is clear, then the principal differential diagnosis in adulthood is multiloculated renal carcinoma. However, as in this atypical case, where cyst septa are not clearly identified it can also masquerade as a solid renal carcinoma.

Recognition of the radiological features of MLCN and, in particular, the intervening septa evident on CT, should raise the possibility of this diagnosis prior to surgery. This recognition has important therapeutic implications—namely, if the tumour is confined and has little or no extension into the renal pelvis, a limited operation (rather than radical nephrectomy) can be performed in adults with *in vivo* inspection of the kidney supplemented by frozen section examination [4]. In children, where the main differential diagnosis is multicystic nephroblastoma, cytotoxic agents can be omitted prior to surgery [3].

References

1. Parienty RA, Pradel J, Imbert M, et al. Computed tomography of multiloculated cystic nephroma. Radiology 1981; 140:135–9.
2. Madewell JE, Goldman SM, Davis CJ Jr, et al. Multilocular cystic nephroma: a radiographic–pathologic correlation of 58 patients. Radiology 1983;146:309–21.
3. Garrett A, Carty H, Pilling D. Multiloculated cystic nephroma: report of three cases. Clin Radiol 1987;38:55–7.
4. Banner MP, Pollack HM, Chatten J, Witzleben C. Multilocular renal cysts: radiologic–pathologic correlation. AJR 1981;136:239–47.
5. Kim SH, Choi BI, Han MC, et al. Multiloculated cystic nephroma: MR findings. AJR 1989;153:1317.

The jockey with a mass in the thigh

A M DAVIES, N EVANS and R J GRIMER

Department of Radiology, Royal Orthopaedic Hospital, Birmingham, UK

A 40-year-old professional jockey presented with a 2 week history of severe pain in the right knee region which commenced whilst riding. Examination revealed a firm mass, 10 cm × 5 cm, within the soft tissues of the medial aspect of the right distal thigh. All laboratory investigations were normal. The radiological investigations of the right femur included plain radiography (Figure 1) and CT (Figure 2). A bone scan showed a solitary, non-homogeneous area of increased uptake in the right distal femur.

What is your diagnosis?

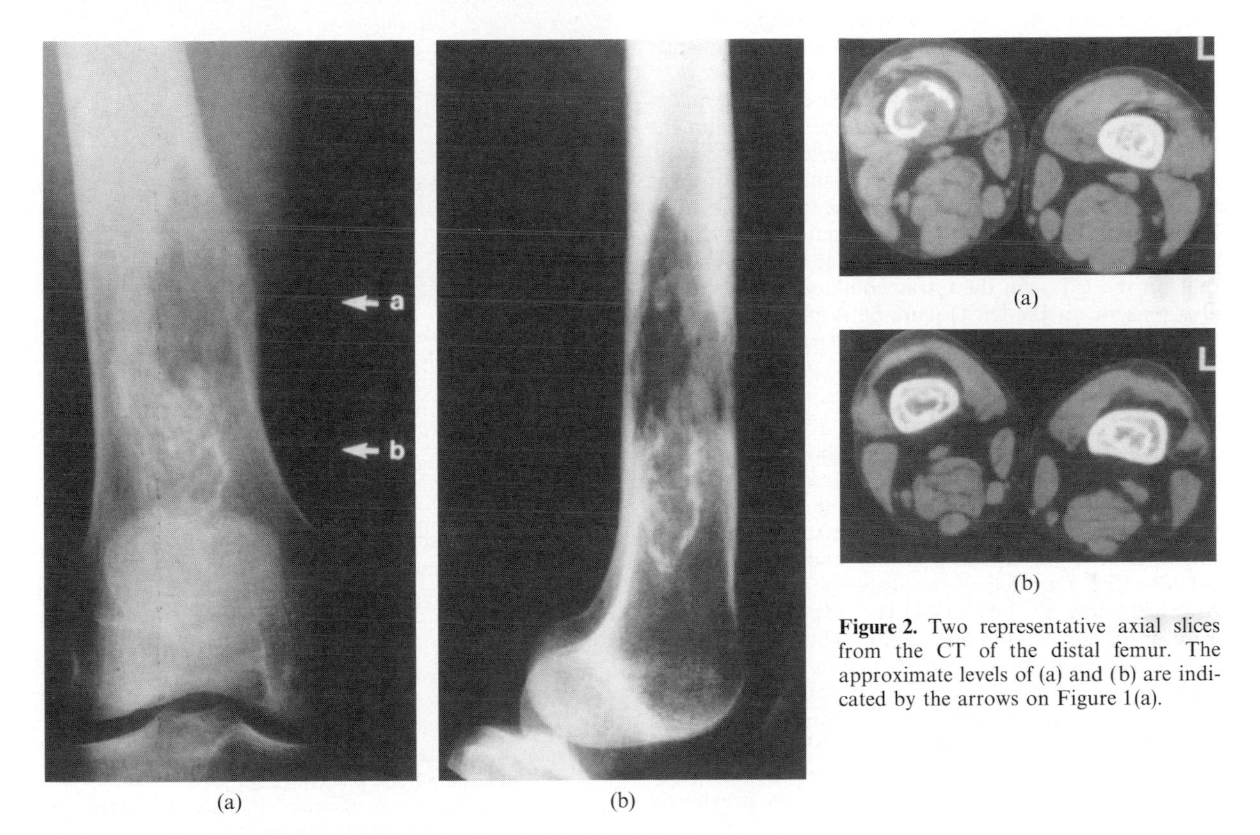

Figure 1. (a) Anteroposterior and (b) lateral radiographs of the right distal femur.

Figure 2. Two representative axial slices from the CT of the distal femur. The approximate levels of (a) and (b) are indicated by the arrows on Figure 1(a).

Based on the case of the month originally published in Br J Radiol 1989;62:183–4.

The plain radiographs (Figure 1) showed an extensive abnormality of the distal femoral metadiaphysis. Superiorly there is a lytic, permeative lesion breaching the medial cortex with minimal periosteal reaction. The cortical defect is associated with a soft tissue mass, confirmed by CT, which also shows soft tissue within the medullary canal (Figure 2(a)).

The radiological features are those of a malignant lesion and the differential diagnosis includes malignant fibrous histiocytoma, fibrosarcoma, lytic osteosarcoma, reticulum cell sarcoma (primary malignant lymphoma) or metastasis. Inferiorly, however, the lesion consists of medullary calcification with a serpiginous margin typical of a long standing medullary infarct. This latter observation effectively reduces the differential diagnosis down to one single probable entity and that is a malignant fibrous histiocytoma (MFH) arising in a bone infarct. This is a rare, but well recognized, complication of chronic medullary infarction and this was subsequently confirmed histologically by biopsy.

Another diagnosis that might be considered is malignant degeneration in a benign cartilage tumour but the medullary calcification would be expected to be central and punctate rather than peripheral and curvilinear as seen in a typical infarct. The presence of symmetrical lesions is also more in favour of infarction than chondroid tumours and the observant reader will have noted that on the CT scan the intramedullary calcification is also present on the left (Figure 2). A plain radiograph of the left femur confirms that the infarcts are bilateral and symmetrical (Figure 3).

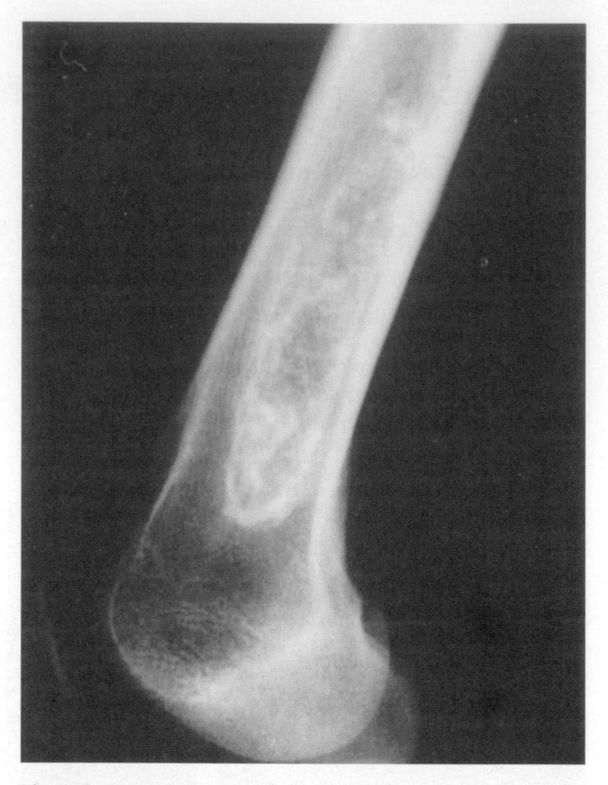

Figure 3. Lateral radiograph of the left distal femur showing a typical medullary infarct.

Malignant fibrous histiocytoma, although a relatively common sarcoma of soft tissues, represents only about 5% of all primary malignant bone tumours [1]. Radiologically this highly aggressive tumour is indistinguishable from a fibrosarcoma and differentiation between the two relies on histological examination. Approximately 20–25% of MFHs have been shown to arise in pre-existing bone abnormalities [2]. These include bone infarction, irradiated bone, Paget's disease, enchondroma, fibrous dysplasia and tissue adjacent to prosthetic joint replacements [2–5]. Those patients with an MFH arising in a pre-existing bone abnormality tend to be older, aged over 40 years and have a poorer prognosis than those with an MFH arising in previously normal bone.

The majority of malignant tumours arising in bone infarcts are MFHs although other tumours such as fibrosarcoma and osteosarcoma have been described [3]. This rare association is not thought to be a coincidental occurrence but to be a true causal relationship. The generally accepted hypothesis is that the MFH arises from primitive mesenchymal cells in the chronic reparative tissue around the periphery of an area of bone infarction [4]. There is a long latent period before such malignant transformation may occur. Three former caisson workers who presented with this complication had all left their employment approximately 20 years before [3].

The aetiology of the bone infarction in the present case is unknown. Chest CT showed no evidence of metastases and treatment consisted of chemotherapy and endoprosthetic replacement of the distal femur. Currently, the patient remains disease free although the quoted 5-year survival for a patient with an MFH arising in a pre-existing bone abnormality is less than 25% [2].

References

1. Boland PJ, Huvos AG. Malignant fibrous histiocytoma of bone. Clin Orthop Relat Res 1986;204:130–4.
2. Capanna R, Bertoni F, Bacchini P, Bacci G, Guerra A, Campanacci M. Malignant fibrous histiocytoma of bone. Cancer 1984;54:177–84.
3. Mirra JM, Bullough PG, Marcove RC, Jacobs B, Huvos AG. Malignant fibrous histiocytoma and osteosarcoma in association with bone infarcts. J Bone Joint Surg 1974;56A:932–40.
4. Heselson NG, Price SK, Mills EED, Conway SSM, Marks RK. Two malignant fibrous histiocytomas in bone infarcts. J Bone Joint Surg 1983;65A:1166–71.
5. Tait NP, Hacking PM, Malcolm AJ. Malignant fibrous histiocytoma occurring at the site of a previous total hip replacement. Br J Radiol 1988;61:73–5.

An opportunity not to be missed

A M BELLI, C ELLIOTT and C W HERON

Departments of Radiology and Pathology, Royal Marsden Hospital, Downs Road, Sutton, Surrey SM2 5PT, UK

A 55-year-old man presented with a 10 day history of breathlessness and productive cough. A chest infection was diagnosed clinically and treated with antibiotics although the chest radiograph was normal.

His past medical history included a renal transplant 7 years previously for end stage membranous glomerulonephritis, following which immunosuppression was continued. 6 months prior to admission he was found to have Stage IIIB nodular sclerosing Hodgkin's disease. Clinical remission was achieved after five courses of chemotherapy. On completion of chemotherapy 3 weeks prior to admission, his white cell count was normal.

The patient initially responded to antibiotics but 4 days later became pyrexial and tachypnoeic and his therapy was changed from cefuroxine and erythromycin to gentamicin, piperacillin and flucloxacillin. The next day he was drowsy with leg weakness but no focal neurological signs. During the next 4 days he deteriorated mentally and his plantar responses became equivocal.

Contrast enhanced cranial CT was performed (Figure 1).

What abnormalities are seen on CT? What is the differential diagnosis and how could the diagnosis be confirmed?

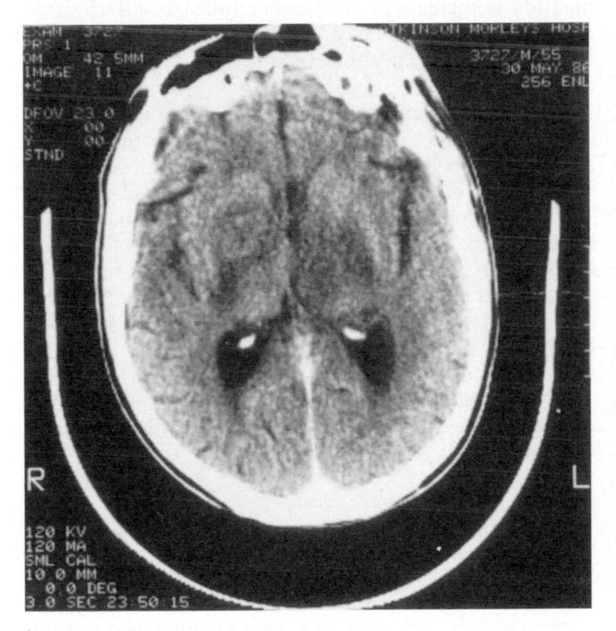

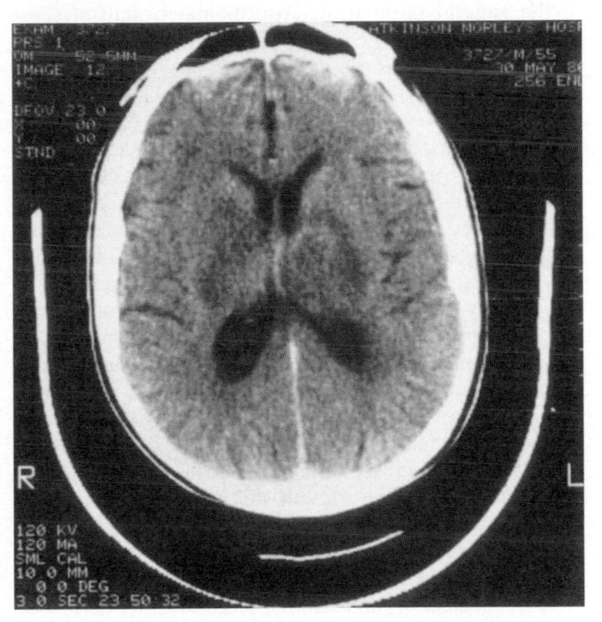

Figure 1. Post-contrast CT sections.

Based on the case of the month originally published in Br J Radiol 1988;61:171–2.

The CT scan showed two major areas of low attenuation situated in the left thalamus and right basal ganglia. There were curvilinear areas of increased density which may have been due to haemorrhage or minimal enhancement following iv contrast medium. Several smaller areas of low attenuation were seen in other parts of the cerebrum. The bilateral lesions have resulted in slight compression and minimal bowing of the third ventricle to the right.

In view of the history, the differential diagnosis includes Hodgkin's disease, non-Hodgkin's lymphoma and an opportunistic infection.

The appearances on CT are compatible with lymphoma. Intracerebral lymphoma involves either the dura and leptomeninges or, rarely, the parenchyma. Parenchymal disease is multicentric in approximately 50% of cases and there is a predilection for the periventricular tissues. Appearances vary but are almost equally divided into poorly defined, low attenuation lesions showing minimal enhancement, and slightly hyperdense enhancing areas.

Non-Hodgkin's lymphoma occurs 50 times more frequently in patients following renal transplantation than in the general population. Approximately half of these tumours arise in the brain. The patient was already known to have Hodgkin's disease but the additional development of non-Hodgkin's lymphoma would have been possible.

Renal transplant recipients are prone to develop cytomegalovirus, fungal and bacterial infections, while patients with Hodgkin's disease show increased susceptibility to the protozoan toxoplasmosis [1]. In immunocompromised patients who are unable to localize infection, cranial lesions are often poorly circumscribed, of low density and may exhibit little contrast enhancement [2]. An opportunistic infection seemed the most likely diagnosis but identification of an organism would have required a biopsy. The patient was considered too unwell for this procedure and he died 5 days later.

A post-mortem examination showed cerebral toxoplasmosis. Coronal sections of the brain revealed a large haemorrhagic necrotic lesion in the left thalamus and smaller haemorrhagic lesions in the right globus pallidus (Figure 2) and the left cerebellar cortex. Microscopic examination of the lesions showed abundant free forms of *Toxoplasma gondii* and pseudocysts. There was residual Hodgkin's disease involving abdominal lymph nodes and the spleen.

There are usually abnormal findings on CT in patients with toxoplasma encephalitis. The appearances are well described although not specific. The corticomedullary junction, thalamus and basal ganglia are the typical sites of involvement. Most frequently there are multiple low attenuation lesions showing ring or nodular enhancement with associated oedema and mass effect. A number of lesions show no contrast enhancement. Optimal visualization is obtained by using double-dose contrast enhancement and delaying scanning for 1 h after the administration of contrast medium [3]. Thin (5 mm) axial sections are also useful. The disease is rapidly progressive without treatment and serial CT scans will demonstrate an increase in the number and size of the lesions. Early diagnosis of intracerebral toxoplasmosis is essential in order that appropriate antibiotic therapy may be instituted.

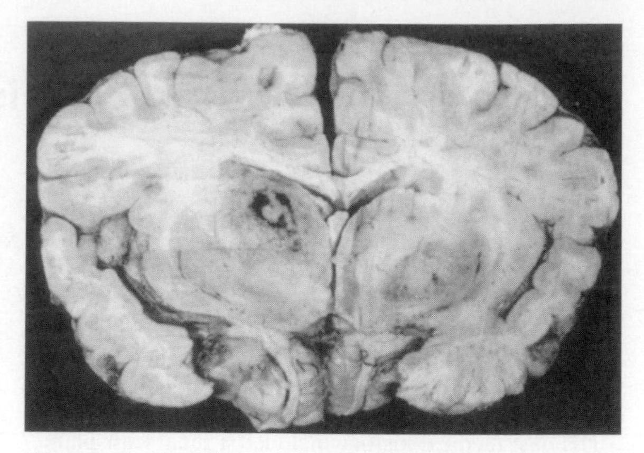

Figure 2. Coronal section of the brain showing lesions in the left thalamus, right globus pallidus and smaller lesions within the cerebral cortex.

MRI is more sensitive than CT in detecting the intracerebral lesions of toxoplasmosis, permitting earlier biopsy and institution of treatment [4]. MRI also permits better visualization of the posterior fossa.

The incidence of intracerebral toxoplasmosis has increased due to AIDS and the diagnosis should always be considered in any immunocompromised patient with vague neurological signs suggestive of intracerebral disease. As effective treatment is available, early MRI and biopsy are indicated when doubt about the causative agent exists.

[*For recent reviews of this subject see [5] and [6], MR proton spectroscopy is helpful in distinguishing abscesses from other mass lesions in AIDS, ED*]

References

1. Carey RM, Kimball AC, Armstrong D, Lieberman PH. Toxoplasmosis. Clinical experiences in a cancer hospital. Am J Med 1973;54:30–8.
2. Enzmann DR, Brant-Zawadzki M, Britt RH. CT of central nervous system infections in immunocompromised patients. AJR 1980;135:263–7.
3. Post MJD, Kursunoglo SJ, Hensley GT, Chan JC, Moskowitz LB, Hoffman TA. Cranial CT in acquired immunodeficiency syndrome: spectrum of diseases and optimal contrast enhancement technique. AJR 1985;145:929–40.
4. Zee C-S, Segall HD, Rogers C, Ahmadi J, Apuzzo M, Rhodes R. MR imaging of cerebral toxoplasmosis: correlation of computed tomography and pathology. JCAT 1985;9:797–9.
5. Martin-Duverneuil N, Cordoliani YS, Sola-Martinez MT, et al. Cerebral toxoplasmosis: neuroradiologic diagnosis and follow-up. Neuroradiology 1995;22:196–204.
6. Chang L, Cornford ME, Chiang FL, et al. Cerebral toxoplasmosis and lymphoma in AIDS. AJNR 1995;16:1653–63.

Getting to the heart of the matter

R S DAVIES, N PANG and J HARPER

Department of Diagnostic Radiology, Princess Alexandra Hospital, Ipswich Road, Woolloongabba 4102, Brisbane, Queensland, Australia

A 65-year-old lady presented with a 48 h history of increasing epigastric pain. She had vomited but had had no haematemesis or melaena. She had had surgery for a peptic ulcer 30 years earlier and two cerebrovascular accidents (CVAs), 21 years and 10 years earlier. She also suffered from angina.

On examination she was haemodynamically stable and had moderate epigastric pain with some guarding. There were no heart murmurs and plain radiographs were unremarkable. At laparotomy there was haemoperitoneum with clot in the free edge of the lesser omentum but no bleeding points were identified. The patient made a rapid recovery.

CT was performed 3 days after admission (Figure 1) and was followed by arteriography (Figure 2). 36 h later the patient suddenly deteriorated and a repeat laparotomy was performed. At operation a large retroperitoneal haematoma was found and a ruptured branch of the superior mesenteric artery (SMA) posterior to the duodenum was identified as the bleeding site and ligated.

The patient made a slow but steady recovery and was commenced on steroids for a presumed vasculitis. However, apart from a moderately raised erythrocyte sedimentation rate (ESR) (55 mm h^{-1}) all immunological markers were unremarkable.

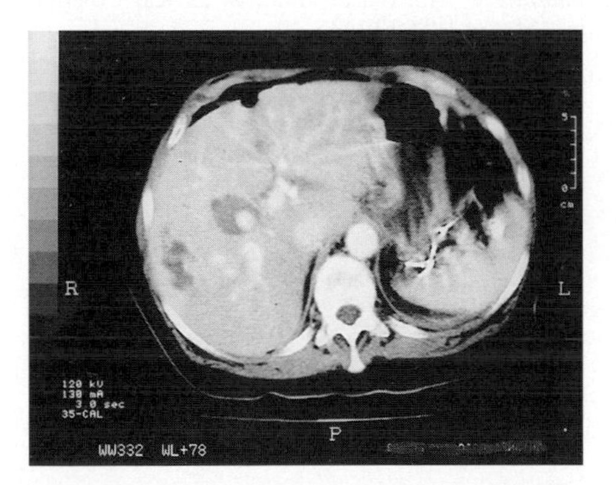

Figure 1. Contrast enhanced CT shows multiple low attenuation areas within the liver, the largest of which shows marked central enhancement.

Based on the case of the month originally published in Br J Radiol 1997;70:659–60.

Echocardiography was performed to exclude endocarditis as a cause for mycotic aneurysms.

What do CT (Figure 1), aortography (Figure 2) and echocardiography (Figure 3) show? What is the diagnosis?

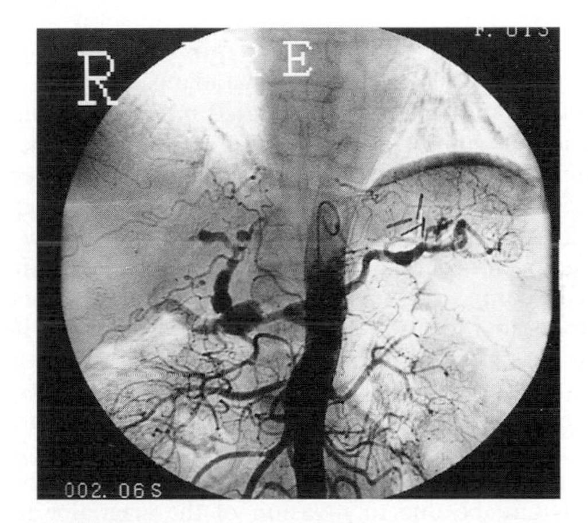

Figure 2. Flush aortogram.

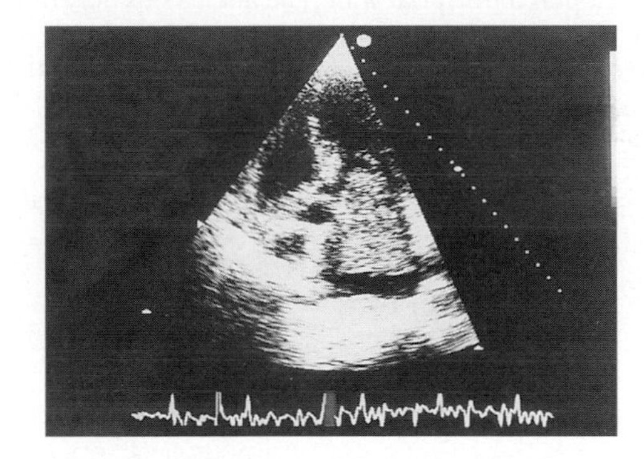

Figure 3. Echocardiogram through the left atrium.

CT showed multiple low attenuation areas within the liver, some with dense central contrast enhancement as demonstrated on Figure 1. Angiography confirmed the presence of multiple aneurysms of both the left and right hepatic arteries. The large aneurysm at the bifurcation corresponded to the lesion shown on CT. These were successfully embolized.

The patient made a slow but steady recovery following the second laporotomy and was commenced on steroids for a presumed vasculitis. However, apart from a moderately raised ESR (55 mm l^{-1}), all immunological markers were normal.

The echocardiogram, which was performed to exclude endocarditis as a cause for mycotic aneurysms, showed a large 4 cm × 4 cm mass in a dilated left atrium. The appearances were typical of an atrial myxoma and this was confirmed at surgery.

Primary cardiac tumours are rare with an incidence of 0.0017% [1]. Most are benign and most are myxomas. Initial symptoms may be separated into three groups.

The commonest symptoms are cardiac and include dyspnoea, chest pain and syncope. These are due to interference with venous drainage and valvular function.

The second group of symptoms are due to embolization which occurs in about 50% of people [2]. Emboli may be composed of myxomatous material or thrombus and the final location of the embolus depends on if the tumour is right-sided (approximately 15%) or left-sided [3]. At least 50% of embolic events involve the central nervous system (CNS). As well as causing symptoms due to vascular occlusion, emboli may also cause multiple aneurysms both in the CNS and elsewhere. This is thought to be due to invasion of the arterial wall by myxomatous material with subsequent weakening and dilatation of the arterial wall. The aneurysms may resolve after resection of the primary tumour [4].

The third group of symptoms are constitutional manifestations such as fever, myalgia, arthralgia and weight loss. There may be a raised ESR, anaemia and leucocytosis and patients may be misdiagnosed as having collagen vascular disease. The clinical picture of atrial myxoma has also been duplicated by the rare antiphospholipid antibody syndrome. Vascular occlusions can mimic emboli and, if an atrial thrombus is present, can simulate a myxoma.

The clinical and radiological findings in this case were of intraperitoneal and retroperitoneal haemorrhage presumed to be secondary to rupture of intraabdominal aneurysms. The causes of multiple abdominal aneurysms include vasculitis (particularly polyarteritis nodosa), mycotic aneurysms and aneurysms occurring in generalized disorders such as Marfan's disease. In the patient presented here a vasculitic cause was felt to be most likely despite the only positive finding being a moderately raised ESR. It was only when echocardiography was performed to exclude an infective source that the atrial myxoma was discovered. In retrospect, the patient had experienced episodes of chest pain in the past and the two CVAs she had suffered may also have been related to the myxoma.

Atrial myxoma is a rare but treatable cause of multiple aneurysms in the abdomen, CNS and elsewhere and should be considered in the differential diagnosis.

References

1. Straus R, Merliss R. Primary tumour of the heart. Arch Pathol Lab Med 1945;39:74–8.
2. Larsson S, Lepore V, Kennergren C. Atrial myxomas. Results of 25 years' experience and review of the literature. Surgery 1988;105:695–8.
3. Harwood-Nash DC, Howard BA, Solsbery DM, et al. Image interpretation seminar. Ischaemic small bowel, arterial embolus and left atrial myxoma. Radiographics 1992; 12:196–8.
4. Krepper LE, Biller J, Adams Jr HP, Bruno A. Neurological manifestations of atrial myxoma. A 12 year experience and review. Stroke 1988;19:1435–40.

The case of the recalcitrant Welshman

K LYONS and C EVANS

Department of Radiology, University Hospital of Wales and Cardiff Royal Infirmary, Cardiff, UK

A 72-year-old retired carpenter presented to his general practitioner with an attack of left renal colic and frank haematuria. He refused hospital admission and settled with antibiotics and analgesia. He also refused investigation at that time, as he looked after an elderly sister. He had had an attack of similar pain 3 months later but with no haematuria on that occasion. He was referred for a urological opinion.

There were no positive findings on clinical examination. Apart from these two attacks he had been well with no relevant past history. Investigations included haemoglobin 16.0 $g\,dl^{-1}$, white blood cell count $8.3 \times 10^9\,l^{-1}$, glucose 5.9 $mmol\,l^{-1}$, serum calcium 2.27 $mmol\,l^{-1}$ (normal range 2.25–2.60 $mmol\,l^{-1}$), urea 7.9 $mmol\,l^{-1}$, creatinine 208 $\mu mol\,l^{-1}$, uric acid 0.38 $mmol\,l^{-1}$ (normal range 0.1–0.4 $mmol\,l^{-1}$). A mid-stream urine specimen yielded no growth. Microscopy showed 0–5 red cells per high-power field.

On intravenous urography (IVU), no calculi or other abnormality were seen on the central radiograph. Appearances on the 15 min urogram (Figure 1) and on tomography (Figure 2) are shown.

What abnormality is shown?

What is the differential diagnosis and how would you investigate the patient further?

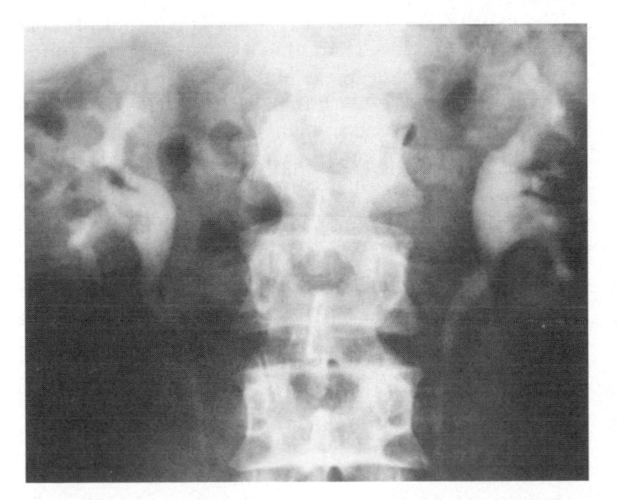

Figure 1. 15 min radiography of the renal area on intravenous urography.

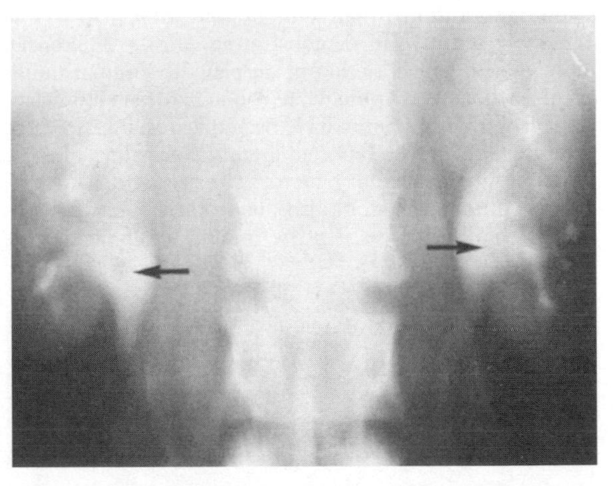

Figure 2. Tomography of the renal area.

Based on the case of the month originally published in Br J Radiol 1987;60:93–5.

The urogram showed two filling defects in the renal pelves.

CT (Figure 3) showed calculi in both renal pelves. The diagnosis of non-opaque stones, probably uric acid, was made. He was treated with Allopurinol, sodium bicarbonate and encouraged to take a lot of fluids. He passed a total of 16 small ureteric stones over the next 6 months, several of which were analysed and were composed of uric acid. He has refused radiological follow-up as he felt well.

Non-opaque filling defects shown in the renal pelvis on an IVU have many different causes, but the main differential diagnosis lies between urothelial tumours, radiolucent calculi, blood clot and sloughed papillae. While clinical history, biochemistry, urinalysis and urine cytology may be helpful, further investigation is frequently warranted. Ultrasound, retrograde pyelography, brush biopsy and angiography have been used with varying degrees of success prior to exploratory surgery. CT both allows these patients to be investigated non-invasively and indicates the most appropriate management.

Radiolucent calculi account for approximately 8% of all urinary calculi. Most are composed of uric acid, while a few are xanthine, matrix or cystine stones. As CT is extremely sensitive in demonstrating density differences, these calculi, which are lucent on plain abdominal radiographs, will appear "pure white" on uncontrasted CT [1]. Calculi as small as 5 mm have been diagnosed [2]. There is discrepancy in the reported attenuation values of these calculi, probably due in part to technical factors, such as partial volume effect, but also due to their heterogeneous composition [1]. This is not of practical significance as

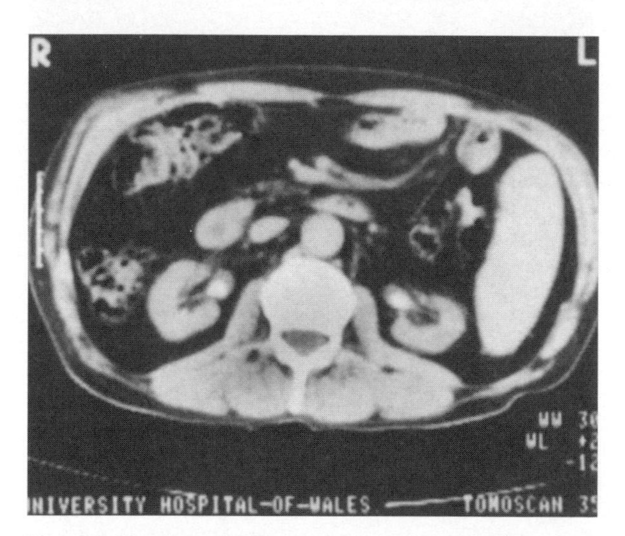

Figure 3. Unenhanced CT scan through the renal pelves showing "pure white" renal calculi.

in vitro studies have shown that, while CT attenuation data confirm the order of density of calculi as seen on plain radiography, it is impossible to predict their chemical composition accurately from their CT attenuation numbers alone [3]. Its role is in distinguishing between radiolucent calculi and other non-opaque filling defects of the pelvicalyceal system. Small calculi may be missed on ultrasound as differentiation from the echogenic pelvis may be impossible if there is no demonstrable acoustic shadowing [4].

Transitional cell carcinoma presenting as a filling defect on urography may be difficult to recognize on uncontrasted CT scans, having a density of 30–40 HU which is greater than that of urine but less than that of renal parenchyma. It will be more clearly visible on post-contrast scans and will show some enhancement [1], although this enhancement will always be less than that of normal renal parenchyma. At the same time it is possible to stage the tumour by identifying extrapelvic spread and metastases to enlarged lymph nodes [5]. Some caution is necessary as 2% of transitional cell carcinomas calcify and it may not always be possible to differentiate between transitional cell carcinoma invading the renal parenchyma and renal cell carcinoma invading the pelvis.

The density of blood clot is higher than that of renal parenchyma but less than that of non-opaque stones, and shows no enhancement after contrast medium [1]. Attenuation will vary with the age of the clot, being less than that of soft tissue when liquefaction occurs and approaching that of calculi when calcified. Blood clots are often transient. Sloughed papillae would be expected to have an attenuation number similar to that of soft tissue although if calcified, differentiation from calculi is difficult.

It may not always be possible to be certain about the presence, or the intrinsic or extrinsic nature, of a filling defect in the renal pelvis on an IVU. Extrinsic lesions such as parapelvic cysts are clearly demonstrated on CT, a differentiation that is not always easy on ultrasound as transitional cell carcinomas are frequently hypoechoic.

References

1. Parienty RA, Ducellier R, Pradel J, Lubrano J-M, Coquille F, Richard F. Diagnostic value of CT numbers in pelvicalyceal filling defects. Radiology 1982;145:743–7.
2. Segal AJ, Spataro RF, Linke CA, Frank IN, Rabinowitz R. Diagnosis of nonopaque calculi by computerised tomography. Radiology 1978;129:447–50.
3. Newhouse JH, Prien EL, Amis ES Jr, Dretler SP, Pfister RC. Computerised tomographic analysis of urinary calculi. AJR 1984;142:545–8.
4. Pollack HM, Arger PH, Banner MP, Mulhern CB Jr, Coleman BG. Computerised tomography of renal pelvic filling defects. Radiology 1981;138:654–51.
5. Baron RL, McClennan BL, Lee JKT, Lawson TL. Computerised tomography of transitional-cell carcinoma of the renal pelvis and ureter. Radiology 1982;144:125–30.

A pulmonary embolus, or what?

[1]R UBEROI, [2]L JENKINS, [2]A J MARSHALL and [1]I P WELLS

Departments of [1]Clinical Radiology and [2]Cardiology, Derriford Hospital, Plymouth, UK

A 36-year-old man who had previously been well, presented with a 7 day history of shortness of breath and sudden onset of left sided pleuritic chest pain. On admission he was apyrexial and not distressed. His pulse and blood pressure (120/85) were normal. There was a soft systolic murmur in the pulmonary area. The chest was clear on auscultation and there was no evidence of lymphadenopathy or abdominal abnormality. He had a normal white count ($4.9 \times 10^9\ l^{-1}$), haemoglobin ($14.8\ g\ l^{-1}$), urea and electrolytes. An electrocardiogram (ECG) demonstrated inversion of T waves in lead 3 only. A portable chest radiograph was performed (Figure 1), followed immediately by a ventilation and perfusion scan (Figure 2).

What do these show? Is there any disparity between the appearances on the two investigations? How would you investigate this patient further?

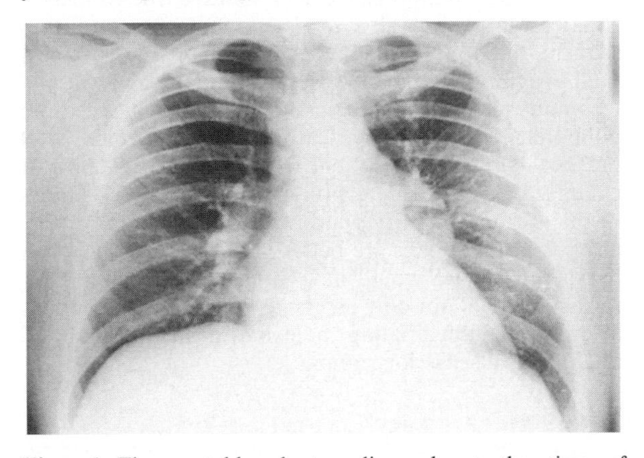

Figure 1. The portable chest radiograph at the time of presentation.

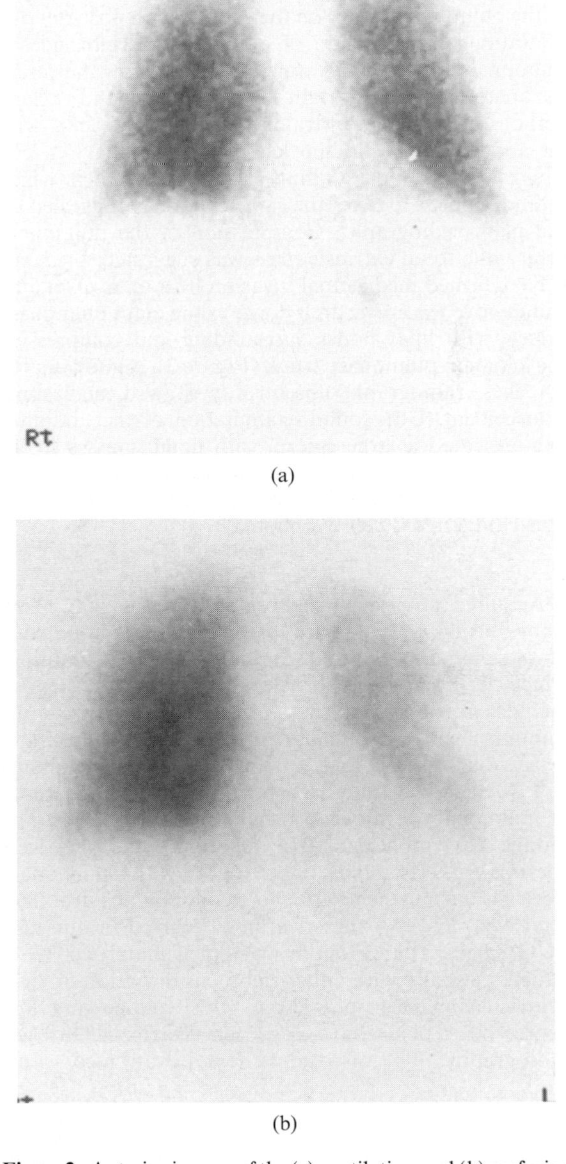

(a)

(b)

Figure 2. Anterior images of the (a) ventilation and (b) perfusion lung scans.

Based on the case of the month originally published in Br J Radiol 1996;69:575–6.

The initial anteroposterior (AP) chest radiograph was taken in expiration and interpreted as showing large central pulmonary arteries and cardiomegaly. The apparent widening of the mediastinum was attributed to the poor inspiration. The perfusion scan demonstrated reduced perfusion to the whole of the left lung with a normal ventilation scan. However, there was a disparity in the appearances of the chest radiograph and perfusion scan. It was difficult to reconcile the bilateral enlargement of the pulmonary arteries with the unilateral oligaemia of the perfusion study. It was felt that this could be due to pre-existing pulmonary arterial hypertension with a superadded large left pulmonary artery embolism. The patient was too well for this to be a reasonable diagnosis. Another possibility, suggested at the time, was stenosis of the pulmonary artery on the left side with post-stenotic dilatation and diversion of blood to the right side. A pulmonary angiogram was performed to show the vascular anatomy, measure right heart pressures and exclude embolism. This demonstrated left-sided oligaemia, with an abnormal flow in the left main pulmonary artery. There was incomplete filling of the vessel lumen, which did not appear to be of the same calibre as suggested on the plain radiographs. Compression of the pulmonary artery due to an extrinsic mass was suggested. Dynamic CT confirmed mediastinal invasion by a mass extending from above the aortic arch down to the main pulmonary artery, with hilar nodes surrounding and compressing the left main pulmonary trunk (Figure 3). A good quality PA chest radiograph subsequently showed mediastinal enlargement. Ultrasound examination of the abdomen demonstrated a large spleen, with nodal masses in the region of the pancreas and porta hepatis. A mini-laparotomy with nodal biopsy confirmed a high grade non-Hodgkin's B cell lymphoma.

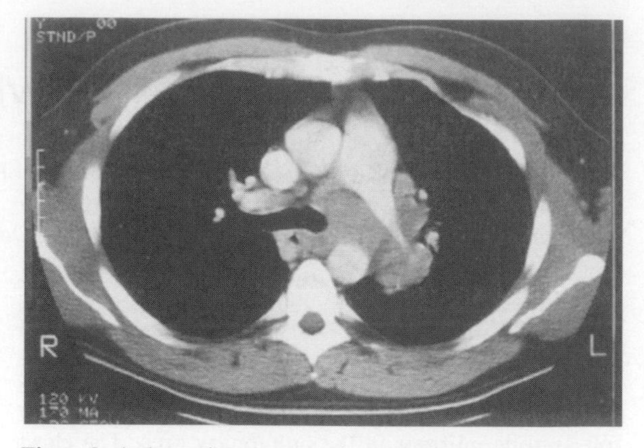

Figure 3. A dynamic contrast enhanced CT scan through the chest demonstrates marked compression of the left pulmonary artery by enlarged hilar nodes.

Acquired pulmonary stenosis is rare and may result from intrinsic valvular disease or extrinsic compression of the pulmonary outflow tract or artery. Conditions which cause acquired extrinsic pulmonary artery stenosis include aortic aneurysms, mediastinal cysts, sternal tumours (benign and malignant), fibrosing mediastinitis, pericardial disease and anterior mediastinal tumours [1]. Mediastinal tumours which most frequently result in pulmonary artery obstruction are teratomas and Hodgkin's lymphoma [2]. Reported symptoms were chest pain (69%) and dyspnoea (60%), with a pulmonary ejection murmur being the most common physical finding (89%) [2]. All these features occurred in our case. ECG changes are found in approximately 60% of patients, usually with either right axis deviation or right ventricular hypertrophy. Low QRS voltage and first degree heart block have also been described. On chest radiography, 70% of patients demonstrate mediastinal or hilar adenopathy [2] with 26% said to have normal radiographs at presentation.

In our patient, pulmonary angiography finally gave the diagnosis of a mediastinal mass which was demonstrated more specifically by dynamic enhanced CT. Echocardiography has also been used not only to diagnose acquired pulmonary artery stenosis due to mediastinal tumours but also to assess the success of subsequent therapy [3, 4]. MRI, although not routinely used in assessing patients with lymphoma, is a very useful technique in assessing mediastinal and hilar masses, and pulmonary vessels can be clearly seen as flow voids. MRI has been shown to be equal to or better than contrast enhanced CT in the detection of hilar nodes [5]. Nodes in the aortopulmonary window, lower left paratracheal and subcarinal nodes are better visualized by MRI than by CT [6]. MRI would have been an alternative non-invasive way of not only assessing the central pulmonary arteries but in evaluating the extent of mediastinal and abdominal disease for staging.

References

1. Dalby AM, Forman R. Acquired pulmonary stenosis. S Afr Med 1979;55:218–20.
2. Marshall EMMS, Trump DM. Acquired pulmonary stenoses caused by mediastinal tumours. Cancer 1982;49:1496–9.
3. Fox R, Pandis IP, Kotler MN, et al. Detection by Doppler echocardiography of acquired pulmonic stenosis due to extrinsic tumour compression. Am J Cardiol 1984;53:1475–6.
4. Israeli A, Rein AJJT, Krivisky M, et al. Arch Intern Med 1989;149:2105–6.
5. Swensen SJ, Ehman RL, Brown LR. Magnetic resonance imaging of the thorax. J Thor Imaging 1989;4:19–33.
6. Webb WR, Jensen BG, Solitto R, et al. Bronchogenic carcinoma: Staging with MR compared with staging with CT and surgery. Radiology 1985;156:117–24.

An underdiagnosed abdominal mass?

R D EDWARDS and W KINCAID

Department of Radiology, Western Infirmary, Dumbarton Road, Glasgow G11 6NT, UK

A 49-year-old woman presented with a 6 h history of severe abdominal pain and a superficial, palpable mass in the right lower abdomen. She was obese and had noted a variable swelling in this area for 4 months. A right inguinal herniorrhaphy had been performed 3 months previously. Views from the initial ultrasound (US) of the anterior abdominal wall and subsequent barium follow-through (FT) are shown (Figures 1 and 2).

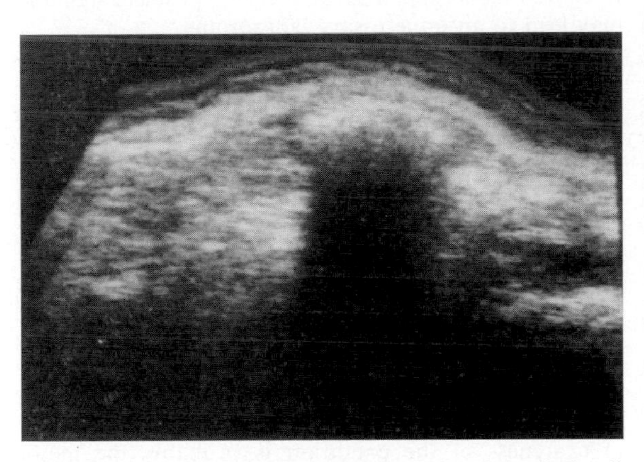

Figure 1. Longitudinal US scan of the anterior abdominal wall.

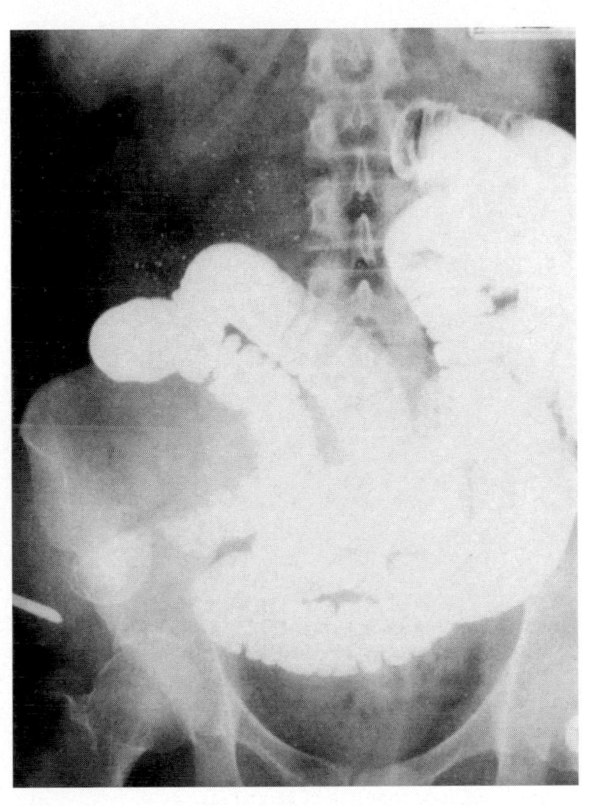

Figure 2. View from barium FT examination.

Based on the case of the month originally published in Br J Radiol 1992;65:453–4.

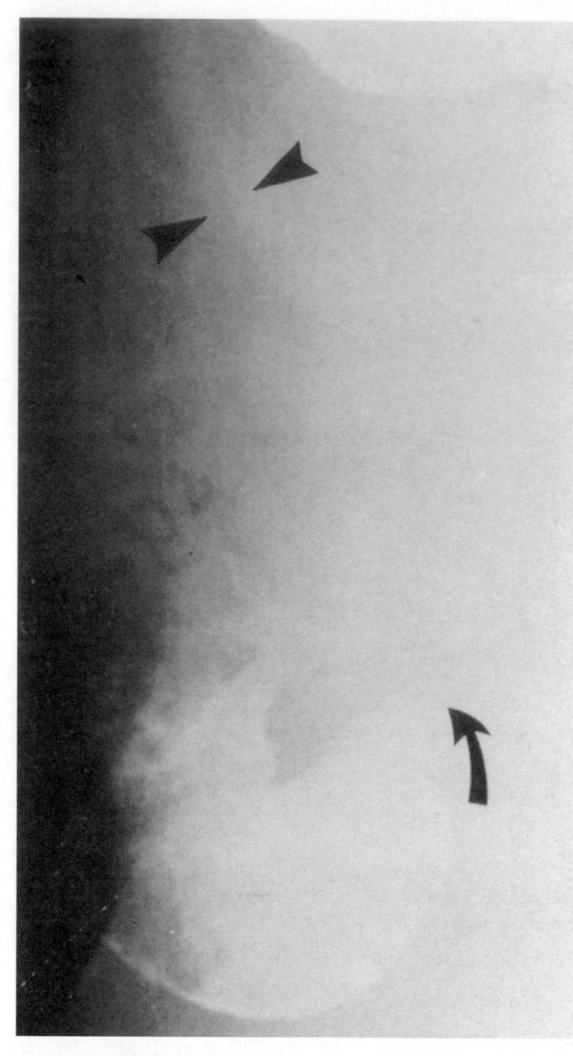

Figure 3. Oblique spot film of hernial sac.

The US showed an oval hypoechoic structure containing gas lying subcutaneously in the anterior abdominal wall. The barium FT showed a dilated proximal small bowel and a herniated loop of bowel in the right lower quadrant. An oblique spot film taken during the barium FT (Figure 3) showed the neck of the hernial sac (curved arrow) and its relationship to the external oblique muscle (arrowheads).

The patient had a Spigelian hernia (also known as a spontaneous lateral ventral hernia). This uncommon hernia consists of a defect in the aponeurosis of the transverse abdominal muscle between the semilunar (Spigelian) line and the lateral border of the rectus muscle. 90% occur between the level of the umbilicus and the anterior superior iliac spine. The hernial sac may dissect the layers of the transverse and internal oblique muscles and present clinically as a mass lateral to the semilunar line. In less than 5% of cases, the sac penetrates the external oblique muscle and lies subcutaneously, as was seen in this patient.

In a review of 744 patients with surgically confirmed Spigelian hernia [1], the mean age was 50 years (range 6–94 years) with a slight female preponderance (male: female ratio = 1 : 1.4). The hernial orifice is usually less than 2 cm in diameter but may reach 8 cm. Incarceration is seen in 21% of cases treated surgically [1]. The hernial sac most often contains omental fat, small bowel or colon, but may consist solely of pre-peritoneal fat. Rarely, the sac may contain stomach, gallbladder, appendix, Meckel's diverticulum, ovary, uterine fibroid or testicle. An association with inguinal or femoral hernia is recognized.

The commonest symptom is pain, which is typically intermittent and is aggravated by prolonged standing or sustained physical effort. A lump, noticed by the patient in 54% of cases [2], may be impalpable as it is normally covered by the external oblique aponeurosis. Localized tenderness may be the only physical sign and may lead to an unnecessary laparotomy.

In one series the correct pre-operative diagnosis was made in only 52% of cases, while the remainder were diagnosed as appendicitis, adhesions, tumours and intestinal obstruction [2].

Ultrasound can identify the defect in the aponeurosis [3], determine the contents of the hernial sac and distinguish it from other causes of an anterior abdominal wall mass [4]. Barium studies are of value only if the hernial sac contains bowel. CT may demonstrate the hernial orifice [5].

Excision of the sac and repair of the defect is the standard surgical treatment. In this case necrotic omentum was found, but the herniated bowel had reduced spontaneously.

Awareness of the condition is probably the major factor in the diagnosis of Spigelian hernia. Ultrasound of the abdominal wall is the diagnostic method of choice and should be considered in a patient with relatively non-specific lower abdominal symptoms with or without a mass in the region of the Spigelian line.

References

1. Spagen L. Spigelian hernia. Surg Clin North Am 1984;64: 351–66.
2. Weiss Y, Lernau OZ, Nissan S. Spigelian hernia. Ann Surg 1974;180:836–9.
3. Deitch EA, Engel JM. Spigelian hernia. An ultrasonic diagnosis. Arch Surg 1980;115:93.
4. Fried AM, Meeker WR. Incarcerated Spigelian hernia. AJR 1979;133:107–10.
5. Pyatt RS, Alona BR, Daye S, Wenzel DJ, Woods E, Alexieva B. Case report: Spigelian hernia. JCAT 1982;6:643–5.

Blindingly obvious

E A TILLEY, E J ADAM and A E A JOSEPH

Department of Radiology, St George's Hospital, Blackshaw Road, London SW17 0QT, UK

A 55-year-old man presenting with a 4 week history of abdominal swelling was found to have hepatomegaly. An abdominal ultrasound scan was performed using a 3.5 MHz transducer and a longitudinal section through the right upper quadrant shown below (Figure 1).

Ultrasound-guided fine needle biopsy of the liver provided a cytological diagnosis which prompted further direct questioning and examination. The patient described how a mild loss of vision in his right eye 3 years earlier had progressed to blindness over a 1 year period. His optician had diagnosed bilateral cataracts 8 months prior to admission. Ultrasound scans of both eyes obtained with a 10 MHz transducer are shown below (Figure 2).

What is the diagnosis? What complication is seen in the right eye?

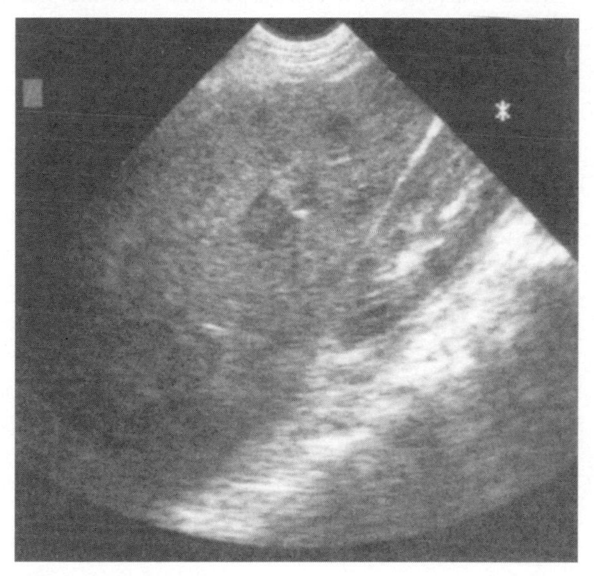

Figure 1. Longitudinal ultrasound scan through the right upper quadrant.

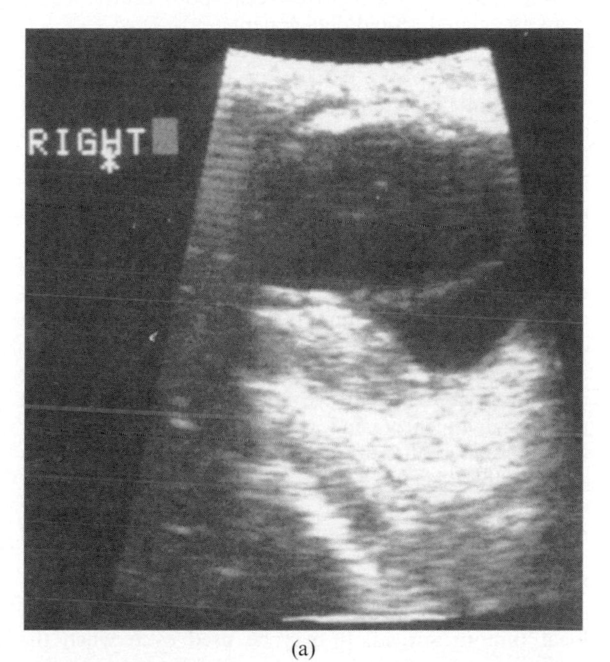

(a)

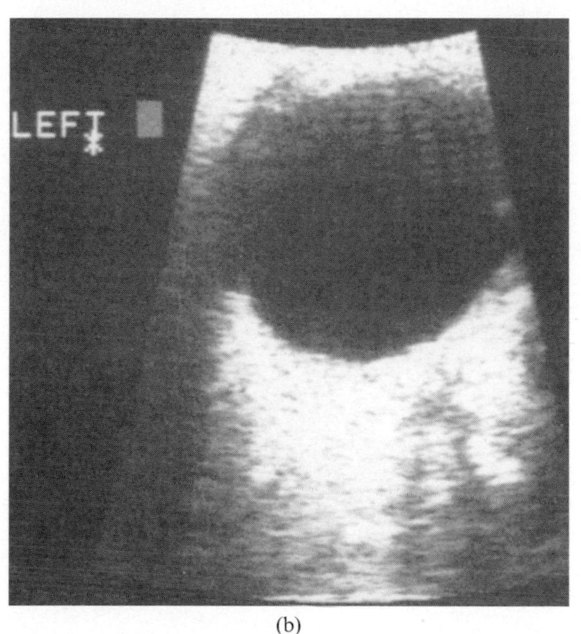

(b)

Figure 2. Ultrasound scan of the right eye (a) with the left (b) for comparison.

Based on the case of the month originally published in Br J Radiol 1988;61:87–8.

Abdominal ultrasound confirmed the hepatomegaly and showed a mixture of echo-poor and target lesions throughout the liver. Cytology obtained from one of these gave the diagnosis of metastatic melanoma. No cutaneous lesions were found and in view of the patient's symptoms his eyes were examined. Unlike fundoscopy, the efficacy of ultrasound is not reduced by cataracts and using this technique the primary choroidal melanoma was demonstrated in the right eye. The tumour is oval in shape with a relatively echo-poor centre. There is an associated retinal detachment.

Malignant melanoma is the primary tumour in approximately 1% of patients with hepatic metastases [1]. Ultrasonically, the metastases are usually of very low echogenicity, but this appearance is not diagnostic and may also be seen in lymphoreticular tumours. Less commonly, the metastases are echogenic [2].

Non-cutaneous malignant melanomas have an incidence rate one sixth that of cutaneous melanomas. 79% of the non-cutaneous tumours occur in the eye and most of these arise in the choroid [3]. Intraocular melanomas are rare ($0.5/10^5$ population per year in England) but they comprise 70% of all eye malignancies. The incidence rate rises with increasing age and is eight times higher in Caucasians, blue eyes being a risk factor. The sexes are equally affected [4].

Fundoscopy, ultrasound and fluoroscein angiography have all proved useful in the diagnosis of choroidal malignant melanoma. Ultrasound is of particular value because it not only provides a 95% rate of tumour detection, but can also assess retinal detachment and local tumour spread. It may be used even when the media are opaque.

A choroidal malignant melanoma may have one of two typical appearances on ultrasound. It will appear oval if confined by the membrane of Bruch, or have a collar stud configuration if the membrane has been breached. The characteristic echo pattern is of a solid mass which may have an anechoic area within it, or in the retro-orbital fat behind [5]. An associated retinal detachment is common and is due to accumulation of exudative fluid beneath an intact retina. Tumour spread is mainly local but metastases to the liver, lung, central nervous system, bone and skin are also found in approximately 50% of patients.

The earliest presentation is with mild loss of vision if the macula is involved. Others may present with retinal detachment, secondary glaucoma or blindness, or with symptoms due to metastatic spread.

Malignant melanoma should be considered in any patient presenting with hepatic metastases, particularly if these are of very low echogenicity, and careful examination made of the skin and eyes.

References

1. Willis RA. The spread of tumours in the human body (3rd edn). London: Butterworths, 1973.
2. Cosgrove DO, McCready VR. Liver metastases. In: Ultrasound imaging: liver, spleen, pancreas. New York: John Wiley & Sons, 1982:149–75.
3. Scotto J, Fraumeni JF, Lee JAH. Melanomas of the eye and other noncutaneous sites: epidemiological aspects. J Nat Cancer Inst 1976;56:489–91.
4. Tucker MA, Hartge P, Shields JA. Epidemiology of intraocular melanoma. Recent Results Cancer Res 1986;102:159–65.
5. Coleman DJ, Abramson DH, Jack RL, Franzen LA. Ultrasonic diagnosis of tumours of the choroid. Arch Opthalmol 1974;91:344–54.

The case of the surplus clues

S PURI, S SHARMA and V N BAIJAL

Department of Radiology, Safdarjang Hospital, New Delhi, India

A 16-year-old girl was admitted with a history of backache, fever and 4 month history of generalized weakness. Examination revealed pallor, sternal tenderness and hepatomegaly. Urine examination and the blood biochemistry were essentially normal. The haematological examination showed: haemoglobin, 5.5 gm%; packed cell volume, 16%; reticulocyte count, 2%; platelet count, 4000 cm^{-3}; total leucocytic count, 9800 cm^{-3}; and differential leucocytic count: 40% segmental neutrophils, 30% bands, 16% lymphocytes, 10% monocytes and 4% lymphoblasts with deeply basophilic cytoplasm containing prominent vacuoles. Subsequently, radiographs of the chest (Figure 1), dorsolumbar spine (Figure 2), skull (Figure 3) and pelvis (Figure 4) were obtained. What is your differential diagnosis?

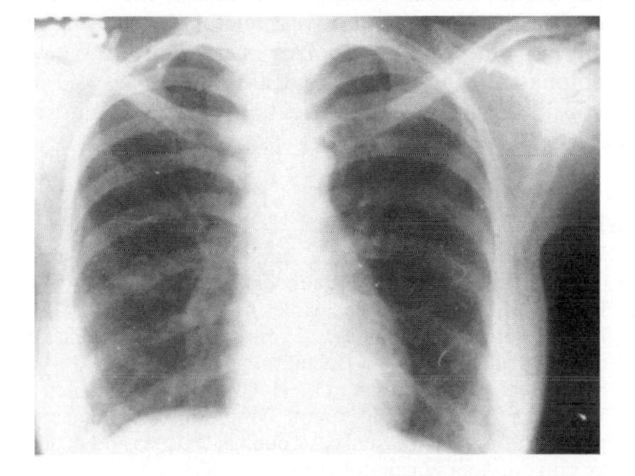

Figure 1. Chest radiograph (posteroanterior view).

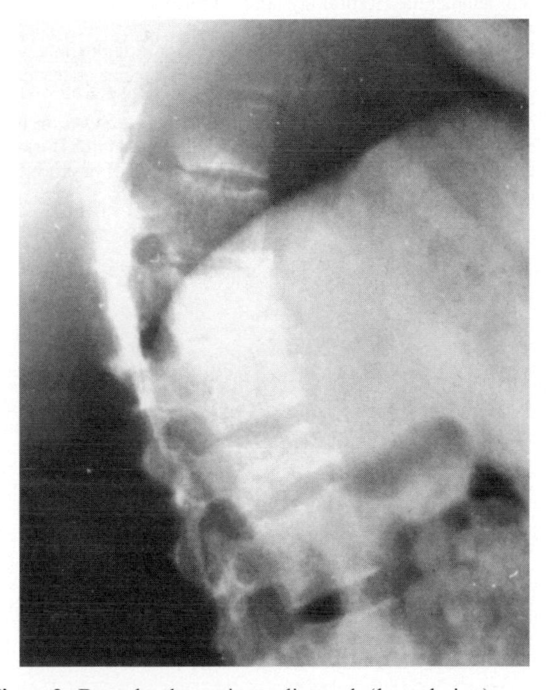

Figure 2. Dorsolumbar spine radiograph (lateral view).

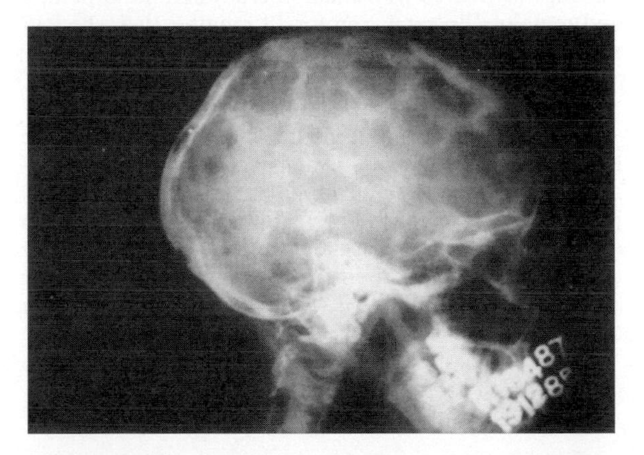

Figure 3. Skull radiograph (lateral view).

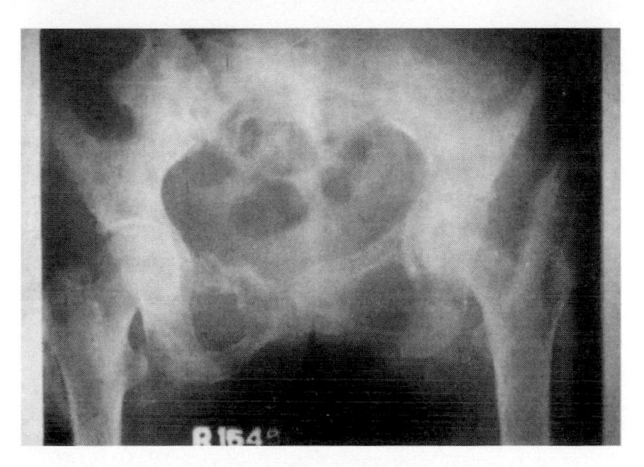

Figure 4. Pelvis radiograph (anteroposterior view).

Based on the case of the month originally published in Br J Radiol 1990;63:227–8.

The chest radiograph (Figure 1) showed a few ill defined osteolytic lesions involving the lateral end of the left clavicle and left scapula. There were vertebral collapses involving the first and third lumbar vertebrae with intact disc spaces (Figure 2). The radiograph of the skull showed widespread destructive lesions involving the vault (Figure 3). The radiograph of the pelvis showed expansile destructive lesions involving the pubic bones (Figure 4). Serum calcium and phosphorus levels were within normal limits and serum alkaline phosphatase was mildly elevated. The radiological differential diagnosis of such skeletal lesions usually includes lymphoma, metastatic deposits, histiocytosis-X, cystic tuberculosis, cystic angiomatosis and hyperparathyroidism [1]. Skeletal involvement secondary to acute leukaemia is unlikely in view of the pattern and extent of radiological involvement.

The lymphoblasts in the peripheral smear showed typical features of Burkitt's cells. Bone marrow examination showed 60% infiltration by these polyvacuolated blast cells. Histochemical stains for Sudan Black, Peroxidase and Periodic Acid Schiff were negative, whereas there was a positive reaction with Oil Red. The diagnosis of L-3 acute lymphoblastic leukaemia (acute leukaemia with Burkitt-type cells) was thus established [2]. The patient was treated with chemotherapy and radiotherapy and remained in remission for 14 months, then she had a relapse and died.

A rare variant among acute leukaemias, L-3 acute lymphoblastic leukaemia is a specific disorder accounting for 1–3% of all acute lymphoblastic leukaemia (ALL) patients [3, 4]. Clinical differentiation of L-3 ALL from other forms of ALL is usually not possible, except that the former runs a more aggressive course and is usually fatal within 6 months [5]. The leukaemic blast cells in these patients are, however, readily recognized by the characteristic cytological and immunological features [6]. It is important to differentiate L-3 ALL from Burkitt's lymphoma, in which the patients usually present with characteristic extranodal tumour masses involving the jaws or the abdominal viscera. These patients of Burkitt's lymphoma can occasionally develop a leukaemic picture in the terminal stages.

Radiological involvement in L-3 ALL has received little attention [4, 5]. Flandrin et al [4] reported isolated lytic lesions in the humerus (one patient), tibia (one patient) and mandible (one patient). Marmary et al [5] described a patient of L-3 ALL with diffuse demineralization and numerous osteolytic lesions in the mandible. The widespread and extensive skeletal destruction seen in this patient has not previously been reported. We wish to emphasize that L-3 ALL, although rare, should also be considered in the radiological differential diagnosis of widespread, destructive skeletal lesions.

References

1. Wilner D. Radiology of bone tumours and allied disorders (Vol II). Philadelphia: WB Saunders & Company, 1982:1388.
2. Bennett JM, Catovsky D, Daniel MT, Flandrin G, Galton DAG, Gralnick HR, Sultan C. Proposals for the classification of acute leukaemias. Br J Haematol 1976;33:451–8.
3. Schlaeffer F, Ziberman D, Hatskelson L, Kaplan H, Vermiqhu T. Burkitt's-like acute lymphoblastic leukaemia—presentation of an unusual case: clinical features and diagnostic criteria. Acta Haematol 1984;72:45–8.
4. Marmary G, Gerfunkel A, Naparstek E. Burkitt's lymphoma cell leukaemia. Radiology and cytotoxic medication. Int J Oral Surg 1981;10:367–70.
5. Flandrin G, Brouet JC, Daniel MT. Acute leukaemia with Burkitt's cells. A study of six cases with special reference to lymphocyte surface markers. Blood 1975;45:183–9.
6. Mangan KF, Ranch AE, Bishop M, Spiers ASO, Lorch C, Scharfman WB. Acute lymphoblastic leukaemia of Burkitt's type (L-3 ALL) lacking surface immunoglobin and 8:14 translocation. Am J Clin Pathol 1985;83:121–6.

An unusual metastatic involvement

M P CALLAWAY, J F FIELDS and J HAWNAUR

Department of Diagnostic Radiology, Manchester Medical School, Stopford Building, Oxford Road, Manchester, UK

A 56-year-old woman presented with a short history of weight loss, epigastric pain and jaundice. On examination there was hepatomegaly, and liver function tests confirmed an obstructive picture. An ultrasound scan showed an inflamed gallbladder containing multiple calculi. The common bile duct was dilated and contained a calculus. Endoscopic retrograde cholangiopancreatography (ERCP) and sphincterotomy were performed to aid drainage, but the patient developed post-ERCP pancreatitis. An abdominal CT scan demonstrated extensive pancreatic inflammation but at this time no focal lesion was seen within the liver. A cholecystectomy and bile duct exploration were performed. Post-operative recovery was uneventful, but the patient was readmitted after 3 months with a history of further weight loss. Examination was normal. A repeat abdominal CT scan was performed, pre- and post-intravenous contrast medium. This showed an irregular mass in the head of the pancreas suggestive of pancreatic malignancy. The liver images are shown, what are the findings? What is the next stage of investigation?

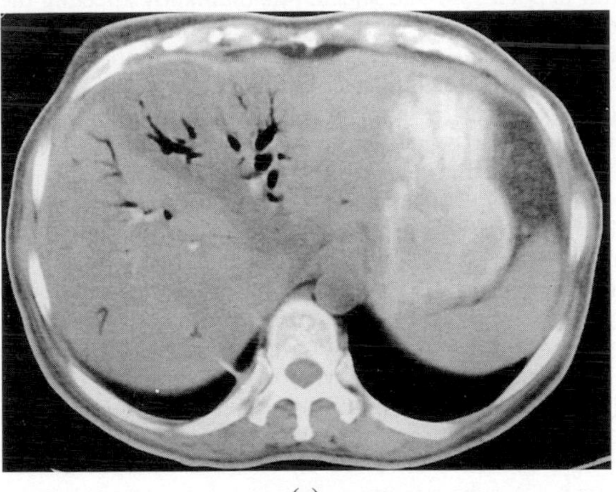

(a)

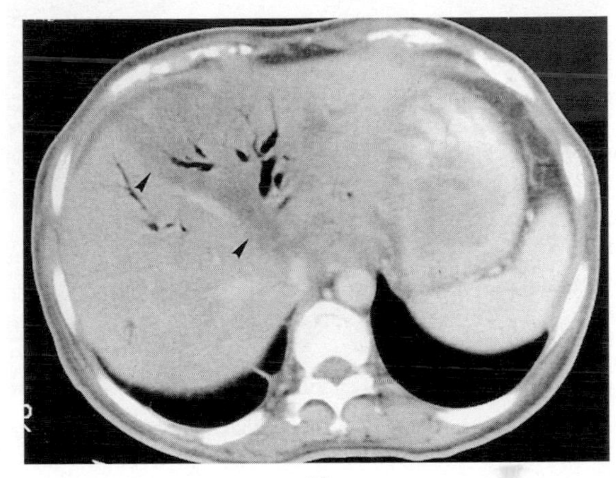

(b)

Figure 1. (a) Pre- and (b) post-contrast abdominal CT.

Based on the case of the month originally published in Br J Radiol 1998;71:239–40.

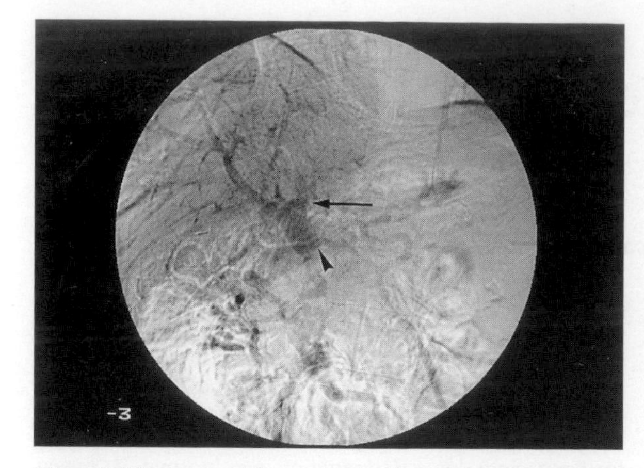

Figure 2. The venous phase of a coeliac angiogram. There is occlusion of the proximal portion of the portal vein at the level of the pancreatic head (arrowhead), with reformation of the distal vein. In addition, there is occlusion of the left intrahepatic portal vein (arrow).

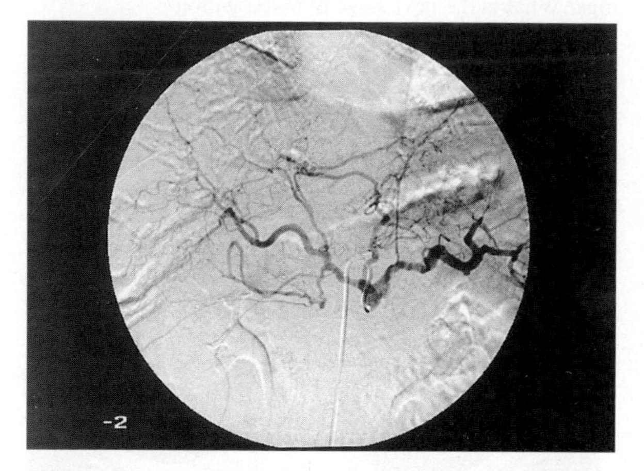

Figure 3. Arterial phase of the coeliac angiogram shows a patent hepatic artery.

The repeat abdominal CT scan, both pre- and post-intravenous contrast medium, showed a diffuse low attenuation of much of the left lobe of the liver, with sharply demarcated borders (black arrowheads). These findings are consistent with segmental infarction and subsequent atrophy of the liver. Angiography subsequently confirmed interruption of the hepatic blood supply. There was occlusion of the proximal portion of the portal vein, at the level of the pancreatic head, with reconstitution of this vessel distally (Figure 2). The left intrahepatic portal vein was also occluded (Figure 2), but the main hepatic artery and its tributaries were patent (Figure 3). On ultrasound examination, the left lobe of the liver was diffusely hyperechoic and contained a 2 cm soft tissue mass closely related to the left portal vein. A second 2 cm mass was superficially located in the right lobe of the liver. In view of the patient's poor clinical condition it was felt inappropriate to biopsy the infarcted area. It was deemed appropriate to biopsy the superficial mass in the right lobe of the liver. The biopsy confirmed infiltrating adenocarcinoma, compatible with pancreatic malignancy and metastatic spread, occluding the hepatic blood supply. The patient died shortly afterwards.

There have been only a few case reports documenting the radiological appearances of hepatic infarction [1–3]. This entity has not been described in association with metastatic disease. It has even been postulated that the presence of tumour would decrease the liver's susceptibility to infarction [4]. Initial reports of the CT appearances of hepatic infarction described a well circumscribed, peripheral wedge shaped area of low attenuation predominantly affecting the right lobe [2]. However, round or oval lesions occurring centrally within the liver parenchyma have also been described [3]. The only consistent finding has been a failure to enhance following intravenous contrast medium. The incidence of hepatic infarcts remains low, a consequence of the dual blood supply. Infarction of the liver has been reported in association with hypotension and shock, predominantly affecting the right lobe [2]. Histopathologically, there is a close correlation between the infarcted region and thrombosis of the peripheral microcirculation of the portal vein. A correlation between small portal vein thrombosis and the area of infarct has been established in post-mortem studies [5]. These findings suggest that disruption of the intrahepatic portal venous system is an important component in the pathogenesis of an infarct. We believe that the combination of occlusion of the extrahepatic portal vein and the left intrahepatic portal vein in this case reduced the hepatic blood supply sufficiently to cause an area of infarction within the liver, despite a patent hepatic artery. This supports the post-mortem study [5] and illustrates clinically that disruption of the portal blood supply leads to both ischaemia and infarction. Surgery was not likely to be a causative factor as all vessels at the porta were patent. The subacute presentation of this case without the pyrexia or leucocytosis normally associated with hepatic infarction is unusual but is probably due to the gradually progressive nature of the infarction.

References

1. Doppman JL, Dunnick NR, Girton M, Fauci AS, Popovsky MA. Bile duct cysts secondary to liver infarction. Radiology 1979;130:1–5.
2. Adler DD, Glazer GM, Silver TM. Computed tomography of liver infarction. AJR 1984;142:315–8.
3. Lev-Toaff AS, Friedman AC, Cohen LM, Radecki PD, Caroline DF. Hepatic infarcts: new observations by CT and sonography. AJR 1987;149:87–90.
4. Seeley TT, Blumenfield CM, Ikede R, Knapp W, Ruebner BH. Hepatic infarction. Human Pathol 1972;3:265–76.
5. Saegusa M, Takano Y, Okidaria M. Human hepatic infarction: histopathological and post mortem angiological studies. Liver 1993;13:239–45.

A geriatric plum

N JEYAGOPAL, F HEARN and E CUMMINS

Department of Radiology, Frimley Park Hospital, Frimley, Surrey GU16 5UJ, UK

A 76-year-old retired manager presented with shortness of breath. On examination he had normal blood pressure and signs of left upper lobe collapse. He was also noted to have a protruberant abdomen and an easily palpable, large mass in the lower abdomen. The patient denied symptoms suggestive of prostatic hypertrophy. Both testes were absent from the scrotum. Blood biochemical tests for liver and renal function were normal.

A chest radiograph showed a left hilar mass and collapse of the left upper lobe. Subsequently, bronchoscopy showed a squamous cell carcinoma in the left upper lobe bronchus. CT showed occlusion of the left upper lobe bronchus by tumour and collapse of the left upper lobe. There was no evidence of pulmonary or hepatic metastases. CT was continued down to the pelvis.

What are the abnormalities seen on the CT scans of abdomen and pelvis (Figures 1 and 2)?

Intravenous urography was performed later and a radiograph at 4 h after injection is shown (Figure 3). Can you make a diagnosis?

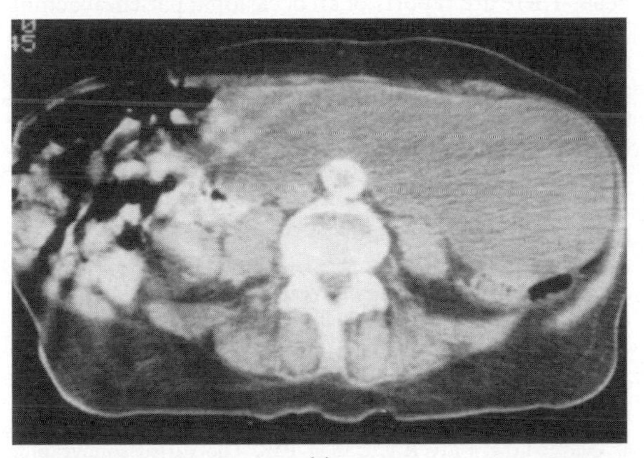

(a)

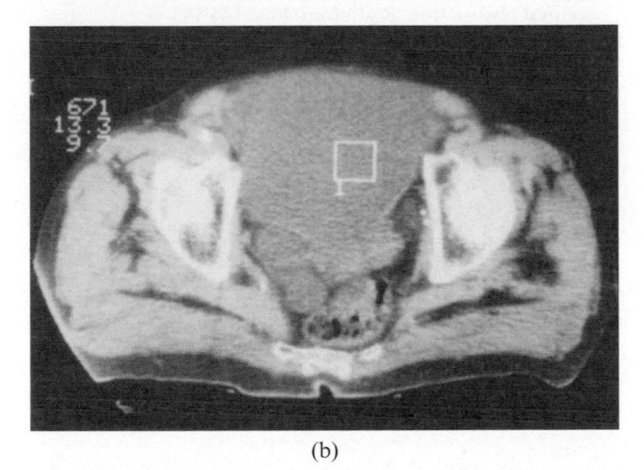

(b)

Figure 1. CT section (a) below the level of kidneys and (b) through the pelvis.

Based on the case of the month originally published in Br J Radiol 1988;61:1085–6.

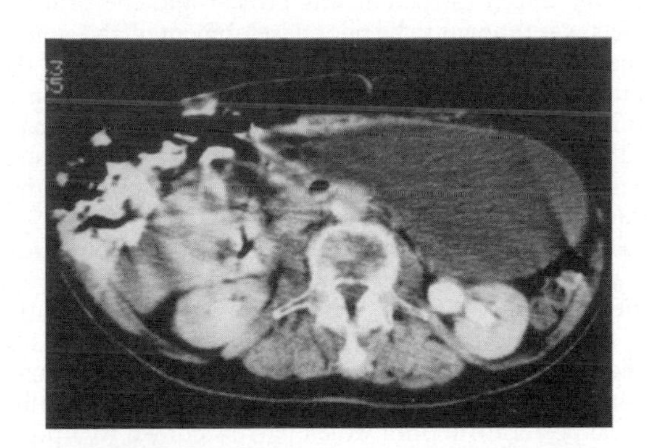

Figure 2. CT section at the level of kidneys after intravenous contrast medium.

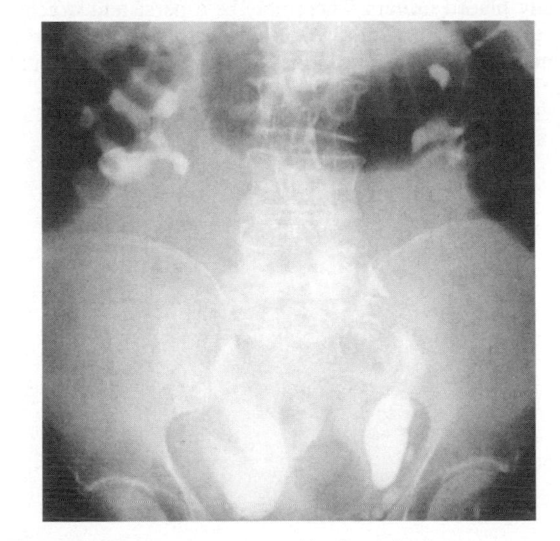

Figure 3. Intravenous urogram 4 h after injection.

CT showed altered contour with general flattening of the abdomen and deficiency of the anterior abdominal musculature, particularly in the lower part. There is also a large cystic mass arising from the pelvis with dilated ureters posteriorly. Both kidneys showed excretion of intravenous contrast medium with some dilatation of the left upper ureter. Figure 3 shows gross dilatation of both ureters and only faint opacification of the urinary bladder at 4 h. The collecting system on the right is bizarre in appearance, suggesting dysplasia of the right kidney. (The filling defect was confirmed to be a non-opaque stone by subsequent ultrasound examination.)

The combination of deficiency of the anterior abdominal wall muscle, urinary tract anomalies and cryptorchidism makes a diagnosis of prune belly syndrome.

Deficiency of abdominal muscles was first noted by Frölich in 1839 and its association with undescended testes, megacystis and hydroureter was reported by Parker in 1895. The incidence of this condition appears to be about 1:40000 births. In the earlier cases, no urinary tract obstruction was proved and the primary defect was thought to be poor development of abdominal muscles. Over 95% of the affected were males and the condition was even thought to be a two-step, autosomal dominant mutation with sex-linked expression that partially mimics X-linkage. Recently it has been suggested that intrauterine urethral obstruction is the primary disorder, the other features being secondary [1].

Deficiency of abdominal muscles may be asymmetrical or partial with involvement below the umbilicus [2]. The patient, classically, has inability to rise from the supine position without using the arms. The most significant associated conditions occur in the genitourinary tract in the form of cryptorchidism, tapering dilatation of the posterior urethra which narrows down to a point at approximately the membranous level, megacystis, vesico-ureteric reflux, tortuous, dilated and rather laterally placed ureters. There may be a persistent urachus or even urachal fistula when there is complete obstruction of the urethra. The kidneys may be normal, although the majority are dysplastic. Other associated conditions include talipes equinovarus, congenital dislocation of the hips, malrotation of the gut, imperforate anus and chest wall deformities [3]. The patients are also more prone to respiratory infection because of impaired ability to cough.

Intrauterine diagnosis is possible with the detection of oligohydramnios, large bladder and dilated ureters. The presence of sonographically identifiable cysts in the kidney on ultrasound is considered to be a direct sign of dysplastic kidneys [4]. When the diagnosis is made early enough in gestation, termination of pregnancy may be considered in severe cases. In both children and adults, CT will demonstrate well features of the syndrome. With better management and the resultant increased survival, malignant changes in the undescended testes are to be expected. As many surgeons wish to bring the testes down, CT may allow location of the often intraabdominal testes in prune belly syndrome pre-operatively [5].

With 20% incidence of stillbirth and a 2-year survival rate of 50%, prune belly syndrome carries a poor prognosis. There are reports of an occasional patient reaching 70 years of age. This patient is 76 years old which would make him the oldest reported survivor with this condition. Although his bronchial carcinoma has responded to radiotherapy it seems likely that his survival will be limited by this, rather than by the usual renal complications of prune belly syndrome.

References

1. Pagon RA, Smith DW, Shepard TH. Urethral obstruction malformation complex: a cause of abdominal muscle deficiency and the "prune belly". J Paedatr 1979;94:900–6.
2. Silverman FN, Huang N. Congenital absence of the abdominal muscles. Am J Dis Child 1950;80:91–124.
3. Welch KJ, Kearney GP. Abdominal musculature deficiency syndrome: prune belly. J Urol 1974;111:693–700.
4. Glazer GM, Filly RA, Callen PW. The varied sonographic appearance of the urinary tract in the fetus and newborn with urethral obstruction. Radiology 1982;144:563–8.
5. Reinig JW, Curry NS, Schabel SI, Holland RD. CT evaluation of the prune belly syndrome. J Comput Tomogr 1981;5:548–9.

Hair raising artefacts in MRI

V C WILLIAMSON

Department of Neuroradiology, Walton Hospital, Rice Lane, Liverpool, UK

A 44-year-old shot blaster from Cammell Lairds ship yard was referred to the neurology outpatients clinic with a history of episodes of diplopia and ptosis. These had occurred over the past 7 years and all had resolved fully. In addition, he had had an episode of weakness in the left leg when aged 8 years old. This had lasted for a few weeks before resolving.

In view of the above history, demyelinating disease was considered, and MRI was performed. Images were obtained on a General Electric Signa 1.5 T scanner using spin echo sequences. A T_1 weighted (TR = 600 ms, TE = 30 ms) sagittal series, and an axial proton density and T_2 weighted sequence (TR = 2000 ms, with dual echoes at 20 ms and 80 ms) were performed.

What abnormality is seen on these sagittal T_1 (Figure 1) and axial proton density (Figure 2) images? What may have caused this appearance?

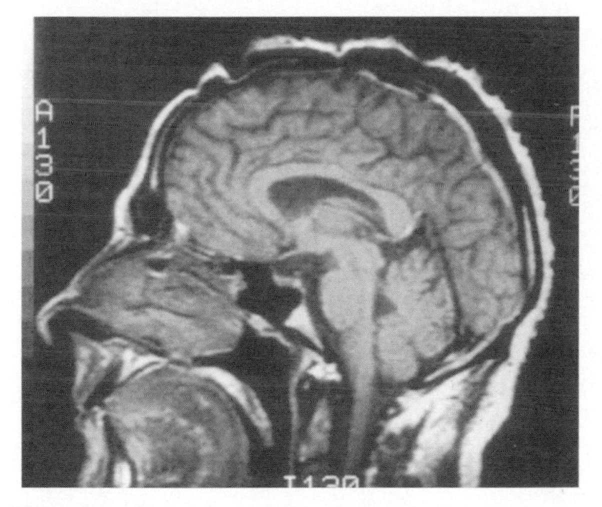

Figure 1. Sagittal T_1 weighted (TR = 600, TE = 30) image through the head.

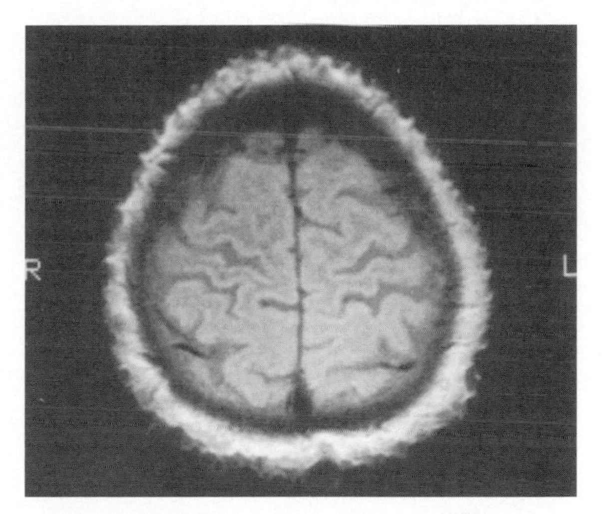

Figure 2. Axial "proton density" (TR = 2000, TE = 20) image through the brain.

Based on the case of the month originally published in Br J Radiol 1993;66:475–6.

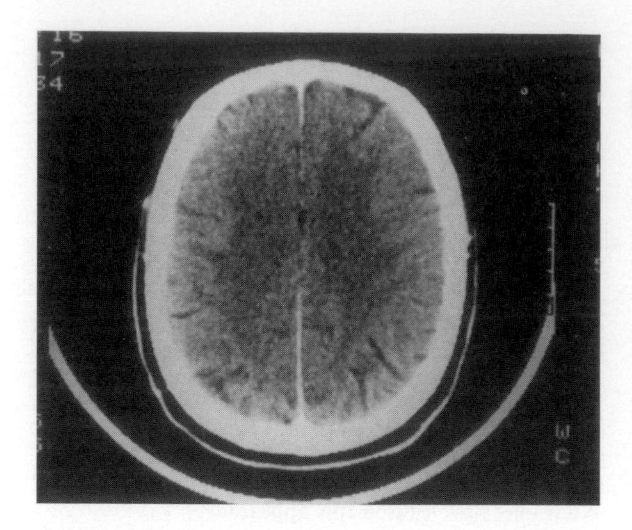

Figure 3. Axial CT section through the brain demonstrating the metal fragments embedded in the scalp.

No intracranial lesion was seen but there was an abnormal appearance to the scalp and hair, which appeared to have undulations and was of high signal (Figures 1, 2).

Physical examination showed no abnormality but, because of his work, he had multiple small fragments of metal embedded in his scalp. These are visible on an otherwise normal CT scan performed 3 years earlier to investigate the same problem (Figure 3).

The artefact was due to the ferromagnetic metal fragments producing localized distortions of the magnetic field. Metal artefacts are well recognized in MRI, even with non-ferromagnetic metals, which leave a signal void. The risk of causing movement of loose metal prostheses, intraocular foreign bodies or cerebral aneurysm clips is an accepted contraindication to MRI in these cases. In our case, however, it just produced an interesting artefact. Although metal artefacts are also common in CT the fragments were too small to be significant, unlike on the MRI scan.

Iceberg in the pleural space

[1]M L SEETHARAMAN and [2]S SALUJA

Departments of [1]Tuberculosis and Chest Diseases, and [2]Radiodiagnosis, Jawaharlal Institute of Post-Graduate Medical Education and Research, Pondicherry 605 006, India

A 50-year-old non-diabetic male subject was admitted with a 4 day history of high grade fever with shaking chills, a cough with scanty expectoration that later turned purulent and a discomfort in the right side of the chest. He denied any history of seizures, trauma to chest and contact with domestic animals. He was a smoker and had consumed alcohol socially. He had no past history of significant respiratory illness.

He appeared to be toxic, was not clubbed, had a heart rate of 110 min^{-1} and rapid respirations. The trachea was deviated to the left and clinically a diagnosis of hydropneumothorax could be detected on the right side. Bronchopleural fistula was indicated by the presence of amphoric breath sounds heard posterolaterally on the right side. Abdomen, cardiovascular and other systems were normal. He had a haemoglobin level of 12 gm% and a marked neutrophilic leucocytosis. Sputum culture grew *Streptococcus pneumoniae*, but blood culture was sterile. Routine serum biochemical parameters and an ultrasound scan of the liver were normal. Sputum acid fast stains were negative on three occasions. A postero-anterior chest radiograph (Figure 1) was obtained. Pleural fluid was found to be putrid on diagnostic tap. The institution of intercostal drainage under water seal, however, was complicated by recurrent tube blocks. What abnormalities are evident in the chest radiograph? What is the most likely diagnosis?

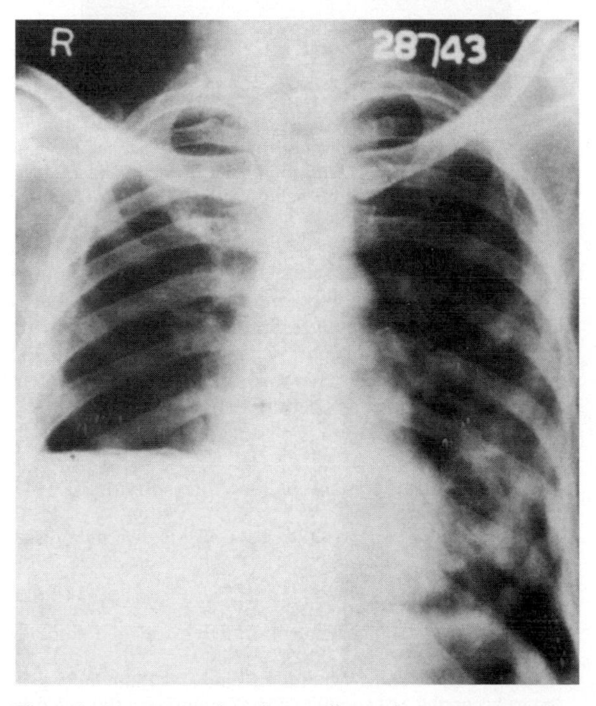

Figure 1. Posteroanterior chest radiograph.

Based on the case of the month originally published in Br J Radiol 1994;67:909–10.

The chest radiograph (Figure 1) demonstrated hydropneumothorax on the right side. The interesting feature is the wavy air–fluid interface suggesting the presence of a floating structure, the iceberg phenomenon, in the pleural fluid. The ill defined patchy shadows evident in the lower zone of the left lung field represent a spillover phenomenon from the right side.

Since the patient was unwilling to have any surgical intervention, a complete evacuation of the pus was attempted by blunt finger dissection through the already existing intercostal wound. There was a spontaneous expulsion of a large mass of fleshy, necrotic and putrid lung parenchyma (Figure 2) along with a gush of pus. The tissue sections studied suggested pulmonary gangrene. Pleural fluid and the necrotic material contained *Streptococcus pneumoniae*. The subsequent clinical course of the patient was uneventful. Bronchography (Figure 3) 12 weeks later, using oily dianosil, demonstrated non-filling and disruption of the bronchus beyond the take off of the right middle lobe bronchus (arrow). However, leakage of the contrast material into the pleural space confirmed the existence of bronchopleural fistula.

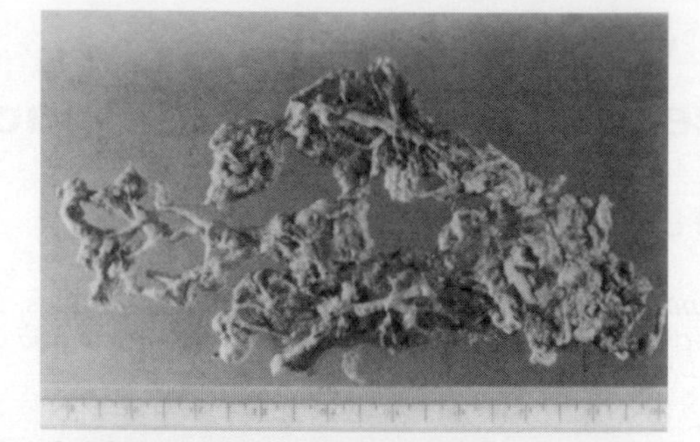

Figure 2. Macroscopic appearance of the spontaneously extruded lung tissue.

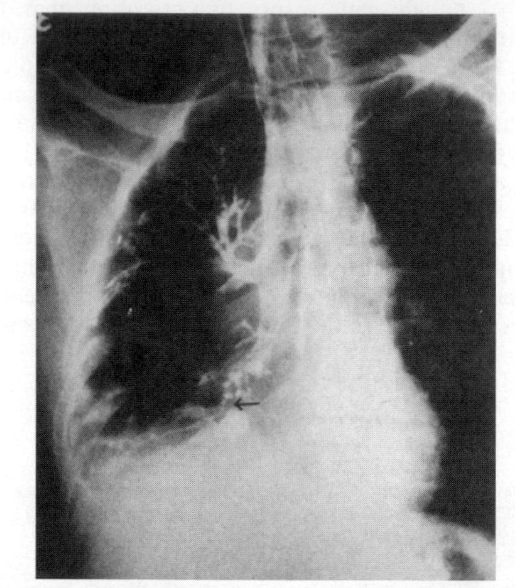

Figure 3. Bronchogram on the right side (left posterior oblique view) showing normal upper and middle lobe bronchial anatomy. There is complete disruption of the bronchus beyond the take off of the middle lobe bronchus, with collection of contrast in the pleural space.

Pulmonary gangrene is a rare but life endangering complication described in association with fulminant infections caused by *Streptococcus pneumoniae*, *Klebsiella pneumoniae*, *Haemophilus influenzae* and *Mycobacteria* [1–4]. Although essentially a pneumonic process, the pathogenesis of pulmonary gangrene involves intense inflammation, arteritis and vascular thrombosis with resultant putrefaction and necrosis of lung parenchyma. The vast majority of cases reported in the literature have demonstrated the characteristic and almost pathognomonic radiographic evolution of the disease [2, 4, 5]. In a typical presentation, pulmonary gangrene is recognized as passing through three distinct phases, progressing from lobar pneumonia, subsequently breaking down into numerous small abscess cavities, the coalescence of which will eventually form one large single cavity. The mobile necrotic lung tissue falls into and floats in the putrid cavitary contents. Pulmonary gangrene has been described under various synonyms such as spontaneous lobectomy, gangrene with spontaneous amputation, massive sequestration of the lung and massive pulmonary gangrene. The synonyms that best describe the sequence of events in the present case are probably gangrene with spontaneous amputation or spontaneous lobectomy. In fact, the clue to the auto-amputated and gangrenous lung floating in the pleural fluid is evident in Figure 1, the iceberg phenomenon described by Danner et al [2] as were also the recurrent intercostal tube blocks. In our experience, ruptured hydatid cyst with hydropneumothorax is one condition that can mimic pulmonary gangrene radiographically and presents similar problems in management. Apart from pyopneumothorax which is an extremely rare turn of events in the course of pulmonary gangrene, the present case evinces clinical interest on two other accounts in (i) being a lower lobe disease as against the commonly observed upper lobe predilection for lung gangrene [2, 5] and (ii) successful management by medical means. The spontaneous evacuation of the necrotic lung parenchyma combined with antibiotic therapy probably allowed our patient to recover. Surgical resection, involving lobectomy or pneumonectomy is considered to be the mainstay of therapy [5]. However, successful management by medical measures has been reported [3, 4].

References

1. Humphreys DR. Spontaneous lobectomy. Br Med J 1945; 2:185–6.
2. Danner PK, McFarland DR, Felson B. Massive pulmonary gangrene. Am J Roentgenol Rad Ther Nucl Med 1968; 103:548–54.
3. O'Reilly GV, Dee PM, Otteni GV. Gangrene of the lung: successful medical management of three patients. Radiology 1978;126:575–9.
4. Khan FA, Rehman M, Marcus P, Azueta V. Pulmonary gangrene occurring as a complication of pulmonary tuberculosis. Chest 1980;77:76–80.
5. Phillips LG, Rao KVS. Gangrene of the lung. J Thorac Cardiovasc Surg 1989;97:114–8.

Hidden trouble

R O I OBARO

Department of Radiology, Newcastle General Hospital, Westgate Road, Newcastle upon Tyne NE4 6BE, UK

A 64-year-old man presented with an 8 week history of dysuria, frequency, haemoptysis, haematuria, weight loss and pyrexia. Urine cytology and bronchoscopy were negative. An intravenous urogram (IVU) was normal. CT examinations of the lower abdomen are shown in Figures 1 and 2.

Plain radiography of the right humerus showed an osteolytic lesion. Abdominal ultrasound demonstrated a right adrenal mass.

What are the possible diagnoses?

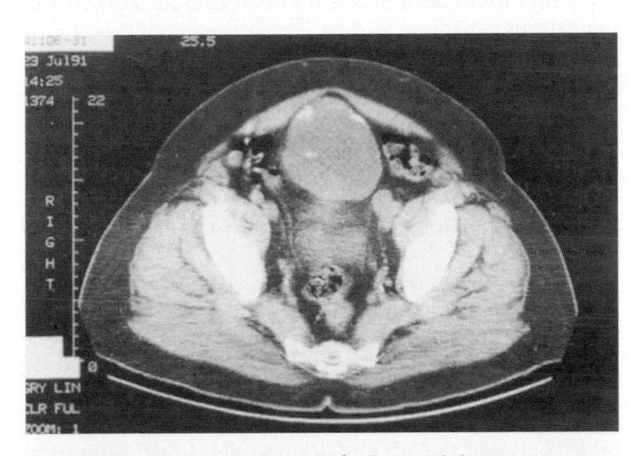

Figure 1. A CT section through the lower abdomen.

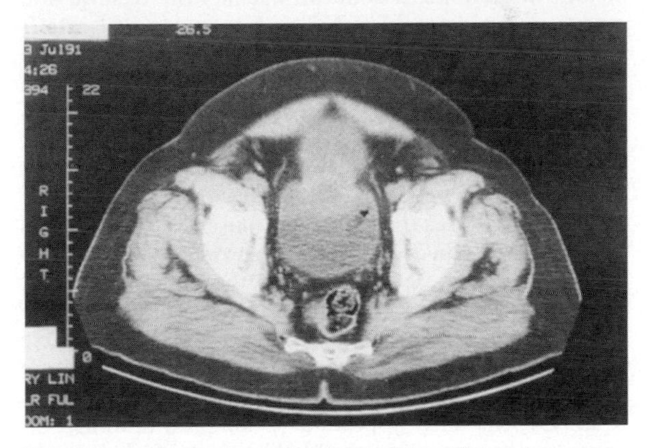

Figure 2. A CT slice immediately caudal to Figure 1.

Based on the case of the month originally published in Br J Radiol 1995;68:1369–70.

Figure 1 shows a soft tissue mass with some discrete areas of calcification along its wall and a small fleck of calcification within it.

The diagnosis is adenocarcinoma of the urachus with metastases to lung, bone and adrenal gland. The other diagnosis to consider is a lung cancer with metastases to the urachus and other sites.

A calcified tumour mass in the midline above the bladder is highly likely to be of urachal origin. Further imaging should be unnecessary in the presence of obvious metastases.

The urachus is the vestigial remnant of the embryonic allantois and cloaca lying in the space of Retzius. It is approximately 5–6 cm long and is divided into supravesical, intramural and intramucosal portions. Tumours of the urachus usually arise from the upper part of the intramural portion or the lower part of the extravesical portion [1].

Urachal carcinomas are rare, constituting 0.01% of all adult malignancies [2] and 0.35–0.7% of all bladder cancers [3] with an annual incidence of one in five million [4]. 85% of all urachal cancers are adenocarcinomas.

Adenocarcinoma of the urachus predominantly affects males between the 5th and 7th decades. Local symptoms include abdominal discomfort, haematuria, dysuria and mucus in the urine [1, 5]. The 5 year survival rate is 6.5–15% [3]. The plain abdominal radiograph and IVU are usually normal, as in this case (Figure 1), although deformity of the bladder dome is the commonest abnormality finding on IVU.

MRI, CT and endovesical ultrasound have been used in the pre-operative diagnosis of urachal carcinoma. MRI demonstrates the lesion as a mass of heterogeneous signal intensity on T_2 [2, 4]. MRI shows the relationship of the tumour to the bladder and the umbilicus, whilst also demonstrating the extent of local disease, by virtue of its multiplanar capability. However, MRI is unable to demonstrate calcification when present, a feature which improves diagnostic specificity.

On CT, the mass appears as a complex, midline, soft tissue mass arising from the bladder dome. Calcification, when present, is demonstrated as a rim around the mass on CT, as demonstrated in this case (Figures 1 and 2). The combination of MRI and CT may improve diagnostic accuracy. In one case, endovesical ultrasound was the first investigation to give a clue as to the urachal origin of a tumour initially diagnosed as a bladder adenocarcinoma on cystoscopy [3].

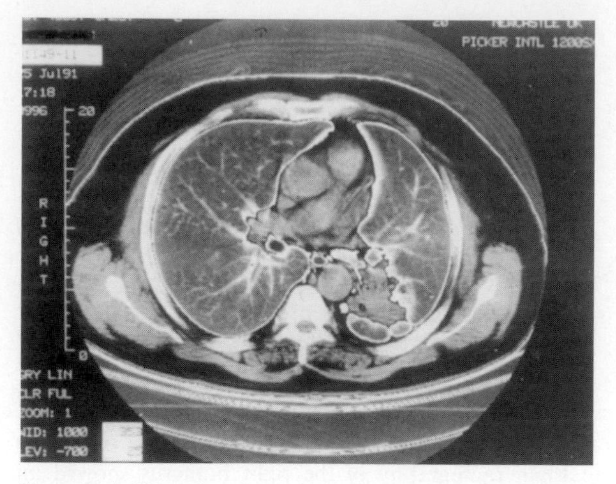

Figure 3. A CT section through the chest at the level of the left lower lobe bronchus.

Urachal adenocarcinoma presents either as an abdominal mass or because of its metastases. Metastases are usually to regional nodes, omentum, liver, lung and bone. This case appears to have metastasized to the adrenal gland. There is a mass lesion in the left lower lobe presumed to be a metastasis in this case (Figure 3).

The differential diagnosis includes tumours of the omphalomesenteric duct, echinococcal cysts, abscesses, desmoid tumours, lipomata, endometrioma, urachal and abdominal cavity cysts.

[*See also a case report of a benign urachal tumour published in the BJR [6], ED*]

References

1. Begg RC. The colloid adenocarcinomata of the bladder vault arising from the epithelium of the urachal canal: with a critical survey of the tumours of the arachus. Br J Surg 1931;18:422–66.
2. Krysiewicz S. Diagnosis of urachal carcinoma by computed tomography and magnetic resonance imaging. Clin Imaging 1990;14:251–4.
3. Wishnow KI. Endovesical ultrasonography of urachal carcinoma. Urol Radiol 1989;11:53–4.
4. Rafal RB, Markisz JA. Urachal carcinoma: the role of magnetic resonance imaging. Urol Radiol 1991;12:187.
5. Beck AD, Gaudin HJ. Carcinoma of the urachus. Br J Urol 1970;42:555–67.
6. Dawson JS, Crisp AJ, Boyd SM, Broderick NJ. Benign urachal neoplasm. Br J Radiol 1994;67:1132–3.

Haemoptysis: a rare cause

J E HYNES and R WHITEHOUSE

Department of Diagnostic Radiology, Manchester Royal Infirmary, Oxford Road, Manchester M13 9WL, UK

A 68-year-old female was referred with a 3 month history of intermittent haemoptysis. She also described recurrent retrosternal discomfort following a coronary bypass and aortic valve replacement 2 years previously for which she had been warfarinized. On examination there was a harsh systolic murmur at the left sternal edge. On investigation an iron deficient anaemia (haemoglobin 8 g dl^{-1}), and abnormal clotting with an INR of 5.2 were found and it was assumed that her haemoptysis was due to abnormal clotting. A chest radiograph demonstrated cardiomegaly and bilateral pleural effusions.

The patient improved following treatment of her cardiac failure and correction of her anaemia and clotting disorder. However, her symptoms recurred over the next year despite well controlled anticoagulation. Her retrosternal pain worsened and she developed a pyrexia of unknown origin. She was readmitted for investigation. On examination there was tenderness over the sternum and again a harsh systolic murmur was heard. Blood cultures, a perfusion scan and bronchoscopy were normal. A thoracic CT scan was performed (Figures 1 and 2).

What are the findings?

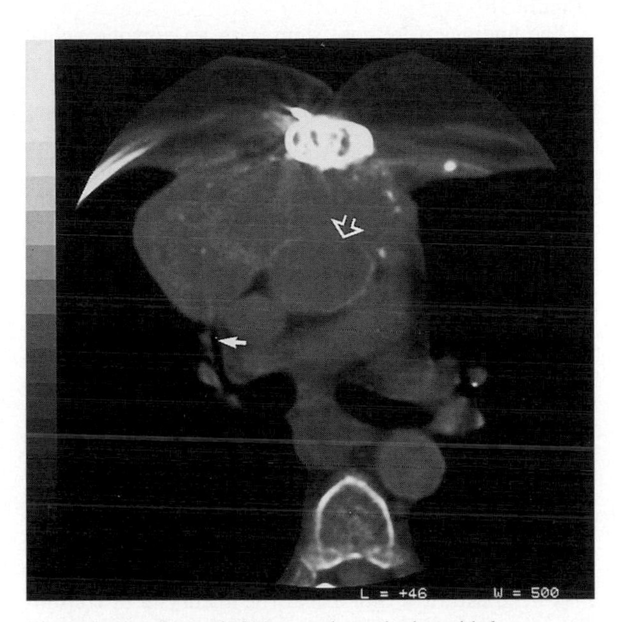

Figure 1. Unenhanced CT scan through the mid-thorax, note the regions indicated by the open and closed arrows

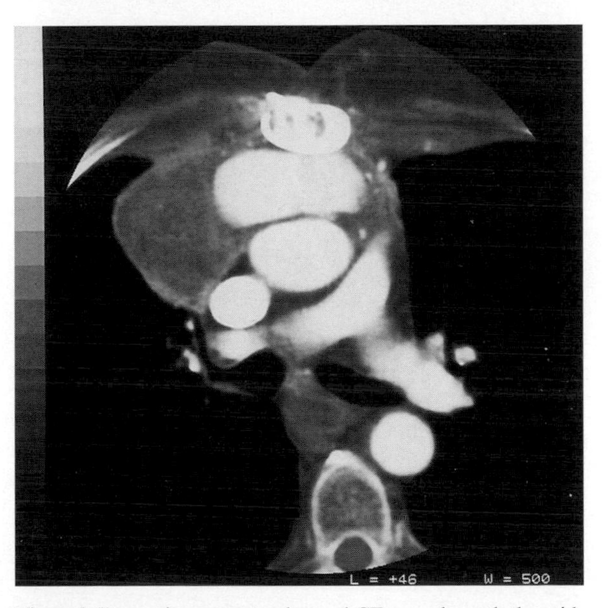

Figure 2. Dynamic contrast enhanced CT scan through the mid-thorax during the arterial phase of enhancement.

Based on the case of the month originally published in Br J Radiol 1997;70:317–8.

The thoracic CT scan demonstrated a marginally calcified mass in the anterior mediastinum. Adjacent to this mass there was sclerosis and irregularity of the cortex at the right sternoclavicular joint and an apparent defect in the anterior wall of the ascending aorta (open arrow). The right middle lobe bronchus (arrow) entered this mass posteriorly (Figure 1). Following iv contrast medium, leakage of contrast medium into a cavity within the mass in the anterior mediastinum was clearly demonstrated (Figure 2).

The findings were consistent with an aortobronchial fistula and a mycotic aneurysm of the ascending aorta associated with sternal osteomyelitis.

Aortobronchial fistulas are rare and usually arise as a complication of aortic surgery or untreated aneurysms of the thoracic aorta [1]. Mycotic aneurysms have been reported as a complication of syphilis and tuberculosis but they are now more likely to arise as a complication of previous cardiac or aortic surgery and have been documented up to 10 years after the original surgery [2]. Intermittent haemoptysis of variable duration may occur and varies from a few days to 1 year before surgical repair [2]. The intermittent nature and varying amount of haemoptysis is thought to be due to repetitive formation and lysis of the clot in the fistula. Bronchoscopy may identify the source of haemorrhage but it has been suggested that it might dislodge the fistulous clot or perforate the aneurysm although there are no documented cases of this occurring [1]. The chest radiograph may demonstrate a thoracic aortic aneurysm or consolidation in the affected portion of the lung from haemorrhage [3]. Aortography is usually negative because the fistula is filled with clot [2]. Surgical intervention is the treatment of choice and usually includes wedge resection of adherent lung and repair or replacement of the affected aorta [4] and is associated with an 80% success rate [3].

Osteomyelitis complicating mycotic aneurysms of the aorta have been documented previously following surgery but it is usually described in relation to the vertebral column and the descending aorta [5]. Osteomyelitis of the sternum with mycotic aneurysm of the ascending aorta is rare [6]. The association of an aortobronchial fistula with sternal osteomyelitis and a mycotic aneurysm of the ascending aorta has not previously been described.

A history of haemoptysis in a patient with a thoracic aneurysm or a history of previous cardiac or aortic surgery should raise the possibility of an aortobronchial fistula and a thoracic CT scan should be performed.

References

1. Coblenz CL, Sallee DS, Chiles C. Aortobronchopulmonary fistula complicating aortic surgery: Diagnosis in four cases. AJR 1988;150:535–8.
2. Graber M, Farrell RM, Neville JF, Parker FB. Successful diagnosis and management of fistulas between the aorta and the tracheobronchial tree. Ann Thorac Surg 1980;29:555–61.
3. Demeter SL, Cordasco EM. Aortobronchial fistula: Key to successful management. Angiology 1980;31:431–5.
4. Paull DE, Keagy BA. Management of aortobronchial fistula with graft replacement and omentopexy. Ann Thorac Surg 1990;50:972–4.
5. McHenry MC, Rehm SJ, Krajewski LP, Duchesneau PM, Levin HS, Steinmuller DR. Vertebral osteomyelitis and aortic lesions; Case report and review. Rev Inf Dis 1991;13:1184–94.
6. Balaji S, Whitehead B, Elliot MJ, Leval MR. Pseudoaneurysm of the aorta after heart–lung transplantation: Diagnosis by colour flow Doppler mapping. J Heart Lung Transplant 1992;11:160–3.

Not another episode of loin pain!

D M A JACKSON and C EVANS

Department of Diagnostic Radiology, University Hospital of Wales, Heath Park, Cardiff CF4 4XW, UK

A 45-year-old female was admitted with a 6 h history of left loin pain. There was no other relevant history except that she had been on the progesterone only contraceptive pill for 5 years. Examination was unremarkable. Routine blood tests and urine microscopy were normal. A plain abdominal radiograph showed no abnormality; in particular no urinary tract calcification. A clinical diagnosis of renal colic was madc. What is the persistent abnormality demonstrated on the intravenous urogram (IVU) (Figure 1)? What diagnosis was reached from the subsequent duplex Doppler ultrasound (Figure 2)?

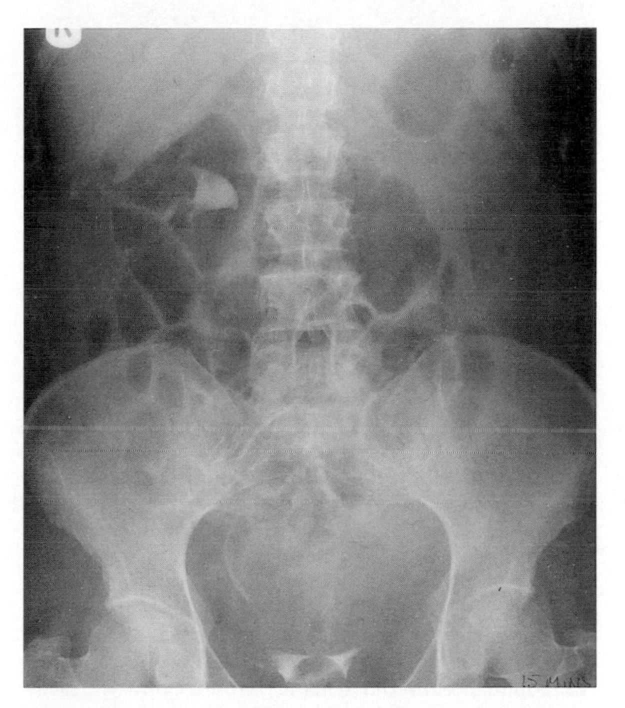

Figure 1. Intravenous urogram 45 min post-intravenous contrast medium.

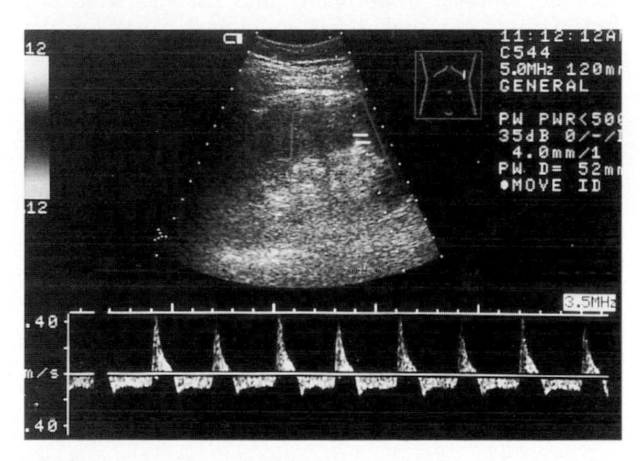

Figure 2. Ultrasound of left kidney, including an arcuate artery Doppler arterial waveform.

Based on the case of the month originally published in Br J Radiol 1998;71:345–6.

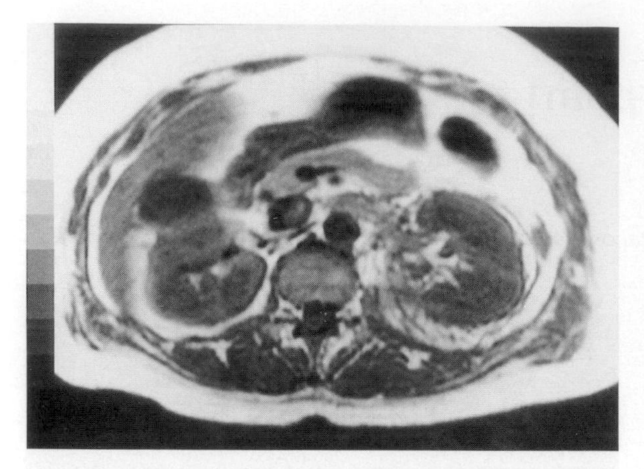

Figure 3. MRI T_1 SE axial image of the abdomen showing an enlarged left kidney with absence of the normal signal void within the left renal vein and the adjacent crescentic portion of the contiguous inferior vena cava (IVC). There remains a small channel of signal void on the right side of the IVC.

The IVU demonstrated an absent left nephrogram over 16 h. The subsequent Doppler ultrasound of a normal size left kidney showed complete reversal of diastolic arterial flow with no Doppler venous signal. Thrombus or expansion of the left renal vein was not visible as the thrombus was anechoic. The infrarenal inferior vena cava (IVC) had a normal Doppler wave pattern but the IVC continuous with the left renal vein was expanded with no recordable Doppler signal. The patient was diagnosed as having a renal vein thrombosis and was anticoagulated. MRI provided confirmation, showing a swollen left kidney and complete thrombosis of the left renal vein extending into the IVC to just below the confluence of the hepatic veins (Figure 3). There remained a narrow channel for blood to return from the lower limbs, explaining why the right kidney was normal with no Doppler abnormality and the legs were not oedematous. No underlying abdominal cause for the thrombosed renal vein was demonstrated.

Renal vein thrombosis (RVT) has two main causes: (1) primary renal disease, especially membranous glomerulonephritis, and (2) renal or adrenal carcinoma extending into the renal vein.

Oral contraceptives predispose to venous thromboembolic disease. They increase the risk three-fold for young, previously healthy, non-pregnant women to approximately three cases per 1000 women years [1]. Activated protein C resistance and Factor V Leiden are strong risk factors for venous thrombosis. A person carrying Factor V Leiden who takes an oral contraceptive pill has a 30-fold increased risk of thrombosis [2].

RVT is also a well recognized, but relatively uncommon, complication in transplant patients. It has been shown in these patients that the absence of venous flow, together with reverse diastolic flow of the arterial waveform, is compatible with RVT [3]. Reverse diastolic flow, however, is not as reliable in a native kidney because acute or severe renal disease can have a similar arterial trace [4]. Venous collaterals can also develop early in a native kidney, preventing the development of absent or reverse diastolic flow [4]. It is, therefore, important to assess the Doppler findings in relation to duration of symptoms and the renal function.

This case illustrates the importance of Doppler assessment with an abnormal nephrogram and apparently normal dynamic real time imaging of a kidney early in the development of loin pain. This ensures that anticoagulation is commenced as soon as possible, maximizing the potential for return of renal function on the affected side. CT or MRI can subsequently be performed to confirm the diagnosis, while anticoagulation is instituted without an unnecessary delay.

References

1. Royal College of General Practitioners' Oral Contraceptive Study. Oral contraceptives, venous thrombosis and varicose veins. J Roy Coll Gen Pract 1978;28:393–9.
2. Vandenbroucke JP, Koster T, Briet E, et al. Increased risk of venous thrombosis in oral-contraceptive users who are carriers of Factor V Leiden mutation. Lancet 1994;344:1453–7.
3. Baxter GM, Morley P, Dall B. Acute renal vein thrombosis in renal allografts: new Doppler ultrasonic findings. Clin Radiol 1991;43:125–7.
4. Platt JF, Ellis JH, Rubin JM. Intrarenal arterial Doppler sonography in the detection of renal vein thrombosis of the native kidney. AJR 1994;162:1367–70.

A persistent offender

D KINSELLA and P NORMAN

Department of Radiology, Derriford Hospital, Derriford Road, Plymouth, UK

A 28-year-old lady presented with a 12 h history of severe occipital headache. The onset of the headache was sudden. On examination there was mild neck stiffness with no focal neurological signs. The initial radiological examination was a CT scan which demonstrated a recent subarachnoid haemorrhage. Cerebral angiography was performed the following day (Figure 1).

What abnormalities are shown and what is the diagnosis?

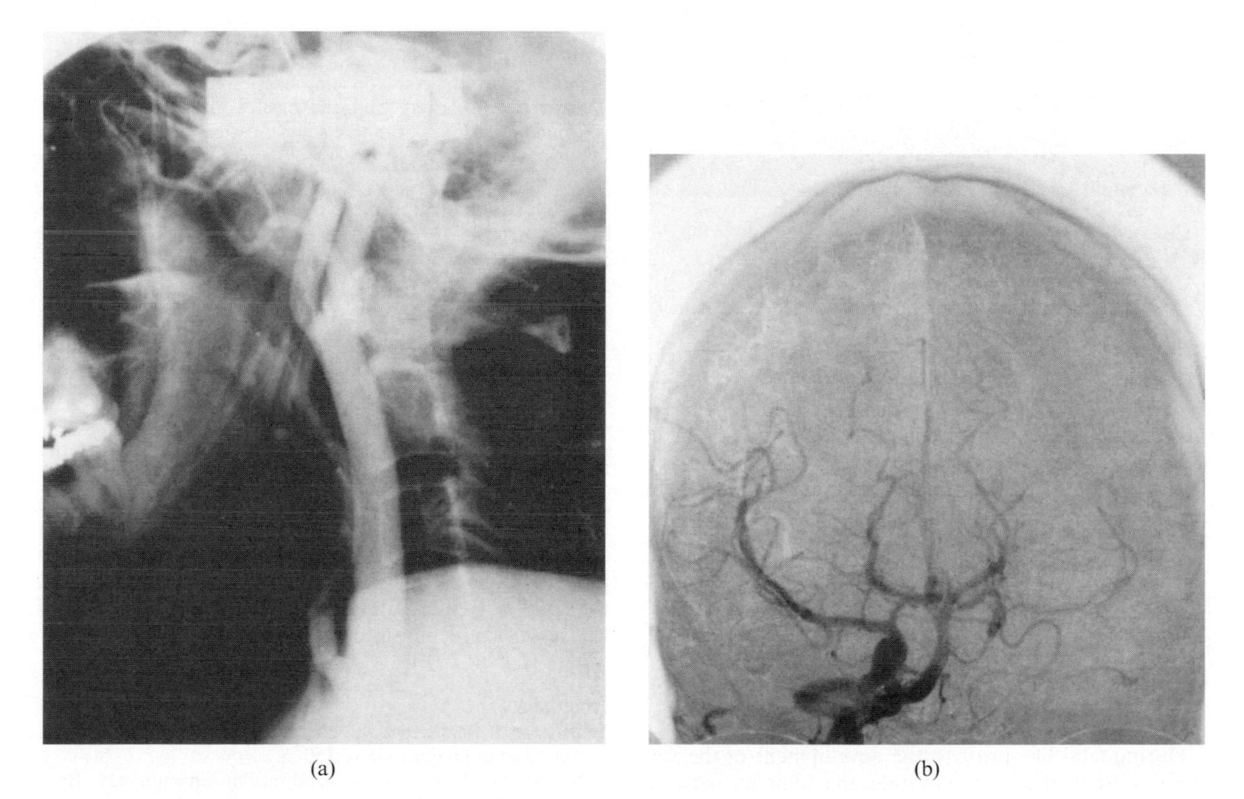

(a) (b)

Figure 1. Two views from the right common carotid arteriogram: (a) lateral cervical and (b) AP cranial.

Based on the case of the month originally published in Br J Radiol 1992;65:85–6.

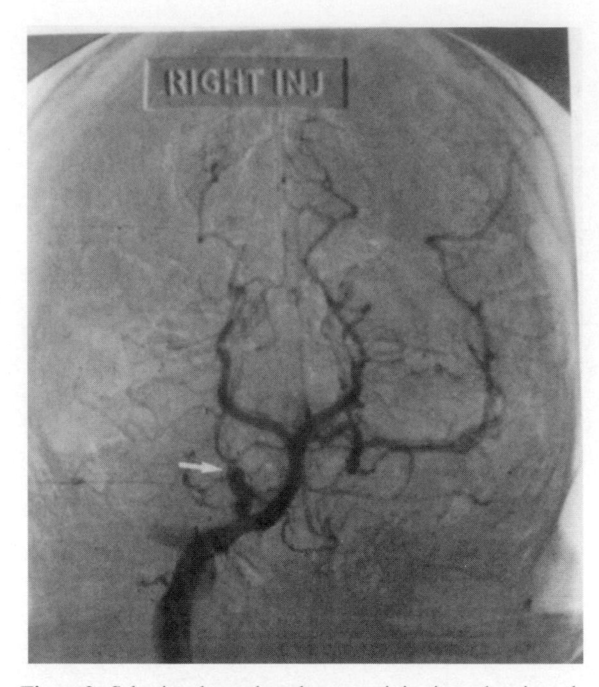

Figure 2. Selective hypoglossal artery injection showing the aneurysmal sac (arrow).

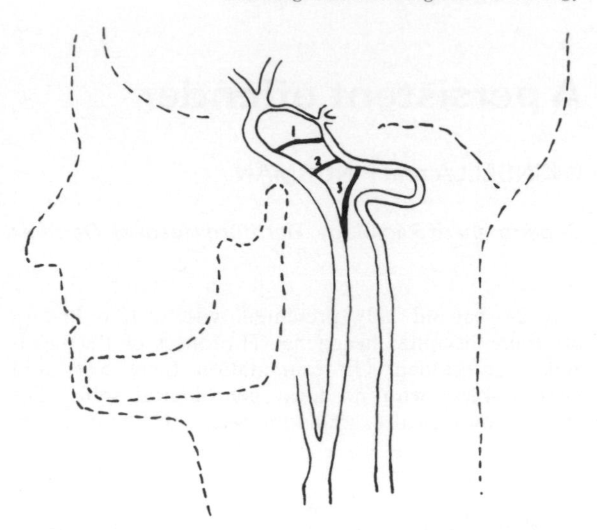

Figure 3. Sites of persistent fetal arteries connecting the right internal carotid artery and the basilar artery: (1) primitive trigeminal artery; (2) primitive acoustic artery and (3) primitive hypoglossal artery.

The right common carotid arteriogram demonstrated a communication between the right internal carotid and the basilar arteries. This is caused by a persistent hypoglossal artery. The hypoglossal artery has a large aneurysmal sac close to its termination in the basilar artery. The sac is projected behind the terminal portion of the right internal carotid artery in Figure 1b. It can be identified clearly following a selective hypoglossal artery injection (Figure 2). There is no retrograde filling of the distal portions of the vertebral arteries following this injection. The origins of the vertebral arteries could not be determined following selective injections into the innominate and left subclavian vessels.

During fetal life, prior to the development of the vertebral system, there are multiple anastomoses between the internal carotid artery and the basilar artery. Usually these anastomoses only function until the end of the first week of post-natal life [1]. However, they may persist as the trigeminal, the hypoglossal or the acoustic arteries (Figure 3). The first angiographic report of a persistent trigeminal artery was published by Sutton [2]. This vessel arises from the internal carotid artery as it enters the cavernous sinus and passes posteriorly to join the basilar artery. In a large angiographic series the frequency of this abnormality is between 0.1 and 0.2% [3]. The persistent hypoglossal artery arises from the cervical portion of the internal carotid artery at C1 or C2. It enters the skull via the hypoglossal canal and terminates as the basilar artery. In the presence of a persistent hypoglossal artery the vertebral arteries are frequently hypoplastic [1].

Less than 5% of cerebral aneurysms occur in the vertebrobasilar system. Although a persistent hypoglossal artery is a rare anomaly, several cases indicating an association with aneurysm formation have been reported [4, 5]. The altered haemodynamic state at the junction of the large persistent hypoglossal artery and the smaller basilar artery could result in weakening of the vessel wall leading to aneurysm formation.

References

1. Brismar J. Persistent hypoglossal artery diagnostic criteria. Acta Radiol Diagn 1976;17:160–6.
2. Sutton D. Anomalous carotid-basilar anastomosis. Br J Radiol 1950;23:617.
3. Lie T. Congenital abnormalities of the carotid arteries. In: Excerpta Medica Foundation. Amsterdam: Elsevier, 1968.
4. Udvarhelyi GB, Lai M. Sub-arachnoid haemorrhage due to rupture of an aneurysm on a persistent left hypoglossal artery. Br J Radiol 1963;36:843–7.
5. Huber P, Rivoir R. Aneurysm on a persistent left hypoglossal artery. Neuroradiology 1974;6:277–8.

A lump on the thigh

M CRONE and I WATT

Department of Radiodiagnosis, Bristol Royal Infirmary, Bristol BS2 8HW, UK

A 50-year-old woman presented with a slightly tender mass on the posterolateral aspect of her thigh. The mass had been present for approximately 10 years and had slowly increased in size, causing a minor degree of discomfort when sitting on a hard seat.

On examination, a diffuse tender swelling, approximately 5 cm × 3 cm, was present on the posterolateral aspect of the thigh. Apart from a small melanoma on the posterolateral aspect of the other thigh, no other abnormality could be found.

Plain radiographs of the femur (Figures 1, 2) are shown.

A radionuclide scan using $^{99}Tc^{m}$-labelled hydroxymethylene diphosphonate (HMDP) showed a normal perfusion phase. The delayed image is shown (Figure 3). What is your differential diagnosis?

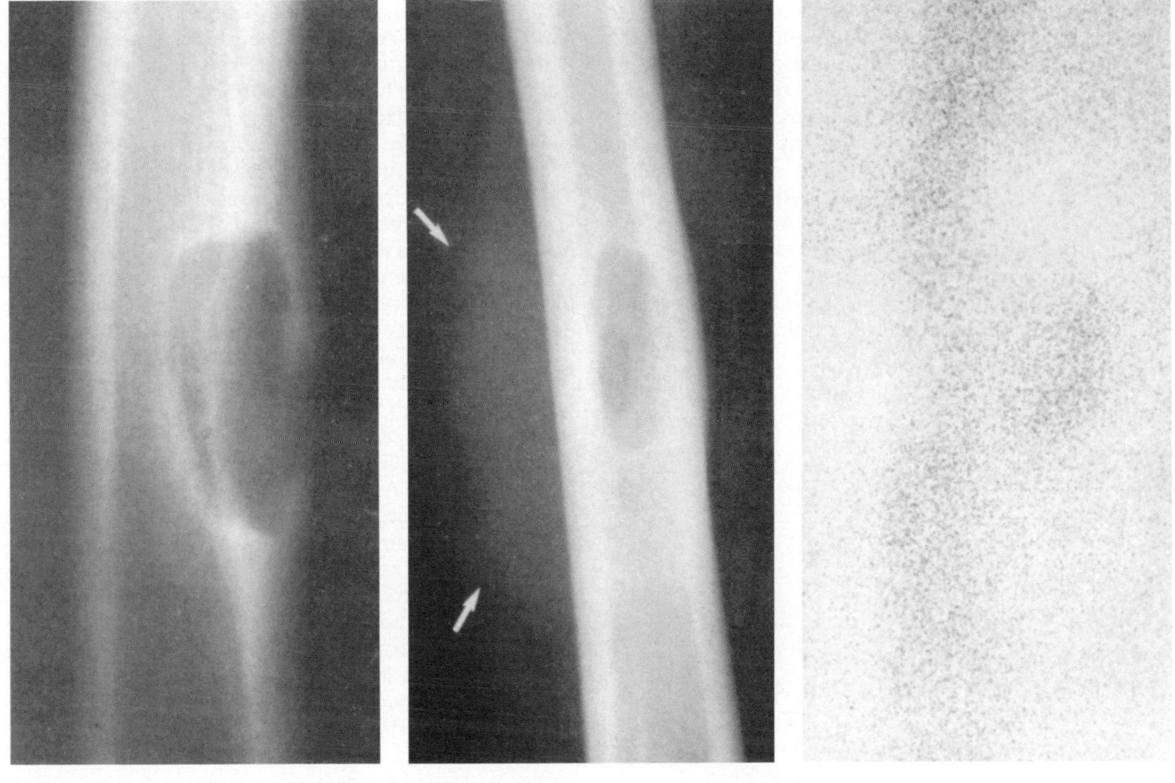

Figure 1. Localized lateral view of the midshaft of the femur.

Figure 2. Localized anteroposterior view of the same area. Note the soft tissue mass (arrows).

Figure 3. Lateral view from an HMDP bone scan (delayed image). Soft tissue accumulation shown dorsal to femur (reader's right).

Based on the case of the month originally published in Br J Radiol 1987;60:1035–6.

Plain radiographs of the femur showed a clearly defined, ovoid lucency in the midshaft with breach of the cortex. A thin rim of sclerosis surrounded this area with a discrete layer of well organized peritoneal reaction on the medial spect of the femur overlying the lesion. A well defined soft tissue mass (arrows, Figure 2) could just be seen. The remainder of the femur was normal and no other lesions were found. The delayed image of the bone scan showed increased uptake of the radiopharmaceutical in the soft tissue mass in the posterolateral aspect of the thigh.

A differential diagnosis of the given radiological appearances includes histiocytosis (eosinophilic granuloma), Brodie's abscess, a chondroma, fibrous dysplasia, or an intraosseous neurilemmoma or neurofibroma.

CT (Figure 4) confirmed the well defined sclerotic margin of the lucency which communicated with the soft tissue mass within the muscles of the thigh through a breach in the femoral cortex. The attenuation value of this mass was lower than the surrounding muscles. The absence of calcification militates against a cartilage tumour. Inactivity on the blood-pool phase of the HMDP scan makes an inflammatory lesion most unlikely, as does the well defined soft tissue mass shown on plain radiographs and CT. Fibrous dysplasia is usually associated with increased avidity on the delayed phase of an HMDP scan, and no soft tissue mass. Histiocytosis can resemble almost anything but the clues to the correct diagnosis lie in the very non-aggressive radiographic features, suggesting very slow progress, and the obvious "dumb-bell"-like nature of a mass arising at the site of a nutrient canal. Thus an intraosseous neurilemmoma is the most probable radiological diagnosis.

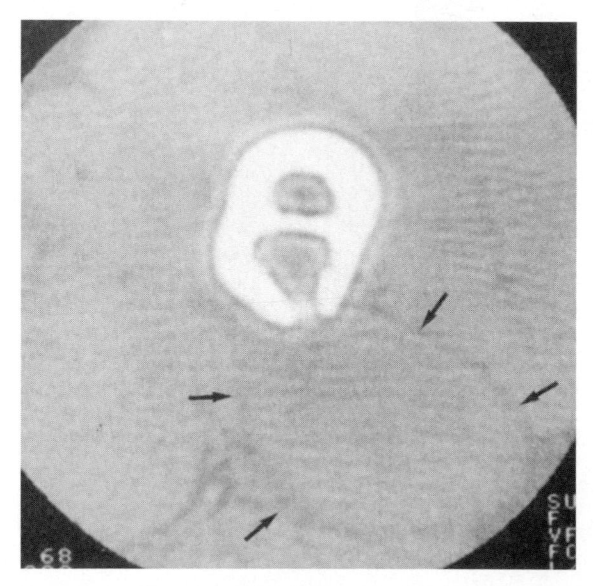

Figure 4. A CT scan of left femur: the soft tissue mass is outlined.

At operation the cavity in the femur was identified and the cloana communicating with the soft tissue demonstrated. Gelatinous material was curetted out from the cavity in the bone, which was very clearly marginated. Similar gelatinous material was removed from the cavity within the muscles which also appeared well encapsulated. Histological examination confirmed the radiological diagnosis.

Intraosseous neurilemmoma is an extremely rare tumour which most often occurs in adult females. It is a benign lesion arising from the Schwann cells of the nerve sheath and appearing with the substance of bone. The major innervation of long bones is by peripheral nerves which enter the bone through the nutrient foramina accompanying the nutrient arteries and veins.

The confusion between neurilemmoma and a solitary neurofibroma makes it difficult to ascertain an accurate incidence. However, it accounts for 1% of all neoplasms that arise in bone. Most pathologists agree that the neurilemmoma and solitary neurofibroma are distinct pathological entities, with the neurilemmoma arising from Schwann cells and the neurofibroma from the connective tissue coats.

Microscopically, the tumour tissue is composed of Antoni Type A areas and a lesser number of Antoni Type B areas, with palisaded nuclei of the Schwann cells, fascicles of closely compacted bundles of spindle-shaped fibres and Verocay bodies.

The neurilemmoma may involve bone in three ways: by central involvement, producing rarefaction of the bone (the majority are of this type); a lesion localized to the nutrient canal with production of a dumb-bell-shaped defect; and an extraosseous tumour eroding the bone secondarily [1, 2].

The diagnosis of the soft tissue tumours in neurofibromatosis using $^{99}Tc^{m}$-labelled diethylenetriamine pentaacetic acid (DTPA) has been described [3] and $^{99}Tc^{m}$-labelled dimercaptosuccinic acid (DMSA) is also known to accumulate in soft tissue tumours. Bone-seeking radiopharmaceuticals are known to localize in extraosseous soft tissue tumours because of calcification and necrosis. One report of a bone-seeking agent accumulating in an extraosseous neurofibroma has been previously made [4]. The present case is thought to be the first case in which the diagnosis of a neurilemmoma has been confirmed by HMDP.

References

1. Gordan EJ. Solitary intraosseous neurilemmoma of the tibia. Clin Orthop Rel Res 1976;117:271–82.
2. Morrison MJ, Ivins JC. Benign intraosseous neurilemmoma of the femur. Skeletal Radiol 1978;2:179–180.
3. Mandell GA, Herrick WC, Harcke HT, Sharkey C, Brooks KM, MacEwan GD. Neurofibromas: location by scanning with Tc-99m DTPA. Radiology 1985;157 803–6.
4. Nolan NG. Intense uptake of 99m Tc diphosphonate by an extraosseous neurofibroma. J Nucl Med 1974;15:1207–9.

An unusual twist

B G BROGDON and B A GEORGY

Department of Radiology, University of South Alabama Medical Center, 2451 Fillingim Street, Mobile, AL 36617, USA

A 17-year-old male sustained a single gunshot wound to the right side of the chest. After evaluation and blood volume replacement in the Emergency Department, he was taken to the Operating Theatre where a right lower lobe lobectomy was performed. Pleural drains were inserted, but there was a persistent post-operative air leak (Figure 1). On the second post-operative day, the patient was referred for CT in order to localize the bullet, which appeared to be lodged in the spinal canal. During this procedure, the patient went into acute cardiopulmonary collapse and the CT scan was aborted before completion. Although the CT scanogram (Figure 2) was available, the definitive diagnostic finding was appreciated neither on the scanogram nor on a subsequent bedside radiograph (Figure 3) obtained before the patient's death. What is the most important diagnostic clue in the chest radiographs? What is the diagnosis?

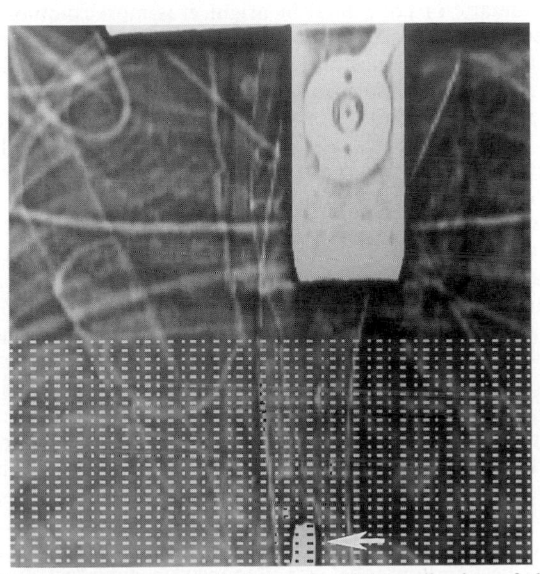

Figure 2. Scanogram of the chest for CT localization of the bullet (arrow).

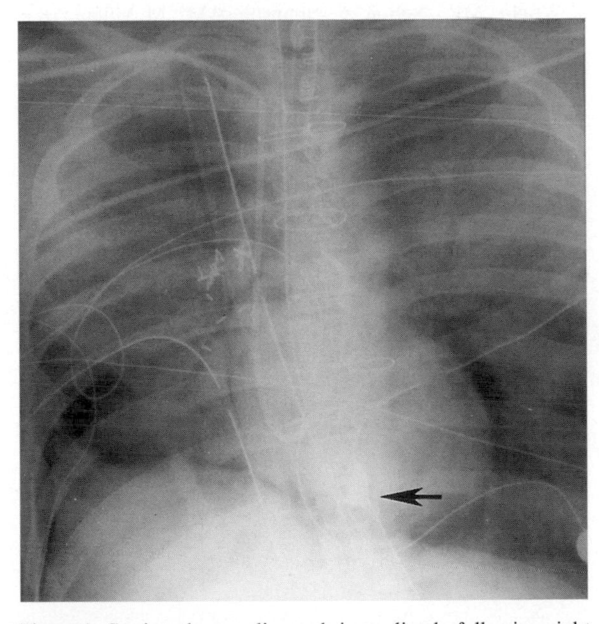

Figure 1. Supine chest radiograph immediately following right intrapericardial lobectomy for a gunshot wound. An arrow marks the bullet.

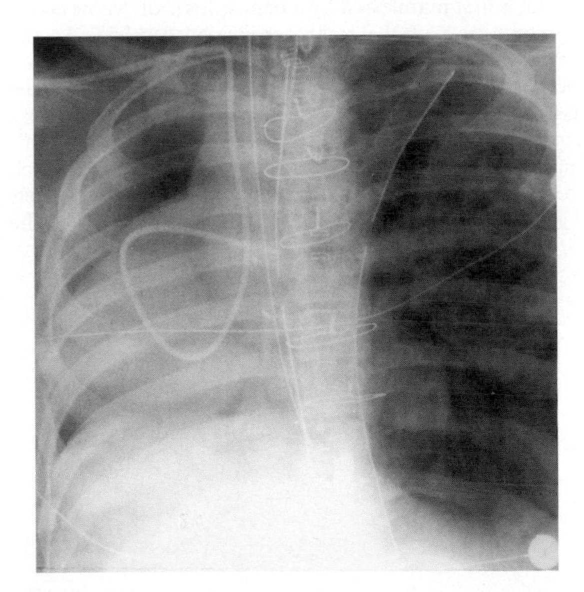

Figure 3. Supine radiograph of the chest obtained at the bedside following aborted CT and preceding the patient's demise.

Based on the case of the month originally published in Br J Radiol 1998;71:691–2.

Both the CT scanogram and the bedside radiograph showed absence of the cardiac shadow in the left hemithorax with a mirror-imaged cardiac shadow on the right (Figures 2 and 3). These findings suggest cardiac herniation and possible volvulus. Furthermore, the loop of the pulmonary artery catheter was now reversed and had a clockwise orientation. This finding is diagnostic of cardiac volvulus, which was confirmed at autopsy.

Although cardiac herniation with volvulus may be traumatic or congenital in origin, it is most commonly seen as a catastrophic complication of right intrapericardial pneumonectomy or lobectomy when it usually occurs in the first 3 post-operative days [1–3]. It may be precipitated by changes in the patient's position (as is probable in this case), the negative pressure in the empty pleural cavity, extubation or cough [1, 3, 4]. The clinical signs and symptoms of cardiac herniation with volvulus are protean in nature and non-specific [1, 2]. They include abrupt cardiac failure, hypotension, tachycardia, superior vena cava obstruction, severe chest pain and cyanosis. Since prompt surgical intervention offers the only hope for survival, a high level of clinical suspicion for cardiac volvulus must exist in the immediate post-operative period following right-sided intrapericardial pneumectomy or lobectomy. Temporary measures to improve or sustain cardiopulmonary function while preparing for surgery include repositioning the patient with the non-surgical side down, avoiding hyperinflation of the remaining lung, and injection of air into the surgical hemithorax [5].

Chest radiography will demonstrate definitive diagnostic findings of cardiac herniation and volvulus. Impending or partial herniation through the pericardial defect is first manifested by a hemispheric or "snow cone" configuration of the right cardiac border [6]. As the majority of the heart herniates through the pericardial defect, it vacates the left hemithorax and projects to the right. The cardiac apex rotates posteriorly to cause organoaxial rotation with kinking in the right atrial-superior vena caval region. This may produce a notch between the rounded cardiac border and the great vessels [7]. The empty cardiac sac may hang to the left of the spine as a curtain or veil-like shadow [4]. Pleural drainage tubes, if present, may be displaced against the right chest wall posteriorly by the shift of the cardiac apex.

Definitive diagnostic evidence of cardiac volvulus is demonstrated if a pulmonary artery catheter is in place. First, there may be a sharp kink or angulation of the catheter at the brachiocephalic venous junction [8] which would make it impossible to pass a pacing catheter into the heart [1]. More important is the direction of rotation of the catheter loop in the right ventricle. In any patient with normal cardiac situs and normal cardiac chambers the inferior loop of the catheter in the right ventricle is always in an anticlockwise direction. This is true regardless of which side is selected for subclavian entry or which pulmonary artery the catheter enters. Contrarily, rotation of the inferior ventricular loop of the catheter in a clockwise direction is diagnostic of cardiac volvulus. This specific sign has been reported only twice before in the English language literature [5, 8]. The fact that this finding was missed by several observers in our department (where one of those previous reports originated) indicates that this sign is not well known and merits re-emphasis.

References

1. Dieraniya AK. Cardiac herniation following intrapericardial pneumonectomy. Thorax 1974;29:545–52.
2. Hidvegi RS, Abdulnour EM, Wilson JAS. Herniation of the heart following left pneumonectomy. J Can Assoc Radiol 1981;32:185–7.
3. Wright MP, Nelson C, Johnson AM, McMillan IKR. Herniation of the heart. Thorax 1970;25:656–64.
4. Castillo M, Oldham S. Cardiac volvulus: plain film recognition of an often fatal condition. AJR 1985;145:271–2.
5. Cassorla L, Katz JA. Management of cardiac herniation after intrapericardial pneumonectomy. Anesthesiology 1984;60: 362–4.
6. Gurney JW, Arnold S, Goodman LR. Impending cardiac herniation: the snow cone sign. Radiology 1986;161:653–5.
7. Tschersich HU, Skorapa V Jr, Fleming WH. Acute cardiac herniation following pneumonectomy. Radiology 1976; 120:546.
8. Brady MB, Brogdon BG. Cardiac herniation and volvulus: radiographic findings. Radiology 1986; 161:657–8.

The man who hated hospitals

D J W MOREWOOD and G H R LAMB

Department of Radiology, Royal Liverpool Hospital, Liverpool, UK

A 40-year-old man who was otherwise well presented to the outpatients department with an intermittent dull ache in the right upper quadrant of his abdomen, which had been present for 1–2 months. On examination, a mass was found at the site of the pain. Ultrasound (using a 3.5 MHz transducer) was performed and a transverse scan at the site of the mass is shown (Figure 1). Further radiological investigation was recommended, but the patient failed to return to hospital. 2 years later he returned with the same symptoms and the abdominal mass was by then larger. He was still otherwise well. His haemoglobin was 14 g dl^{-1}, white cell count 660/mm^3 and his ESR 27 mm h^{-1}. Ultrasound was again performed and a longitudinal scan from this examination is shown (Figure 2). CT was then carried out (Figure 3).

From where is the mass arising and what is your differential diagnosis?

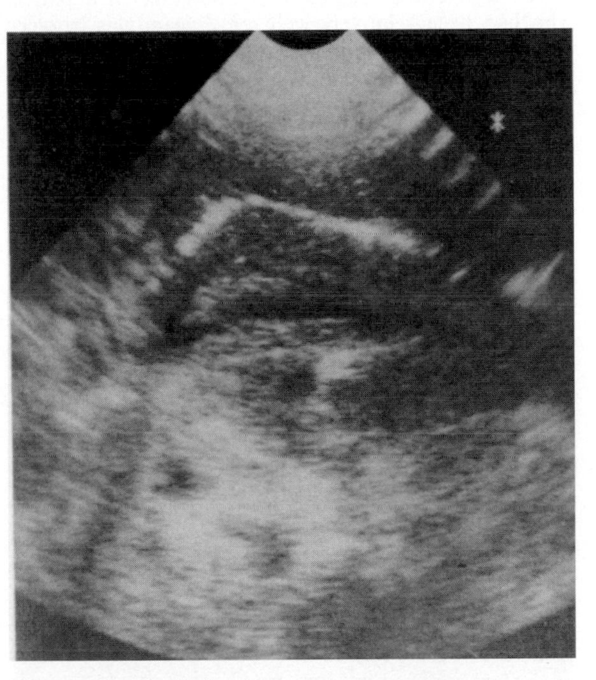

Figure 2. Longitudinal ultrasound scan obtained at the patient's attendance 2 years later. The transverse scan was little changed.

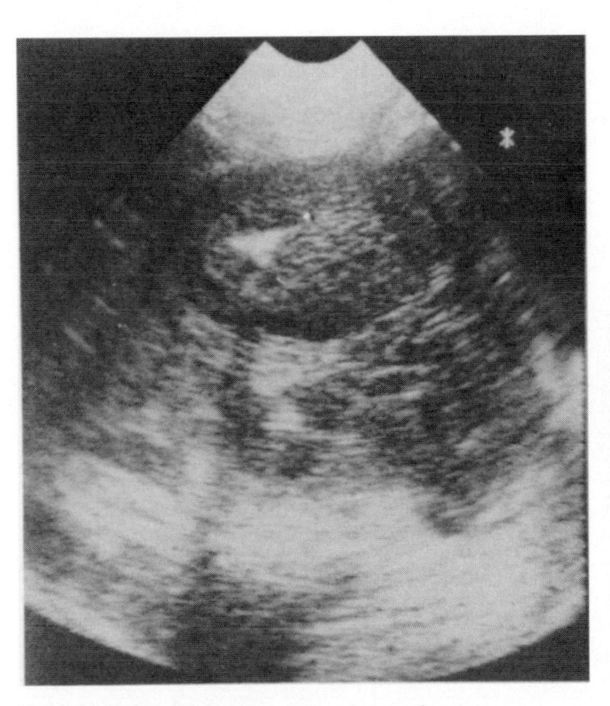

Figure 1. Initial transverse sonogram over the mass.

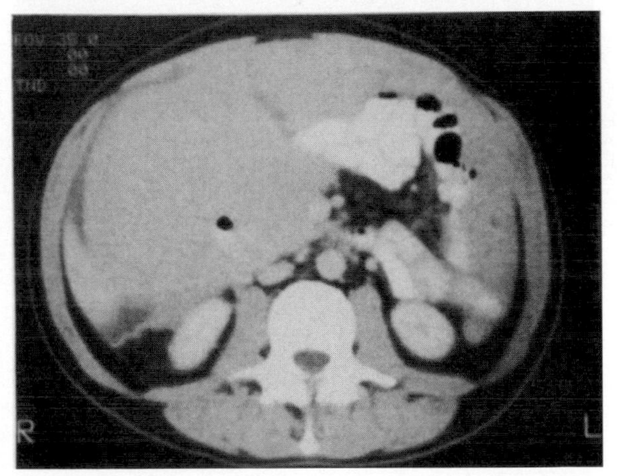

Figure 3. CT section through the abdominal mass.

Based on the case of the month originally published in Br J Radiol 1986;59:793–4.

The typical "bull's eye" or "target" appearance produced on the transverse ultrasound scan by an eccentric triangular echogenic centre within a surrounding irregular echolucent area is a sign of gas within a surrounding soft tissue mass. The site suggests that it may be a colonic lesion. The longitudinal scan shows a long echogenic centre with surrounding echolucency. These appearances were confirmed by CT (Figure 3), which showed a large mass surrounding a narrow, gas-containing lumen.

The differential diagnosis at this stage in a patient who had been relatively well for 2 years was between colonic lymphoma and a benign tumour, such as a leiomyoma. A barium enema was performed and showed a stricture in the right side of the colon, beyond which no barium passed. Some rapid-transit barium was given orally and a radiograph made 1 h later (Figure 4) shows the extent of the constricting soft tissue mass. The next step was to obtain tissue for diagnosis and a Trucut biopsy was performed under local anaesthetic with fluoroscopy. The histology showed a diffuse centroblastic, centrocytic lymphoma (a low grade non-Hodgkin's lymphoma). The patient was then treated with chemotherapy.

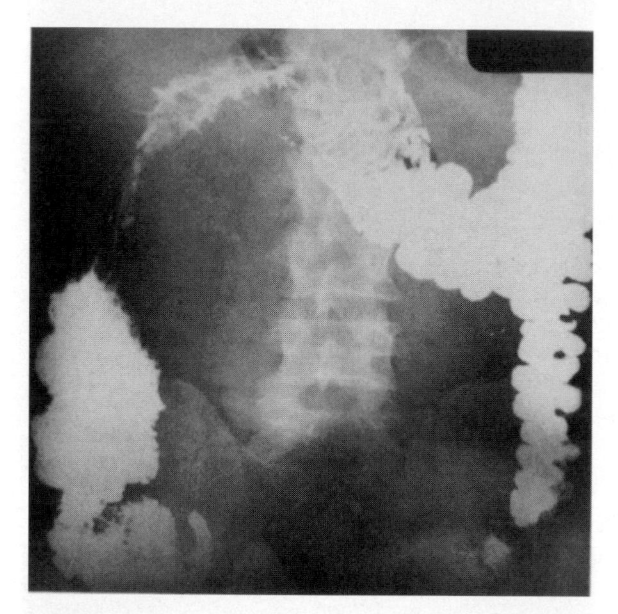

Figure 4. Radiograph after combined barium enema and oral barium.

The most common symptom of colonic lymphoma is abdominal pain over the site of the tumour, a palpable mass occurring in over 60% [1]. Lymphoma of the gastrointestinal tract has a tendency to remain localized to the gut wall with subsequent spread to draining lymph nodes [2]. The caecum is the most common site for primary colonic lymphoma [3].

Any condition producing bowel-wall thickening, such as carcinoma, lymphoma, benign intestinal tumour or Crohn's disease, may be demonstrated by ultrasound and will cause a "target" or "bull's eye" lesion [4]. However, on CT, lymphoma showed the greatest thickening of the bowel wall [5].

Colonic lymphoma produces a spectrum of appearances on barium enema related to whether the lymphoma originates in the bowel or involves it secondarily. This case of primary lymphoma presented as a large mass, which is the most characteristic finding [3], and the most effective way of making a definite diagnosis is to obtain tissue for histology when the mass has been localized.

[*Colonic lymphoma is often associated with prominent retroperitoneal and mesenteric lymphadenopathy, ED*]

References

1. Zornoza J, Dodd GD. Lymphoma of the gastrointestinal tract. Semin Roentgenol 1980;15:272–87.
2. Brady LW, Asbell SO. Malignant lymphoma of the gastrointestinal tract. Radiology 1980;137:291–8.
3. O'Connell DJ, Thompson AJ. Lymphoma of the colon: the spectrum of radiologic changes. Gastrointest Radiol 1978;2:377–85.
4. Fleischer AC, Muhletaler CA, Everette JA. Sonographic patterns arising from normal and abnormal bowel. Radiol Clin North Am 1980;18:145–9.
5. Megibow AJ, Balthazar EJ, Naidich DP and Bosniak MA. Computed tomography of gastrointestinal lymphoma. AJR 1983;141:541–7.

A pain in the neck

[1]A SAIFUDDIN and [2]I G H RENWICK

[1]*St James's University Hospital NHS Trust, Leeds, and* [2]*Middlesbrough General Hospital, Middlesbrough, UK*

A previously healthy 24-year-old man injured his neck in a rugby match and complained of neck pain. There was no history of previous neck trauma. On examination his neck was diffusely tender and there was generalized reduction in neck movements. Plain radiographs of the cervical spine were obtained (Figures 1a, b). What do they show and what is the diagnosis? How would you confirm this?

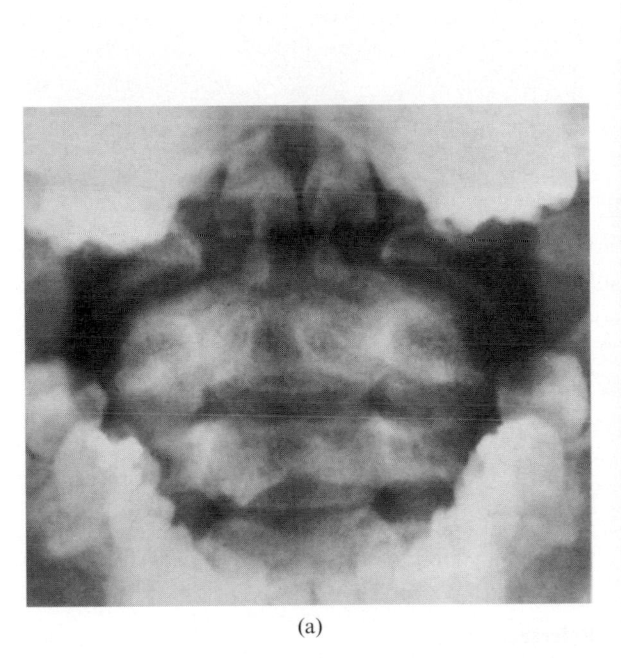

(a)

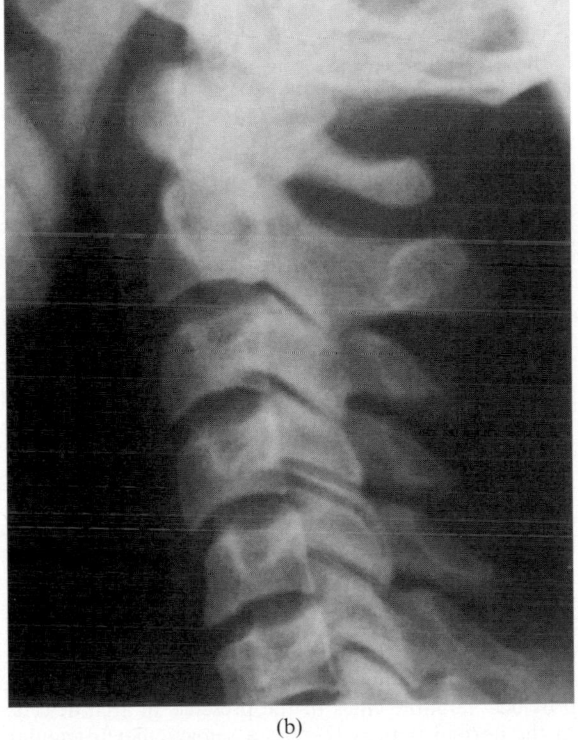

(b)

Figure 1. (a) AP and (b) lateral radiographs of the upper cervical spine.

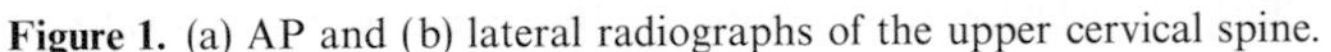

Based on the case of the month originally published in Br J Radiol 1993;66:379–80.

The anteroposterior (AP) radiograph of the upper cervical spine (Figure 1a) showed bilateral atlantoaxial offset of 4 mm. The initial diagnosis was of a burst fracture of the atlas (Jefferson fracture) and CT was performed to confirm this (Figure 2). CT demonstrated a well defined, smooth, corticated anterior cleft and a midline posterior defect. No fracture was seen. A diagnosis of bipartite atlas was made. Following CT, the plain radiographs were reviewed and several abnormalities observed which had not been previously appreciated. On the lateral radiograph (Figure 1b) there was absence of the cortical outline to the anterior tubercle of the atlas and similarly there was no arch–canal line posteriorly. Careful evaluation of the AP radiograph revealed the midline vertical defect of the anterior arch of the atlas. The diagnosis of bipartite atlas could therefore have been made on the plain radiographs.

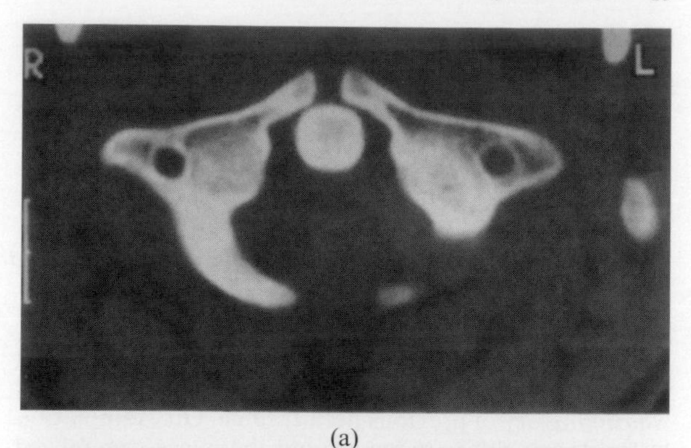

(a)

R L

(b)

Figure 2. Axial CT scans of the atlas showing well corticated (a) anterior cleft and (b) posterior defect.

Bipartite atlas is a rare congenital anomaly of the atlas vertebra caused by incomplete ossification of the anterior and posterior arches with resultant cartilage filled defects. Up until 1971 only 25 cases had been reported [1]. Since then a further 15 cases have been recorded in three separate reports [2–4]. Of this total of 40 cases, clinical details of symptoms and signs are available in only 15 cases. 10 patients were either asymptomatic or had cervical pain secondary to trauma which resolved without treatment. None had neurological deficit. Four others had suffered epileptic seizures.

Gehweiler et al [3] reviewed 36 patients with atlas malformations over a period of 10 years and compared the radiological findings, with particular emphasis on the degree of bilateral atlantoaxial offset, with 10 patients who had sustained Jefferson fractures. 13 of their cases had combined anterior and posterior ossification defects (bipartite atlas) and eight of these had 1–2 mm of bilateral atlantoaxial offset demonstrated on the AP radiograph. This finding was also noted with other anomalies such as total or partial aplasias of the posterior arch and isolated posterior arch clefts. In no case was the degree of offset greater than 2 mm. The authors also noted several abnormalities on the lateral radiograph which provided valuable clues to the presence of arch defects. In the normal patient there is a semicircular/triangular cortical outline to the anterior tubercle of the atlas and a cortical line marking the posterior limit of the cervical spinal canal (arch–canal line). Absence of the former indicates a failure of fusion of the anterior arch and absence of the latter indicates a posterior defect. A combination of these findings therefore indicates bipartite atlas. Prager [4] also stated that bilateral atlantoaxial offsets of greater than 2 mm were not seen with congenital defects. In this respect the present case is atypical.

The CT features of bipartite atlas [3] are a thin midline anterior cleft with well corticated margins and a well defined posterior defect, identical to this case (Figure 2).

The finding of bilateral atlantoaxial offset in patients who have suffered cervical spine trauma raises the possibility of a burst fracture of C1. However, such an appearance may also be due to congenital anomalies and careful evaluation of the lateral cervical spine radiograph can allow a diagnosis to be made from plain radiographs.

References

1. Childers Jr JC, Wilson FC. Bipartite atlas. J Bone Joint Surg 1971;53A:578–82.
2. Lipson SJ, Mazur J. Anteroposterior spondyloschisis of the atlas revealed by computerized tomography scanning. J Bone Joint Surg 1978;60A:1104–5.
3. Gehweiler Jr JA, Daffner RH, Roberts Jr L. Malformations of the atlas vertebra simulating the Jefferson fracture. AJR 1983;140:1083–6.
4. Prager PJ. Differential diagnosis and radiological work-up in bilateral lateral atlantoaxial offset. Eur J Radiol 1983;3: 309–13.

Atypical chest pain!

S EUSTACE, J G MURRAY and E BREATNACH

Radiology Department, Mater Misericordiae Hospital, Eccles Street, Dublin 7, Ireland

A 42-year-old woman presented with sudden onset of severe central chest pain. The patient had been previously well and there was no history of trauma. She had a long history of smoking 20 cigarettes a day, and reported early onset of menarche at 8 years. On physical examination she was mildly distressed. Several "café au lait" areas of skin pigmentation were noted over her trunk and abdomen. There was no other clinical abnormality.

Electrocardiography and routine haematological and biochemical blood tests were normal. Chest radiograph taken on admission (Figure 1) is shown. CT of the chest was subsequently performed (Figure 2).

What abnormalities are demonstrated and what are the possible diagnoses?

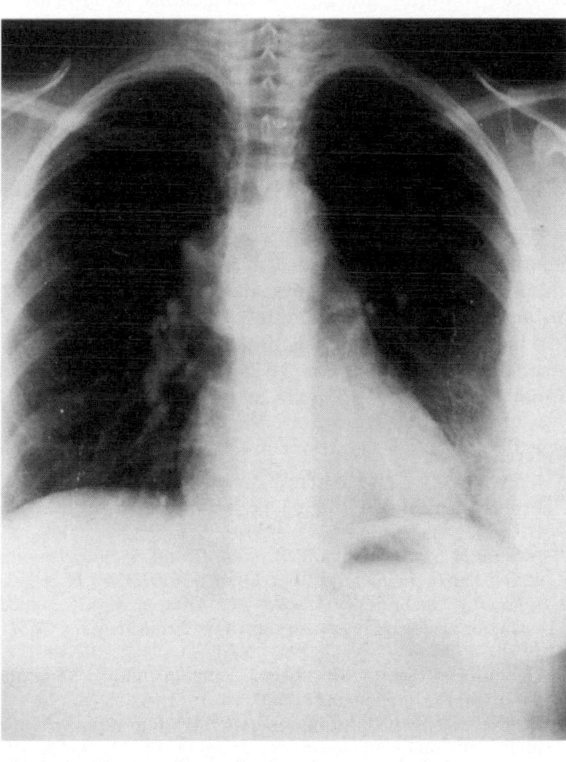

Figure 1. Chest radiograph of patient on admission.

Based on the case of the month originally published in Br J Radiol 1995;68:1261–62.

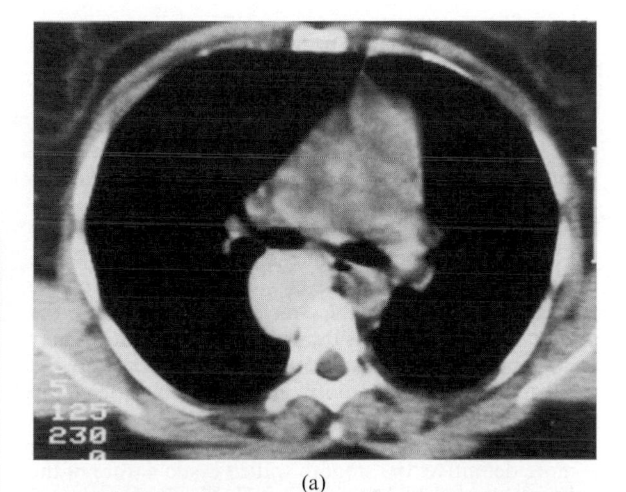

(a)

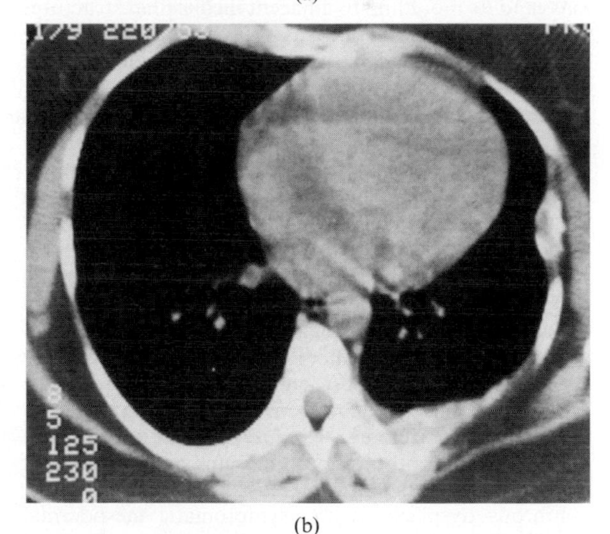

(b)

Figure 2. (a,b) CT of the chest.

The chest radiograph showed a smooth walled homogeneous non-calcified mediastinal mass projected over the lower trachea and right main bronchus. The posterior aspect of ribs 7–10 on the left were not visualized, and a laterally situated soft tissue extrapleural opacity is seen at this level. CT showed a well defined middle mediastinal mass of high attenuation, intimately related to the carina and right main stem bronchus. A section at a lower level showed lytic endosteal bone expansion of ribs 7–10 on the left. There is replacement of the normal marrow by a matrix of uniform soft tissue density.

Under CT guidance fine needle aspiration of the mediastinal mass produced 10 ml of blood stained mucoid material. Cytological examination revealed haemorrhage and epithelial cells. No inflammatory or malignant cells were identified.

A diagnosis of chest pain secondary to haemorrhage into a bronchogenic cyst with incidental Albright's syndrome was made.

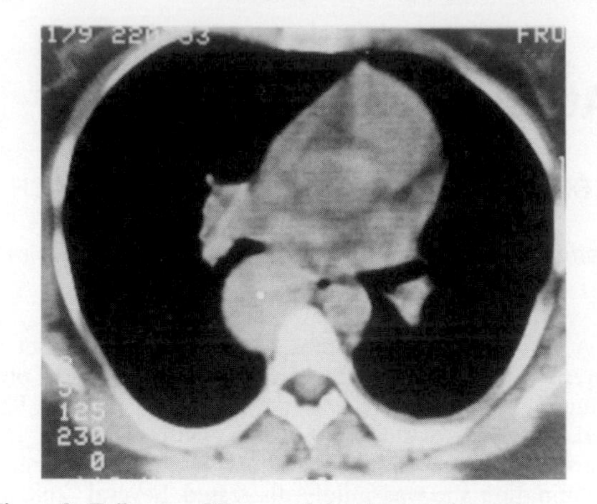

Figure 3. Follow-up CT scan of the chest at 6 months.

Bronchogenic cysts are uncommon thin walled cavities which represent cystic reduplication of the tracheobronchial tree. The majority of cysts are asymptomatic and encountered as chance findings before the fourth decade. They may become manifest clinically as a result of infection or haemorrhage into the cyst. Complications as a result of compression of adjacent structures, *e.g.* superior vena cava or bronchi, are relatively rare despite the central location of bronchogenic cysts [1]. While cysts may occur at any level along the course of the trachea and main bronchi, over 80% are located in the middle mediastinum at subcarinal level. Cavitation may occur and is frequently a complication of infection of cyst contents. The diagnosis should be considered on plain radiographs when a mass is identified in a characteristic location with a smooth outer wall. CT scanning is more definitive: the smooth walled cystic nature of the mass and its moulding to adjacent mediastinal structures are better defined. Cyst densities (20–80 HU) are usually higher than water [2], reflecting their proteinaceous content. In up to 50% of patients cysts have an attenuation coefficient similar to soft tissue and indistinguishable from tumour [2]. In these circumstances surgery or CT guided extrapleural drainage [3] may be necessary to confirm the diagnosis. Calcification, although uncommon, may be curvilinear and confined to the wall or permeate through the cyst as "milk of calcium" [4]. This suspended calcium, or recent haemorrhage as in the case reported here, may further increase the density of the mass at CT. On MRI the high concentration of mucin has a short T_1 relaxation time and the lesion may appear intense on both T_1 and T_2 weighted images [5]. The central mass in this case is unlikely to represent a bronchogenic carcinoma because of its uniform high attenuation, smooth margins, and lack of infiltration of the surrounding mediastinal structures.

Fibrous dysplasia is an asymptomatic mesodermal bone disorder characterized by replacement of cancellous bone by fibro-osseous tissue. In 2–3% of patients, polyostotic bony involvement is associated with sexual precocity and "café au lait" spots—Albright's syndrome [6]. Flat bones are most commonly involved, typically the skull, ribs and pelvis although involvement of long bones, particularly the femur, is well described. In this case the apparent rib destruction on the chest radiograph was confirmed on CT as bony replacement by a uniform soft tissue density matrix. This finding, associated with cortical thinning and bony expansion, is typical of fibrous dysplasia. The uniformity of bony involvement (ribs 7–10), the intact bony cortex and the lack of periosteal reaction are further helpful features in differentiating the condition from lytic metastases. The clinical history of precocious puberty, the presence of multiple "café au lait" pigmentations in association with characteristic CT findings rendered a diagnosis of Albright's syndrome without recourse to bone biopsy.

The patient's symptoms settled with conservative treatment. Follow-up CT at 6 months (Figure 3) showed a marked decrease in the cyst density due to resorption of haemorrhage. No change in cyst size or extension of the bony abnormality was noted. Although bronchogenic cysts and fibrous dysplasia are both developmental anomalies there is no known association.

References

1. Bankoff MS, Daly BDT, Johnson HA, Carter BL. Bronchogenic cyst causing superior vena cava obstruction: CT appearance. JCAT 1985;9:951–2.
2. Nakata H, Sato Y, Nakama T, et al. Bronchogenic cyst with high CT numbers: analysis of contents. JCAT 1986;10:360–2.
3. Adam A, MacSweeney JE, Whyte MKB, et al. CT guided extrapleural drainage of bronchogenic cyst. JCAT 1989;13:1065–8.
4. Cubillo E, Rockoff SD. Milk of calcium fluid in an intrapulmonary bronchogenic cyst. Chest 1971;60:608.
5. Gamsu G. The mediastinum in computed tomography of the body with magnetic resonance imaging. In: Moss, Gamsu, Genant, editors. Philadelphia: WB Saunders, 1992:85.
6. De George AM. Albright syndrome: is it coming of age? J Pediatr 1975;87:1018–20.

A painful big toe

J R COOPER and N A BARRINGTON

Department of Diagnostic Radiology, Royal Hallamshire Hospital, Glossop Road, Sheffield S10 2JF, UK

A 30-year-old student presented to the accident and emergency department with a 1 month history of vague discomfort of the big toe that he had attributed to the strains his keen participation in volleyball had placed upon it. The day before presentation he developed acute onset of pain, swelling and tenderness of his right first toe. He was otherwise well and had no significant past medical history. The only abnormality on examination was swelling and erythema over the first interphalangeal joint. A radiograph was obtained (Figure 1). What abnormality is shown?

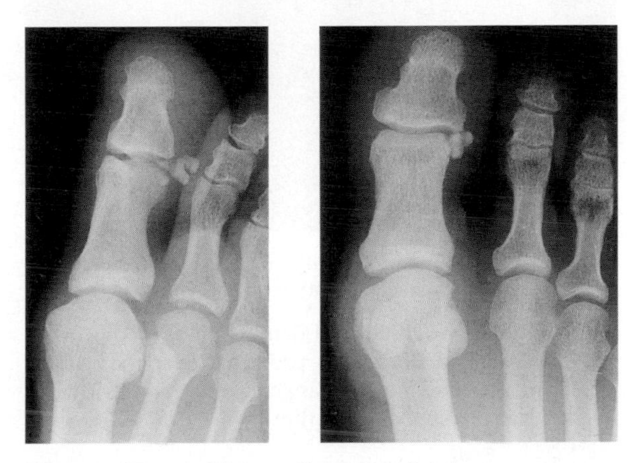

Figure 1. AP and oblique radiographs of right toes.

Based on the case of the month originally published in Br J Radiol 1997;70:223–4.

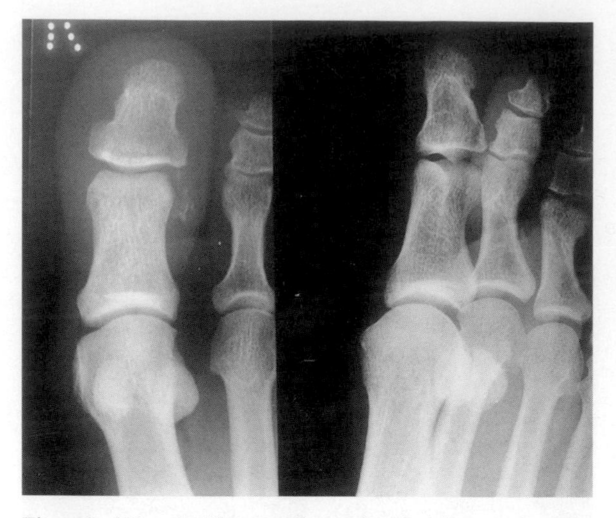

Figure 2. AP and oblique radiographs of right toes 3 weeks after Figure 1. The calcific density has almost entirely resolved.

In Figure 1, a well defined dense, homogeneous opacity with rounded borders is projected over the plantar aspect of the first interphalangeal joint. This is due to hydroxyapatite depostion within the flexor tendon of the big toe.

The symptoms resolved over the next 2 days. On review 3 weeks later, no abnormality was found on examination and a further radiograph showed that the calcification density had almost disappeared (Figure 2).

Calcific tendonitis, hydroxyapatite deposition disease, or peritendonitis calcarea is well recognized in the shoulder, hip, wrist, hand and neck, but reports involving the foot are far rarer although in our experience it is not uncommon [1–3]. This case illustrates the aetiological factors, clinical course and characteristic radiological features of the condition.

Although these calcific deposits have been long recognized radiologically it was not until the 1950s that X-ray diffraction techniques allowed the identification of the material as calcium hydroxyapatite. Hydroxyapatite crystals are found not just in tendons but also in bursae, other periarticular tissues and in joint fluid. Pathogenic mechanisms are poorly understood, but it has traditionally been assumed that hydroxyapatite deposition occurred in damaged or avascular tissues as a consequence of trauma, with subsequent inflammatory changes secondary to the hydroxyapatite deposition. Recent reports of familial cases, polyarticular involvement, and HLA antigen associations are suggestive of systemic and possibly metabolic aetiological factors [3, 4].

Radiological appearances vary but initially thin poorly defined opacities located in tendons, their attachments and/or periarticular tissues are seen, becoming dense, homogeneous, sharply defined with a rounded configuration. Although they sometimes remain unchanged, the usual pattern is for resolution, which may or may not be complete.

Clinically, there is often an association with mild and repetitive trauma involving the affected tendon. In hydroxyapatite deposition in the flexor tendons of the foot repeated forceable plantar flexion has been reported from such insults as stiff brake pedals and ladder climbing [2]. Although some calcific deposits are asymptomatic, the typical pattern is intense pain of acute or semi acute onset with swelling, erythema and tenderness which resolves spontaneously. Other than a mild fever no systemic symptoms have been reported [4, 5].

This case illustrates most of these features: the association with repeated plantar flexion, acute pain, swelling and redness, typical calcification at the site of the flexor hallucis longus tendon and the interphalangeal joint tissues, with rapid resolution of both symptoms and radiographic signs. We believe that foot involvement is probably underdiagnosed but with greater awareness can be readily recognized, and unnecessary treatment for such conditions as gout and soft tissue infections should be avoided.

References

1. Rhodes RA, Stelling CB. Calcific tendonitis of the flexors of the forefoot. Ann Emergency Med 1986;15:751–3.
2. Gruneberg R. Calcifying tendonitis in the forefoot. Br J Radiol 1963;36:378–9.
3. Weston WJ. Peroneal tendinitis calcarea. Br J Radiol 1959;32:134–5.
4. Resnick D. Calcium hydroxyapatite crystal deposition disease. In: Resnick D, Niwayama G, editors. Diagnosis of bone and joint disorders. Philadelphia: WB Saunders, 1988:1733–64.
5. Holt PD, Keats TE. Calcific tendonitis: A review of the usual and unusual. Skeletal Radiol 1993;22:1–9.

A fishy tale?

W J TAYLOR, A D PLATTS and G HAMILTON

Departments of Radiology and Academic Surgery, Royal Free Hospital, London NW3, UK

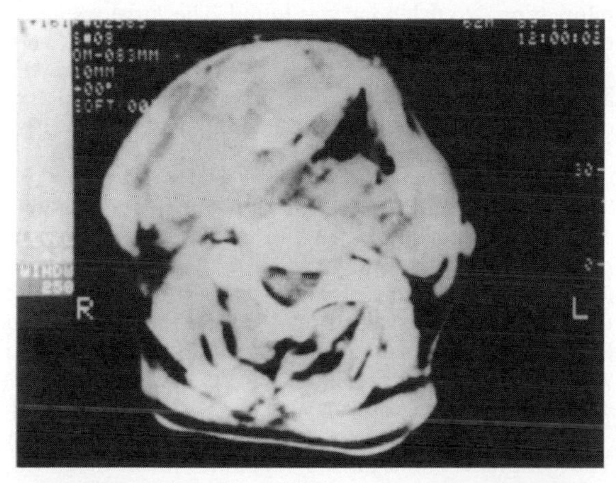

(a)

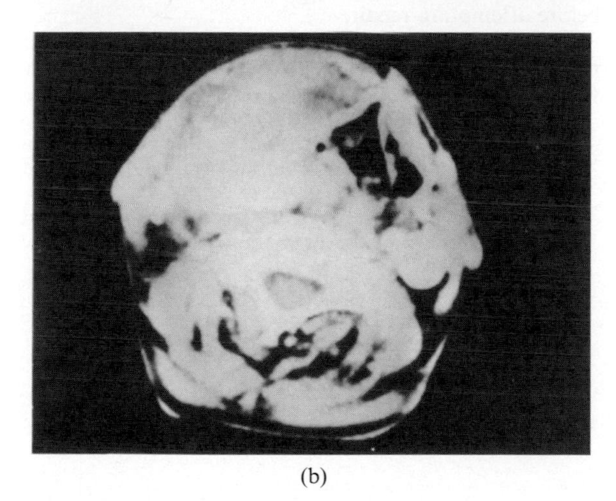

(b)

Figure 1. (a) Pre-contrast and (b) post-contrast CT scans.

A 63-year-old man was admitted to hospital complaining of progressive neck swelling, with bruising and increasing difficulty in swallowing. These symptoms were preceded by a severe bout of coughing. The night prior to admission he had eaten a meal of haddock, had slept well but then experienced the bout of coughing. He had a past medical history of polycythaemia which had been treated with busulphan and regular venesection.

Examination revealed a distressed patient with massive pulsatile swelling on the right side of his neck. The overlying skin was bruised. His blood pressure measured 150/80. His voice was soft, but there was no stridor. The rest of the examination was unremarkable. A contrast enhanced CT examination was performed (Figure 1). The patient proceeded to angiography (Figure 2). What is the diagnosis?

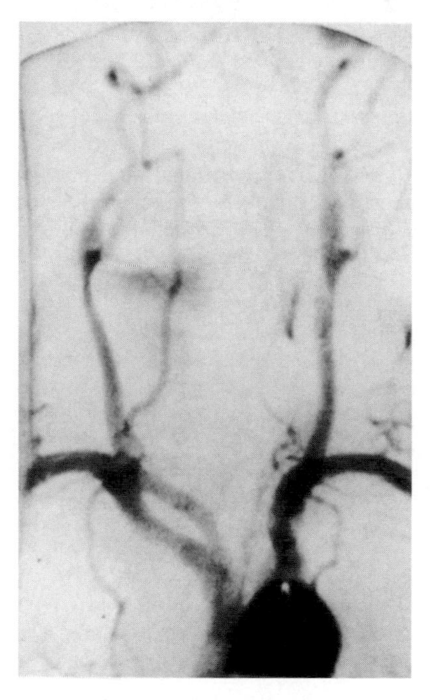

Figure 2. Arch aortogram.

Based on the case of the month originally published in Br J Radiol 1994;67:825–6

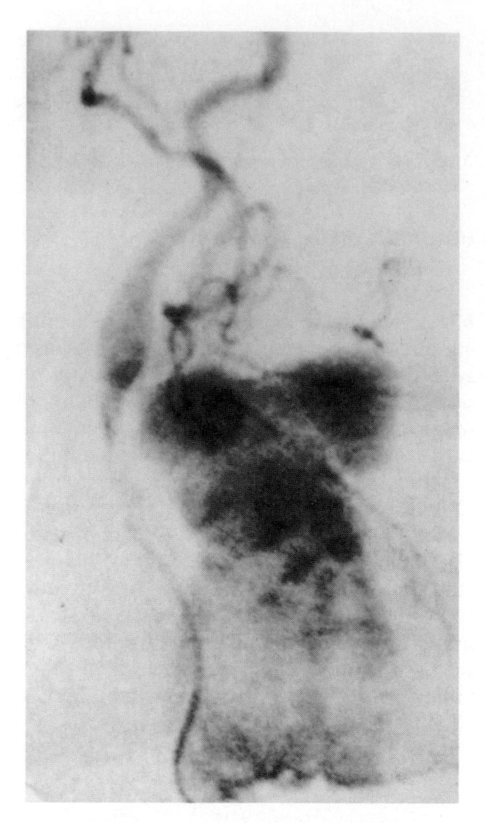

Figure 3. PA view—right common carotid injection.

The CT examination demonstrated a large, slightly hyperdense collection in the region of the right carotid sheath. It showed bright contrast enhancement. The surrounding soft tissues were stretched and the internal jugular vein was deviated laterally. The upper airway was also slightly impinged upon and deviated, but patent.

An arch aortogram and selective study of the right common carotid artery are shown. A jet of contrast medium streamed medially at the level of the common carotid bifurcation (Figure 2) and progressive accumulation of contrast medium in a collection was demonstrated (Figure 3).

At operation a 2 mm hole in the medial wall of the common carotid artery was located just proximal to the bifurcation. No fish bone was found. The surgeons noted that the superior horn of the thyroid cartilage was very sharp and seemed very close to the puncture in the artery. The hole was repaired and the false aneurysm drained. The patient made an uncomplicated recovery.

The real cause of the perforation was never definitely established. In a review of the literature, it has never been reported that the thyroid cartilage has caused such an injury. In a review of 2394 cases of foreign body in the oesophagus carried out in 1978, only two developed the complication of oesophago–aortic fistula and both were fatal [1]. Other isolated reports of arterial perforation by a variety of objects also resulted in death [2, 3].

Carotid artery perforation is a surgical emergency. The symptoms and signs are suggestive of the diagnosis, but definitive imaging is most helpful for the surgeon before attempting repair.

References

1. Nandi P, Ong GB. Foreign body in the oesophagus; review of 2394 cases. Br J Surg 1978;65:5–9.
2. Russo SS, Taff ML. Sudden death resulting from chicken bone perforation of the oesophagus. Am J Forensic Med Pathol 1986;7:263–5.
3. Weaver AD, Brown TP. Fatal transoesophageal carotid arterial perforation by thorns in a calf. J Am Vet Med Assoc 1988;193:1415–6.

What a blow!

G KUMAR, P J BRADLEY and M L WASTIE

Department of Radiology, University Hospital, Nottingham NG7 2UH, UK

Figures 1 and 2 are coronal and axial T_1 weighted images of the neck in a 22-year-old male. What is happening?

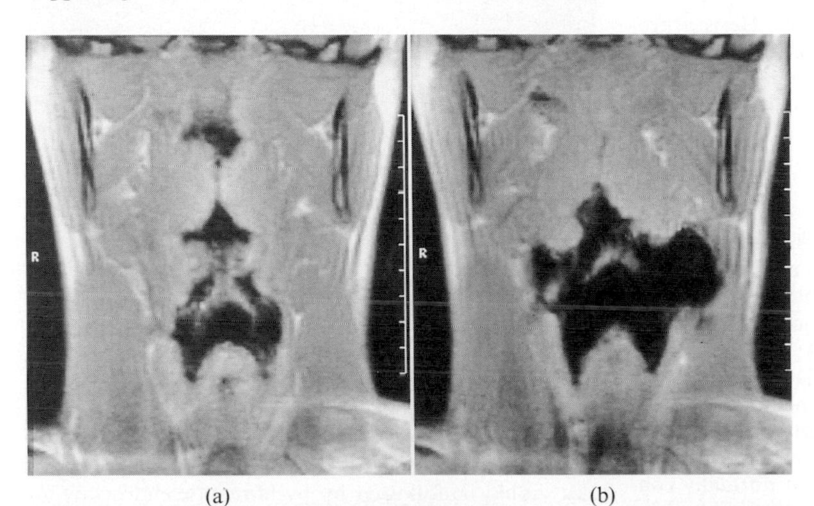

(a) (b)

Figure 1. Coronal T_1 weighted images of the neck.

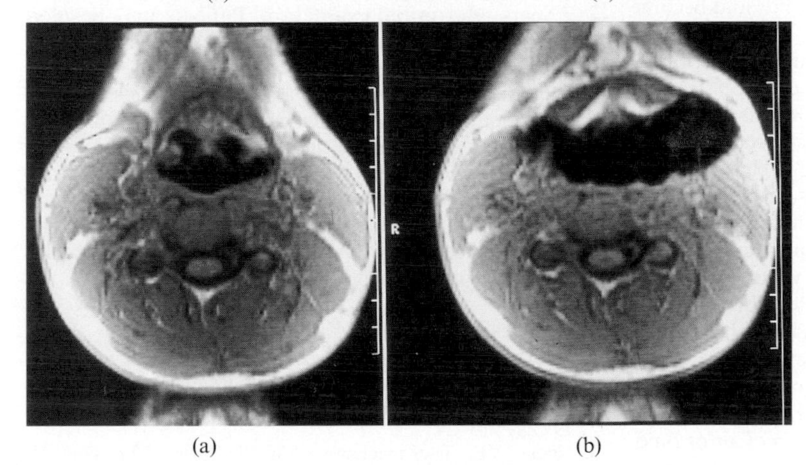

(a) (b)

Figure 2. Axial T_1 weighted images of the neck.

Based on the case of the month originally published in Br J Radiol 1998;71:799–800.

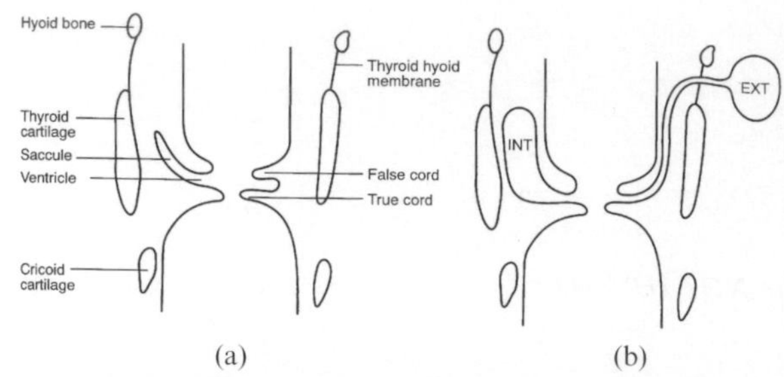

Figure 3. (a) Diagram of normal larynx. On the right side the saccule is unusually large. (b) Internal (INT) and external (EXT) laryngocoeles.

The patient has bilateral laryngocoeles. He is a professional trumpeter who complained of swelling of the neck when playing his instrument. Figures 1a and 2a were taken during shallow breathing. Figures 1b and 2b were taken while performing the Valsalva manoeuvre, when the laryngocoeles appeared.

A laryngocoele is a dilatation of the laryngeal saccule. The saccule is a narrow blind pouch arising from the anterior end of the laryngeal ventricle, extending superiorly into the paralaryngeal space and bounded laterally by the thyroid cartilage. A laryngocoele is defined as internal if it lies within the larynx or external if it protrudes through the thyrohyoid membrane. Mixed laryngocoeles, which are the commonest type, have both internal and external components (Figure 3). As the laryngocoele communicates with the larynx it normally contains air but may be filled with mucus or pus and become fluid filled.

There is diversity of opinion regarding the aetiology of laryngocoeles. A congenital predisposition is considered a likely possibility, a laryngocoele developing if the intraglottic pressure is raised such as occurs in glass blowers and brass instrument players [1]. However, this history is not present in many reports of laryngocoele and laryngocoeles are commonly unilateral.

The saccule is a vestigial structure in humans. Large lateral air sacs arise from the laryngeal ventricles in apes and are thought to enable the animal to rebreath while holding its breath [2, 3]. It has been postulated that laryngocoeles are phylogenic remants of these air filled sacs.

There is an association between laryngocoeles and carcinoma of the larynx [4, 5], the tumour obstructing the outflow of the saccule and causing retention of air or fluid. It is therefore important to investigate fully patients with laryngocoeles. Plain radiography (Figure 4), linear tomography and contrast laryngography were previously performed [6]. CT is much superior to these methods, especially in fluid filled laryngocoeles [7]. Nowadays MRI, because of its multiplanar capability and superior soft tissue resolution, is the investigation of choice for showing the laryngocoele and any associated tumour.

The majority of laryngocoeles are asymptomatic, usually presenting in the fifth decade. All patients with laryngocoeles should undergo direct laryngoscopy and biopsy of the ventricle because of the association with laryngeal cancer. Patients with asymptomatic laryngocoeles should be followed up by fibreoptic endoscopy for 2–3 years after initial evaluation. Patients may develop respiratory distress if the air filled pouch becomes blocked and develops into a mucus filled mass. This may become infected and become a laryngopyocoele.

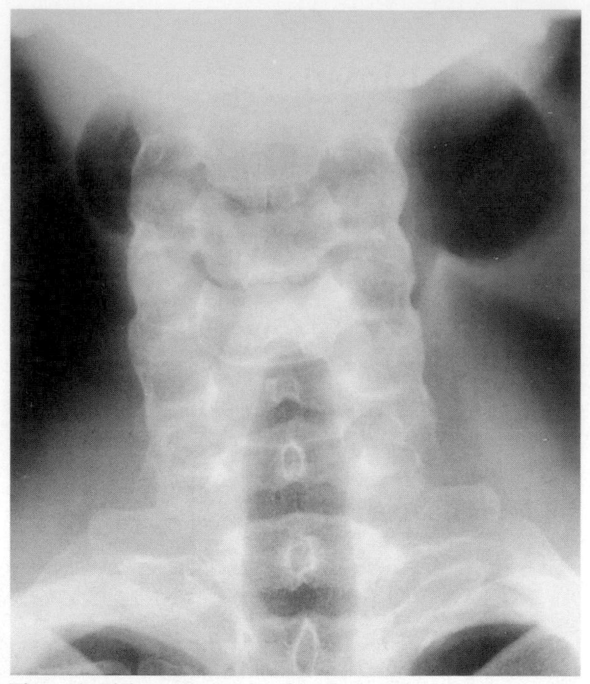

Figure 4. Plain radiograph with the patient performing the Valsalva manoeuvre, showing the laryngocoeles as air filled sacs on either side of the neck.

Treatment of laryngocoeles is surgical excision of the sac by either endoscopic or open techniques. Hemi or total laryngectomy may be indicated in patients with a laryngocoele secondary to malignant disease.

Surgery was avoided in this patient because he changed his technique to avoid producing laryngocoeles when he played his trumpet.

References

1. Hubbard C. Laryngocoele—A study of five cases with reference to the radiological features. Clin Radiol 1981;38:639–43.
2. Stell PM, Maran AGD. Laryngocoele. J Laryngol Otol 1975;89:915–24.
3. Negus VE. The mechanism of the larynx. London: W Heineman, 1929:96–105.
4. Close GL, Merkel M, Deaton WC, Burns DK, Schaffer SD. A symptomatic laryngocoele: incidence and association with laryngeal cancer. Ann Otol Rhinol Laryngol 1987;96:393–9.
5. Harvey RT, Ibrahim H, Yousley DM, Weinstein GS. Radiological findings in a carcinoma associated laryngocoele. Ann Otol Rhinol Laryngol 1996;105:405–8.
6. Trapnell DH. The radiological diagnosis of laryngocoeles. Clin Radiol 1962;13:68–72.
7. Morgan NJ, Emberton P. CT scanning and laryngocoeles. J Laryngol Otol 1994;108:266–8.

A pain in the neck!

R RAJAH, A BOOTHROYD and W R LEES

Department of Radiology, The Middlesex Hospital, Mortimer Street, London W1N 8AA, UK

A 36-year-old female presented with a 24 h history of constant severe pain in the left side of her neck. On clinical examination there was marked tenderness and swelling within the left anterior triangle of the neck. She had documented polycystic ovarian disease and her two previous pregnancies were induced by Clomiphene and an LHRH pump, respectively. 2 months prior to this presentation she had received 10 000 u of human chorionic gonadotrophin (HCG) and her ovaries were monitored regularly. 3 weeks later she developed abdominal distension, nausea, weight gain, pleural effusion, low blood pressure and a tachycardia. A frontal chest radiograph was taken (Figure 1). At this stage a clinical diagnosis was made and treatment commenced. 3 weeks later she presented with neck pain and an ultrasound examination was performed (Figures 2a and b) using 5 MHz linear probe.

What abnormalities are demonstrated on the chest radiograph and ultrasound? What is your diagnosis?

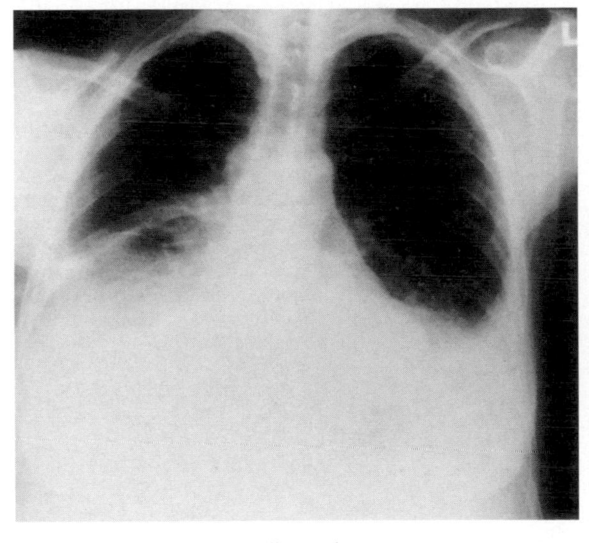

Figure 1. A frontal chest radiograph.

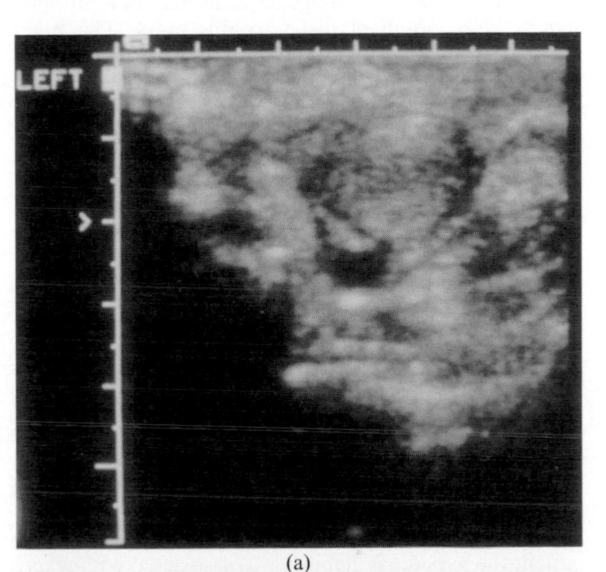

(a)

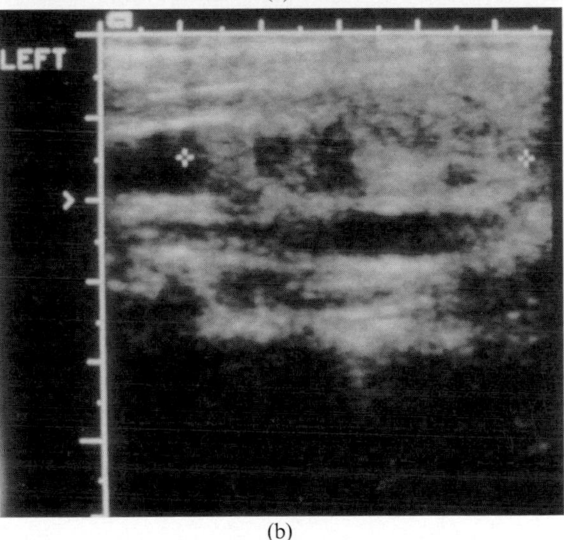

(b)

Figure 2. (a, b) Ultrasound examination of the neck.

Based on the case of the month originally published in Br J Radiol 1991;64:867–8.

The chest radiograph showed bilateral pleural effusions which were compatible with the hyperstimulation syndrome. Diagnosis of a pulmonary embolism was also made, but in view of the strong clinical evidence and early pregnancy an isotope ventilation/perfusion scan was not performed. The patient was heparinized for 7 days after which anticoagulation was discontinued.

The ultrasound examination showed a markedly distended left internal jugular vein. The lumen was completely occluded by echogenic material. No Doppler signals were obtained distal to this mass. The other structures in the neck and the right internal jugular vein were normal. The appearance of the left internal jugular vein was consistent with thrombosis.

The appearances are those of a thrombosis of the left internal jugular vein. These thrombotic episodes are presumed to be caused by hypercoagulability secondary to ovarian hyperstimulation and pregnancy.

Thrombosis of the internal jugular vein is relatively uncommon but is most frequently associated with central venous catheterization [1, 2]. The incidence is gradually rising with the increase in the use of catheters for intravenous feeding, venous pressure measurement, chemotherapy and rapid fluid administration. Spontaneous thrombosis is extremely rare but occasional cases [3] have been reported. In these cases factors such as reduced blood flow (*e.g.* chronic heart failure) or hypercoagulability (*e.g.* oral contraceptives) may play a role. In this patient the hypercoagulability was associated with severe ovarian hyperstimulation, *i.e.* massive ovarian enlargement, ascites and pleural effusion [4], secondary to her treatment for infertility. In the absence of recent venous catheterization the diagnosis is often not considered [5] and a high degree of clinical suspicion is required in the presence of non-specific clinical findings. Other less frequent causes include contiguous head and neck infection [6] and intravenous drug abuse [7].

The diagnosis can also be made using phlebography [8], scintigraphy [9], CT [1] and magnetic resonance [10]. The advantage of ultrasound is that it provides a non-invasive, accurate method of establishing the diagnosis and may exclude other causes of neck swelling.

Doppler studies are valuable in demonstrating reduced or absent flow and are particularly helpful if there is a very recent thrombosis, since fresh clot has identical acoustic properties to liquid blood.

[*One study has shown that jugular vein thrombosis was a long-term complication in a quarter of newborn patients who underwent jugular vein catheterization [11], ED*]

References

1. Krespi YP, Komisar A, Lucente FE. Complications of internal jugular vein catheterization. Arch Otolaryngol 1981;107:310–2.
2. McNeill R. Internal jugular vein thrombosis. Head Neck Surg 1981;3:247.
3. Witte R de B, Lameris JS. Real-time ultrasound diagnosis of internal jugular vein thrombosis. J Clin Ultrasound 1986;14: 712–7.
4. Painvain E, Barlese MG, Mastrojanni F, Bolzano Gaglione R, Dragone L, Ferrarott M, Taramanni C. Ultrasound evaluation of the ovarian hyperstimulation syndrome. Acta Eur Fertil 1987;18:39–43.
5. Albertyn LE, Alcock MK. Diagnosis of internal jugular vein thrombosis. Radiology 1986;162:505–8.
6. Yau PC, Norante JD. Thrombophlebitis of the internal jugular vein secondary to pharyngitis. Arch Otolaryngol 1980;106:507–8.
7. Mehar GL, Colley DP, Clark RA, Herwig SR. Computed tomographic demonstration of cervical abscess and jugular vein thrombosis. A complication of intravenous drug abuse in the neck. Arch Otolaryngol 1981;107:313–5.
8. Chastre J, Cornud F, Bouchama A, Viau F, Benacerraf R, Gibert C. Thrombosis as a complication of pulmonary artery catheterization via internal jugular vein: Prospective evaluation by phlebography. N Engl J Med 1982;306: 278–81.
9. De Navdo SJ, De Navdo GL. Iodine 123. Fibrinogen scintigraphy. Semin Nucl Med 1977;7:245–52.
10. Braun IF, Hoffman JC, Malko JA, Pettigrew RI, Daniels W, Davies PC. Jugular venous thrombosis: MR imaging. Radiology 1985;157:357–60.
11. Rand T, Kohl Hauser C, Popow C, et al. Sonographic detection of internal jugular vein thrombosis after central venous catheterization in the newborn period. Paediatr Radiol 1994;24:577–80.

An unusual cause of gastrointestinal haemorrhage

R C TRAVIS

Department of Radiology, Greenlane Hospital, Auckland, New Zealand

An 18-year-old girl was referred for angiography of a lump under her right heel (Figures 1–3) which was painful on weight-bearing and limited her choice of footwear. On examination, four similar lesions were found elsewhere. She had had four substantial gastrointestinal bleeds requiring transfusion, as well as laparotomies for persistent gastrointestinal blood loss and suspected intussusception at which 27 bowel lesions were resected. See also Figure 4. What is the diagnosis?

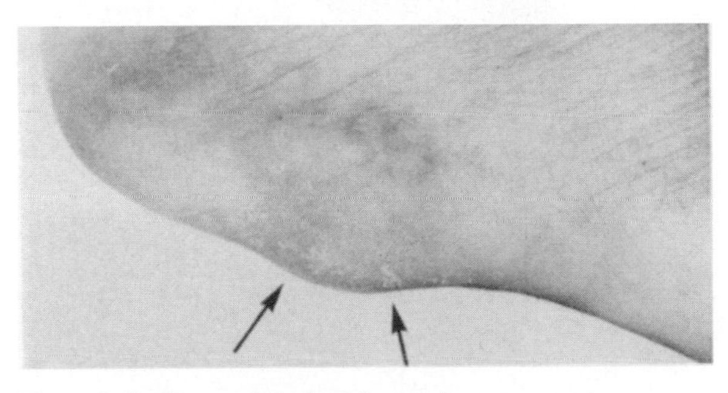

Figure 1. Lesion on right heel (arrows).

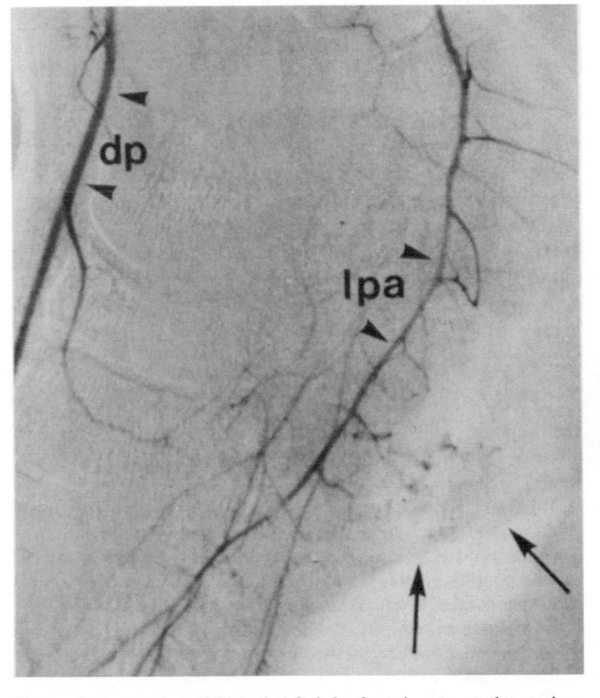

Figure 2. Lateral radiograph of right foot in external rotation. Arterial phase subtraction. (lpa, lateral plantar artery; dp, dorsalis pedis).

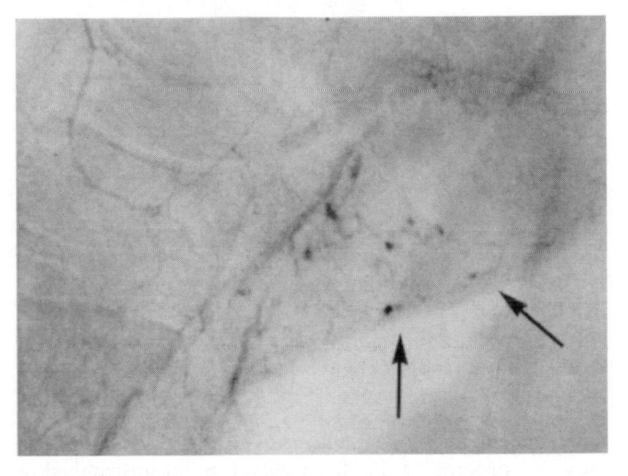

Figure 3. Venous phase subtraction.

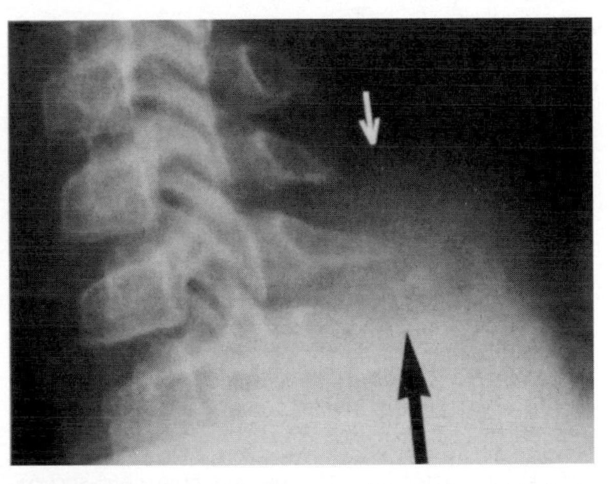

Figure 4. Lateral cervical spine at age 12 years (arrows indicate abnormality).

Based on the case of the month originally published in Br J Radiol 1987;60:933–4.

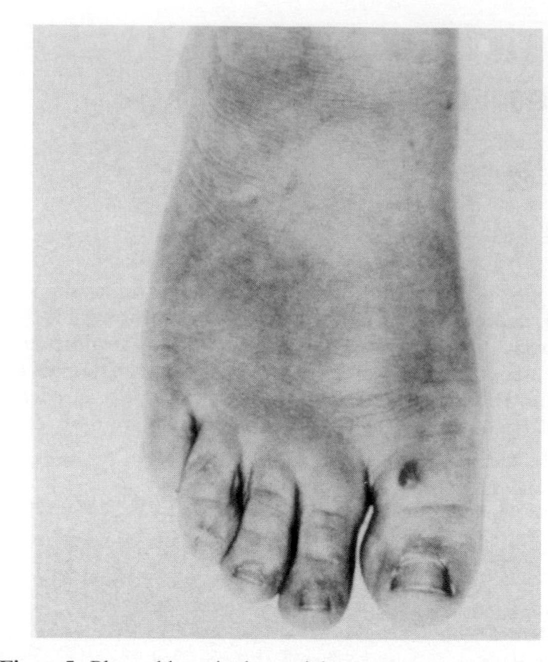

Figure 5. Blue rubber nipple on right great toe.

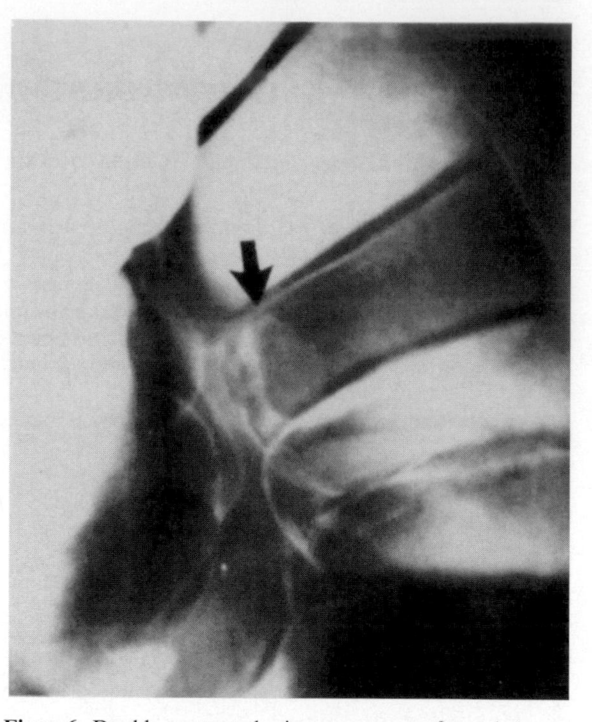

Figure 6. Double-contrast barium enema, performed 1 year after second laparotomy, showing a polyp (arrow) in the sigmoid colon.

The diagnosis is blue rubber bleb naevus syndrome (BRBNS).

In his original description, Bean [1] described three characteristic skin lesions: Type 1, large disfiguring haemangiomas (Figure 1); Type 2, blue rubber nipples that are compressible (Figure 5); and Type 3, irregular blue-black macules. The lesions may be painful and associated with local hyperhidrosis. Lesions of the skin and bowel may be present at birth or develop on normal skin, and vary in number from one to several hundreds. Histologically, they are all cavernous haemangiomas.

Patients usually present for cosmetic reasons and/or gastrointestinal blood loss. The haemangiomas can occur throughout the gastrointestinal tract from mouth to anus but are more common in the small bowel. In association with BRBNS, cavernous haemangiomas have been described in virtually every organ and coelomic cavity [2]. The lesions are not pre-malignant but isolated cases of associated malignancies have been reported [3].

Radiology can assist the diagnosis by demonstrating phleboliths (Figure 4), polyps on barium studies (Figure 6) and the characteristic angiographic appearance (Figures 2, 3) of a cavernous haemangioma, *i.e.* early opacification which then increases in the venous phase.

Angiography and radionuclide studies may help to localize gut lesions which are actively bleeding.

Carbon dioxide laser therapy has been used successfully to remove the cutaneous manifestations [4] and, with the development of endoscopic laser techniques, the need for multiple laparotomies may be obviated.

Blue rubber bleb naevus syndrome is an example of a rare dysembryoplasia; an autosomal dominant inheritance has been reported [5] but most cases are sporadic. It is included in the differential diagnosis of gastrointestinal polyposis syndromes with skin manifestations, namely Peutz–Jeghers, Osler–Weber–Rendu, Gardner's, Kaposi's, Cronkhite–Canada and Cowden's syndromes.

[*Blue naevi are included in the Carney complex. This includes the NAME syndrome (naevi, atrial myxoma, myxoid neurofibroma and ephelides, and a variant of it called the LAMB syndrome: lentigines, atrial myxoma, mucocutaneous myxoma, blue naevi [6], ED*]

References

1. Bean WB. Vascular spiders and related lesions of the skin. Illinois: Charles C Thomas, 1958.
2. Rice JS, Fischer DS. Blue rubber bleb naevus syndrome. Arch Dermatol 1962;86:163–71.
3. Hoffman T, Chasko S, Safai B. Association of blue rubber bleb naevus syndrome with chronic lymphocytic leukaemia and hypernephroma. Johns Hopkins Med J 1978;142:91–4.
4. Olsen TG, Milroy SK, Goldman L, Filder JP. Laser surgery for the blue rubber bleb naevus syndrome. Arch Dermatol 1979;115:81–2.
5. Munkrad M. Blue rubber bleb naevus syndrome. Dermatologica 1983;167:307–9.
6. Taybi H, Lachman RS. Radiology of syndromes, metabolic disorders, and skeletal dysplasias (4th edn). St Louis: Mosby, 1996.

Common symptom: uncommon cause

K T TUNG and G F WILSON

Department of Radiology, St Thomas' Hospital, Lambeth Palace Road, London SE1, UK

A 48-year-old Bangladeshi man presented with a 2 month history of low lumbar back pain radiating down the right leg. He otherwise felt well and in particular had no cough, fever or weight loss.

Examination showed local tenderness over the lower lumbar spine with decreased range of movements but no neurological deficit. The remainder of the physical examination was normal.

The chest radiograph (Figure 1), lateral radiograph of the lumbar spine (Figure 2) and ultrasound scan of the porta hepatis (Figure 3) are shown below.

What is the most likely diagnosis?

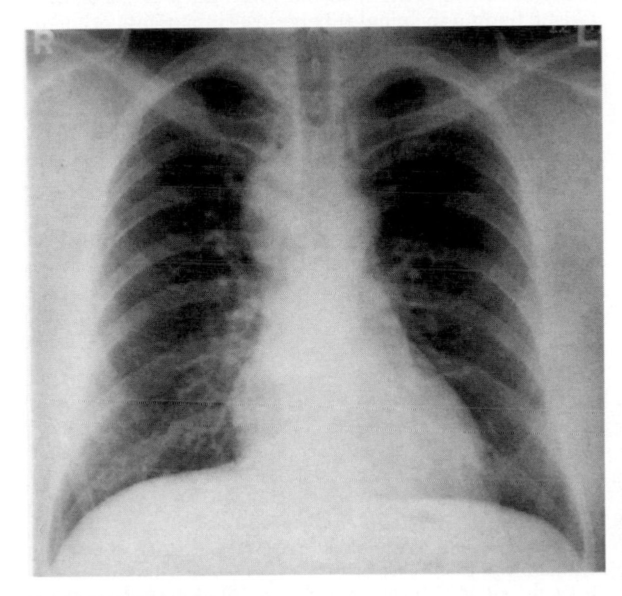

Figure 1. Chest radiograph.

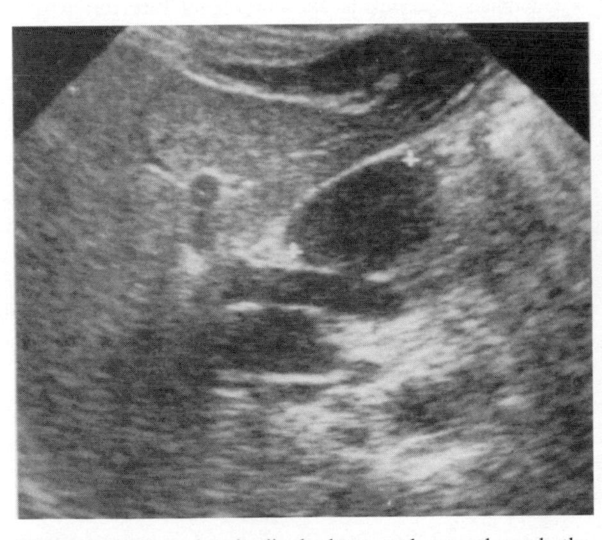

Figure 3. Oblique longitudinal ultrasound scan through the porta hepatis; remainder of abdomen was normal.

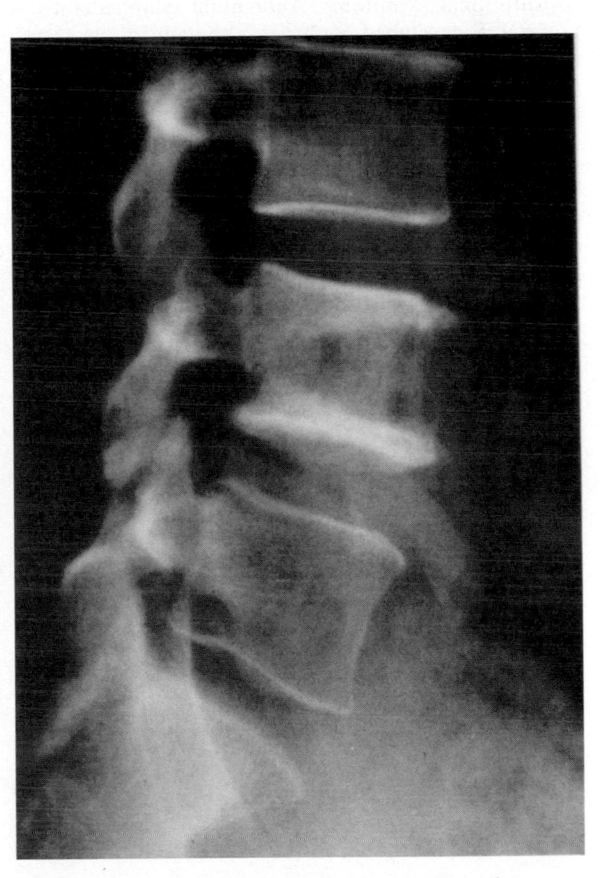

Figure 2. Lateral radiograph of the lower lumbar spine.

Based on the case of the month originally published in Br J Radiol 1989;62:1029–30.

The chest radiograph showed right paratracheal lymphadenopathy with normal hila and clear lungs. The radiograph of the lumbar spine showed a wedge-shaped lytic defect with sclerotic margins in the anterior part of the body of L4 with normal adjacent end-plates and disc spaces. The ultrasound scan of the porta hepatis showed a round, hypoechoic mass typical of an enlarged lymph node lying anterior to the portal vein, which was seen entering the liver and dividing into right and left branches. Posterior to the portal vein, the inferior vena cava runs obliquely through the plane of the section.

Mediastinoscopy and biopsy of the paratracheal nodes demonstrated giant cell granulomata and acid-fast bacilli on Ziehl–Nielson staining, confirming tuberculous lymphadenitis. The patient was started on anti-tuberculous therapy comprising rifampicin, isoniazid and ethambutol. A follow-up chest radiograph at 3 months showed reduction in size of the paratracheal lymphadenopathy but the lumbar spine appearances were not significantly changed.

Tuberculous lymphadenitis is still the most common form of non-pulmonary tuberculosis in England and Wales [1], most often involving the cervical nodes. These patients usually present with neck swelling or minor constitutional symptoms. Abdominal lymphadenitis is unusual in developed countries, although in one survey of abdominal tuberculosis using CT evaluation, adenopathy, including enlarged porta hepatis nodes, was the most common finding [2].

Skeletal tuberculosis accounts for almost 15% of non-pulmonary cases and lesions in the thoracic and lumbar vertebrae predominate. Infection is presumed to have spread by a haematogenous route from an infected focus elsewhere or alternatively from involved paraaortic lymph nodes in direct contact with vertebral bodies.

The most common radiological appearance is that of disc space narrowing with erosion of the adjacent end-plates, but the subligamentous erosion of the anterior part of the vertebral body without disc involvement is a well recognized form [3]. Such anterior erosions may produce "gouge" defects similar to those occasionally seen in lymphoma. A destructive lesion with or without marginal sclerosis confined to a single vertebral body with normal adjacent discs and vertebrae is also a characteristic finding in spinal tuberculosis in patients originating from India, Africa and the Caribbean.

The differential diagnosis in our case includes lymphoma although the distribution of involved nodes with no peripheral lymphadenopathy and the unifocal bone involvement at presentation make this diagnosis less likely.

In conclusion, the diagnosis of tuberculous lymphadenitis must be considered in Asian patients who present with unusual lymphadenopathy and destructive spinal lesions.

[[4] is a good review of current imaging of TB, ED]

References

1. National Survey of Tuberculosis in England and Wales 1978–79. Report from the Medical Research Council Tuberculosis and Chest Diseases Unit. Br Med J 1980;281:895–8.
2. Hulnick DH, Megibow AJ, Naidich DP, Hilton S, Cho KC, Balthazar EJ. Abdominal tuberculosis: CT evaluation. Radiology 1985;157:198–204.
3. Chapman M, Murray RO, Stoker DJ. Tuberculosis of the bones and joints. In: Felson B, editor. Radiology of tuberculosis. New York: Grune and Stratton, 1979:80–96.
4. Goodman PC, Jinkins JR. Imaging of tuberculosis and craniospinal tuberculosis. Radiol Clin N Am 1995;33:4.

A nasty shock on awakening

[1]W C G PEH, [2]F S K CHU and [3]T K HO

Departments of [1]Diagnostic Radiology and [3]Orthopaedic Surgery, University of Hong Kong, and [2]Department of Diagnostic Radiology, Queen Mary Hospital, Hong Kong

A 52-year-old man awoke one morning to find, to his distress, that he had become paraplegic. There was no known history of trauma. The motor and sensory deficits were subsequently confirmed on physical examination. He had no significant past medical history other than having a chronically stiff and aching back for several years.

A lumbar myelogram was done and contrast medium was run up the thoracic spine (Figure 1). This was followed by CT starting from T6 level (Figure 2). What findings are demonstrated and what is the likely diagnosis?

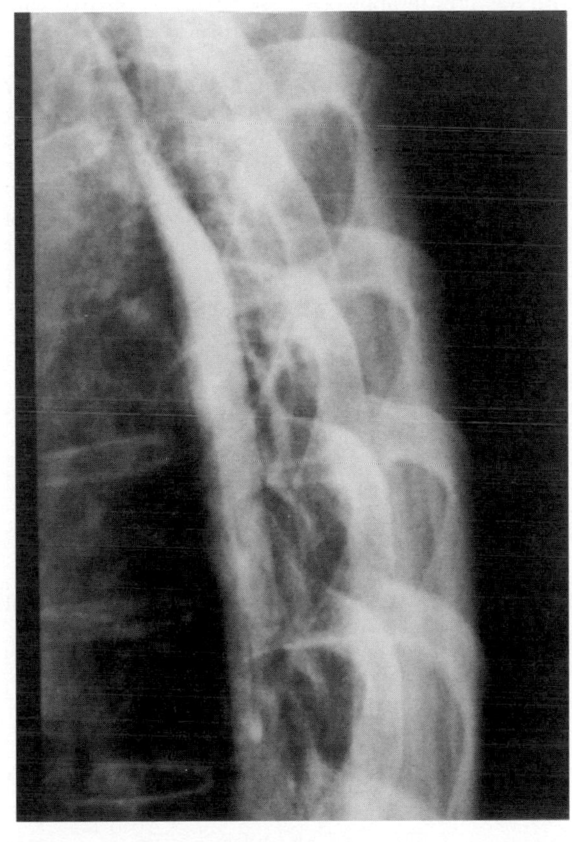

Figure 1. Myelogram of thoracic region, with patient in head down position.

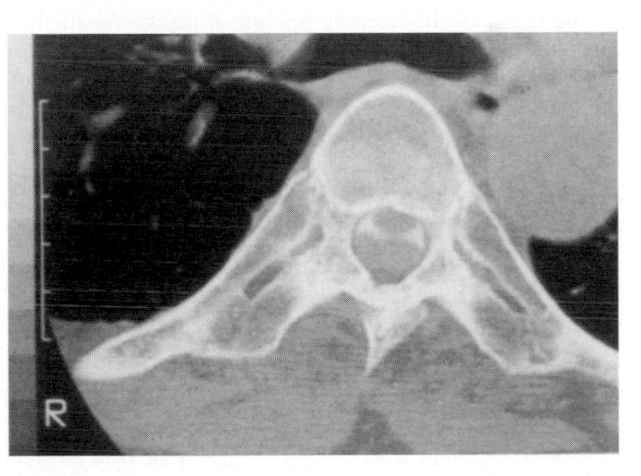

Figure 2. CT scan at level of T6 vertebral body.

Based on the case of the month originally published in Br J Radiol 1994;67:1141–2.

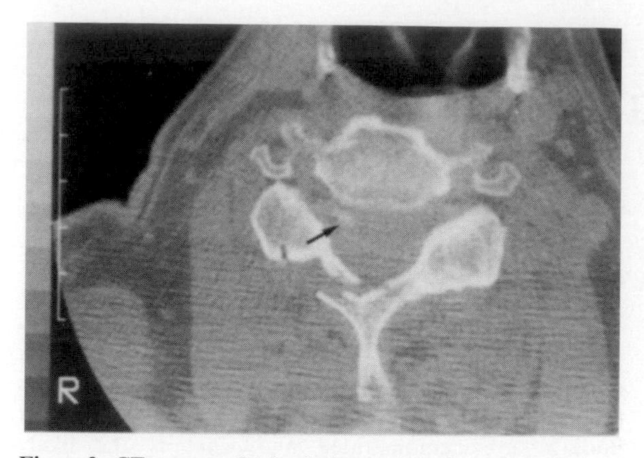

Figure 3. CT scan at C6 level shows right facet and bilateral laminar fractures. Small amount of contrast medium within the displaced dural sac is arrowed.

The myelogram showed obstruction to contrast flow at T6 level. CT demonstrated a posterior intradural extramedullary lesion compressing the spinal cord. Extradural fat is well preserved at this level. There is fusion of the costotransverse and costovertebral joints bilaterally. These appearances are suggestive of ankylosing spondylitis with a subdural haematoma.

The cause of the haematoma was a transverse fracture through the upper C7 vertebral body with C6 laminar and C6/7 facetal fractures (Figure 3). At the level of fractures, the haematoma was extradural. There was gradual transition from an extradural to a subdural haematoma at the cervicothoracic region. Radiographs of the sacroiliac joints and the cervical, thoracic and lumbar spine showed typical changes of advanced ankylosing spondylitis.

These findings were confirmed when the patient underwent decompressive laminectomy and haematoma evacuation.

Fracture of the cervical spine is one of the rare recognized complications of longstanding ankylosing spondylitis. Although sacroiliac and thoracolumbar spine involvement are more common in this disease, fractures when they do occur, tend to do so in the cervical spine [1].

The rigid spine of patients with advanced ankylosing spondylitis is more prone to fractures as it lacks the mobility to accommodate any excessive movement or stress. In such a spine, even trivial forces tend to be magnified. The amount of trauma which causes fractures in these spines is often minor [1, 2]. Conversely, it is well recognized that cervical spine trauma may be the presenting feature of occult advanced ankylosing spondylitis [2].

The site of fracture has been related to the neurological outcome. In the study of Harding et al [2], patients whose fracture line ran through the disc space had significantly less neurological injury and had a much better prognosis. A chalkstick fracture occurring through the vertebral body, however, tended to cause severe neurological damage, as was the case in our patient. A fracture through the vertebral body is probably of significance as bleeding from the cancellous bone and damaged epidural and perivertebral veins may lead to further neurological damage and this is recognized as a particular hazard of fractures in ankylosing spondylitis [3, 4]. Spinal epidural haematomas also occur more frequently with fractures in ankylosing spondylitis compared with fractures of normal cervical spines [1, 4].

Spinal subdural haematoma in the absence of fracture has been reported in ankylosing spondylitis [5]. In our case, presence of haemorrhage on both sides of the dura suggests tearing of the dura mater during or after the traumatic episode, with tracking of blood from the epidural into the subdural space.

Management of these injuries is aimed at reduction of the fracture and stabilization of the spine, by surgical or conservative means. Laminectomy is usually reserved for decompression of the spinal cord.

References

1. Hunter T, Dubo HIC. Spinal fractures complicating ankylosing spondylitis. Arth Rheumat 1983;26:751–9.
2. Harding JR, McCall IW, Park WM, Jones BF. Fracture of the cervical spine in ankylosing spondylitis. Br J Radiol 1985;58:3–7.
3. Farhat SM, Schneider RC, Gray JM. Traumatic spine extradural hematoma associated with cervical fractures in rheumatoid spondylitis. J Trauma 1973;13:591–9.
4. Bohlman HH. Acute fractures and dislocations of the cervical spine. J Bone Joint Surg 1979;61A:1119–42.
5. Sokoloff J, Coel, Ignelzi RJ. Spinal subdural hematoma. Radiology 1976;120:116.

An inevitable progression?

D M HANSELL

Department of Radiology, Westminster Hospital, London, UK

At the age of 56 years the patient, a previously healthy woman, complained of dysphagia and regurgitation. A radiograph from a barium meal examination at that time is shown (Figure 1), and she was treated surgically. 17 years later, now aged 73 years, she returned with an 8-month history of increasingly painful dysphagia and weight loss.

On examination she appeared pale and wasted, but had no lymphadenopathy or other abnormal physical signs. A full blood count and chest radiograph were normal. A barium swallow was performed and is shown (Figure 2).

She then received treatment, following which another barium examination was performed (Figure 3).

She improved symptomatically but developed a cough with purulent sputum. After a chest radiograph the barium meal examination was repeated (Figure 4).

What was the original diagnosis and treatment and what occurred 17 years later? How inevitable is this sequence of events?

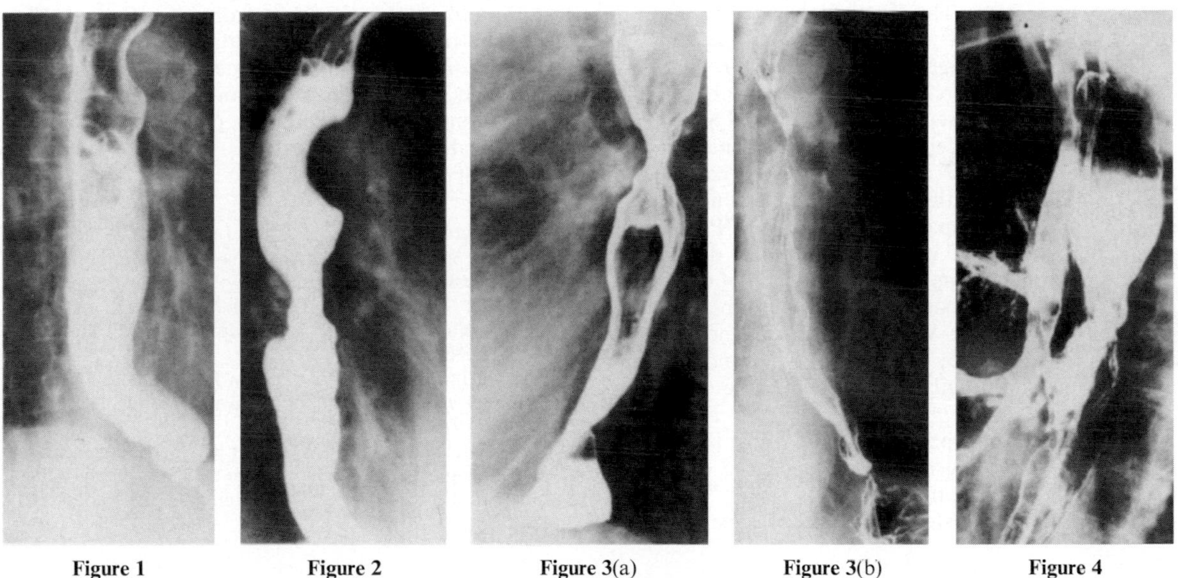

Figure 1 **Figure 2** **Figure 3**(a) **Figure 3**(b) **Figure 4**

Figure 1. Barium swallow radiograph at first presentation. **Figure 2.** Barium swallow study at second presentation, 17 years later. **Figure 3.** a,b Appearances after treatment. **Figure 4.** Barium swallow study after the patient developed a cough, 4 months after treatment.

Based on the case of the month originally published in Br J Radiol 1986;59:521–2.

Figure 1 showed a tapering lower end of a dilated oesophagus with a short, narrowed segment below the diaphragm (typical of achalasia). This was successfully treated by a Heller's myotomy.

Figure 2 showed a short, eccentrically narrowed segment of oesophagus with irregular margins and a sharp transition to normal width: the radiological signs of a carcinoma. Endoscopy and biopsy showed a poorly differentiated squamous cell carcinoma and over the next 7 weeks the patient was treated with radical radiotherapy. A three-field planned technique was used with daily fractions of 200 cGy. The total effective tumour dose was 5400 cGy in 27 fractions.

After radiotherapy (Figure 3a) there was a narrowed segment with a gradual transition to normal width. In Figure 3b (ulceration has now occurred) and in Figure 4 perforation into the bronchus is shown. An Atkinson tube was inserted endoscopically, but the patient died soon afterwards, 7 months after the diagnosis of carcinoma of the oesophagus was made.

The differential diagnosis of dysphagia in a patient known to have had achalasia largely depends upon the time interval between the diagnosis of achalasia and the recurrence of dysphagia. Reflux oesophagitis with consequent stricture formation occurs in up to 52% of patients following myotomy, usually within 4 years, and many surgeons combine a Heller's myotomy with an anti-reflux procedure to prevent this [1]. The typical post-myotomy appearances of the lower oesophagus are clearly seen in Figure 3a where a fluid level is present within the mucosal herniation. This is often visible in only one projection.

The differential diagnosis of dysphagia in an elderly patient is between carcinoma, stricture, neuromuscular and "other" causes. Pseudobulbar palsy and myasthenia gravis manifest themselves as widespread neurological disturbances and are almost exclusively confined to abnormalities of initiation of swallowing and upper oesophageal function. Virtually all patients with Parkinson's disease have abnormal oesophageal motility disorder on cineradiography and up to 20% complain of dysphagia. Other causes of dysphagia in this age group are scleroderma, the Plummer–Vinson syndrome and extrinsic compression caused by mediastinal lymph nodes or an aortic aneurysm, usually readily identifiable on barium swallow studies.

The history of this patient and the recognized association between achalasia and oesophageal carcinoma make malignant change the most likely cause of dysphagia. The reported incidence of squamous cell carcinoma in patients with achalasia varies between 1.7% and 29% [2]. The treatment of achalasia does not appear to reduce the risk of subsequent development of carcinoma of the oesophagus. The carcinoma is often at the site of the fluid level seen in the oesophagus prior to treatment. The prognosis of patients with achalasia who develop carcinoma is particularly poor since the tumour will have reached a considerable size before obstruction occurs. In addition, early detection by endoscopy or barium swallow may be hindered by the presence of fluid or food residue in the oesophagus.

The association between achalasia and oesophageal carcinoma has been questioned [3]. A group of 91 patients with achalasia was followed up for periods ranging from 6 months to 23 years. None of these patients developed oesophageal carcinoma. In another part of the study there was no convincing history of previous achalasia in 153 patients with oesophageal carcinoma. It is likely that oesophageal carcinoma is an extremely rare complication of achalasia and there is no justification for repeated barium swallow studies or endoscopies to detect early carcinoma.

Some patients with the typical radiological features of achalasia may have a carcinoma of the oesophagogastric junction [4] and this should be suspected in any patient over 40 years old with recent onset of oesophageal symptoms and the radiological signs of achalasia.

The complication of tracheo-oesophageal fistula is more commonly seen as a result of a primary bronchogenic carcinoma invading the oesophagus. Because of the relative mobility of the oesophagus, a carcinoma of the oesophagus is more likely to spread along the submucosa than to involve the surrounding mediastinal structures. The treatment with radical radiotherapy almost certainly contributed to the formation of the fistula in this case. It is important to perform a barium swallow examination with the patient prone if a tracheo-oesophageal fistula is suspected.

References

1. Black J, Vorbach AN, Leigh Collis J. Results of Heller's operation for achalasia of the oesophagus. The importance of hiatal repair. Br J Surg 1976;63:949–53.
2. Wychulis AR, Woolam GL, Anderesen HA, Ellis FH. Achalasia and carcinoma of the esophagus. J Am Med Assoc 1971;215:1638–41.
3. Chuong J, Du Bovik S, McCallum RW. Achalasia as a risk factor for esophageal carcinoma: a reappraisal. Dig Dis Sci 1984;29:1105–8.
4. Ott DJ, Gelfand DW, Wu WC, Kerr RM. Secondary achalasia in esophagogastric carcinoma: re-emphasis of a difficult differential problem. Revista Interamer de Radiol 1979; 4:135–9.

Multiple mystifying melaenas

[1]J PRICE, [2]L J MCGUIRE and [1]M S Y CHAN

Departments of [1]Diagnostic Radiology and [2]Morbid Anatomy, Prince of Wales Hospital, The Chinese University of Hong Kong, Shatin, NT, Hong Kong

A 40-year-old Chinese woman was admitted for investigation of recurrent episodes of melaena, which had required multiple admissions to other hospitals over a 6-year period. Repeated upper gastrointestinal endoscopies and barium meals, a recent small bowel follow-through examination and a $^{99}Tc^{m}$ Meckel's scan had all been negative. Barium enema and colonoscopy were also normal. The patient was referred for selective coeliac and mesenteric angiography, with a suggested diagnosis of angiodysplasia. On routine examination, there was suspicion of a mass in the left subcostal region, and an abdominal ultrasound examination was therefore performed. This confirmed the presence of a mobile, rounded, anterior abdominal mass, separate from the left kidney and spleen, but closely related to the pancreatic tail. CT with contrast enhancement was then performed (Figure 1). What are the possible diagnoses and what do you anticipate will be shown on angiography?

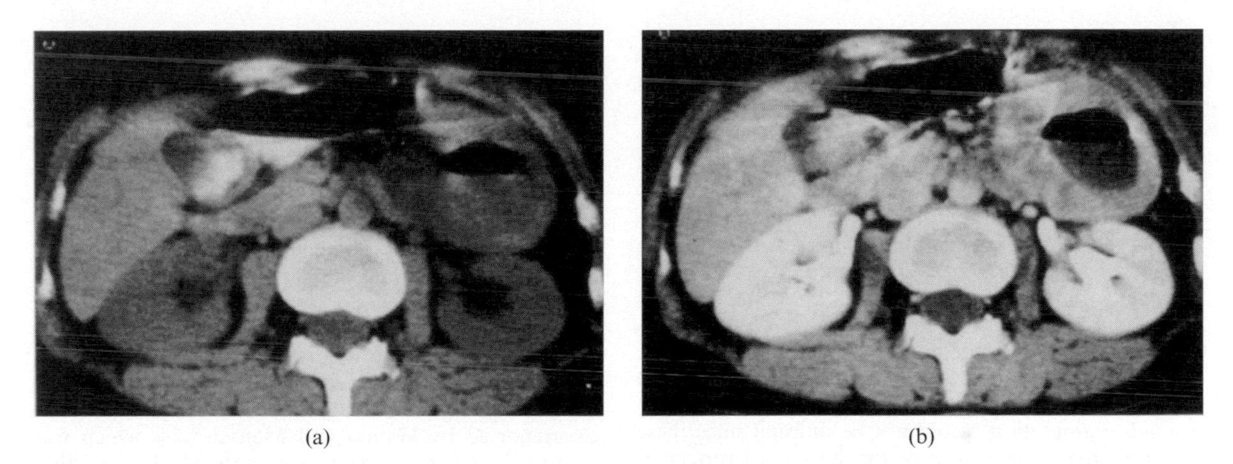

(a) (b)

Figure 1. (a) Pre-contrast and (b) enhanced CT images of the upper abdomen.

Based on the case of the month originally published in Br J Radiol 1988;61:521–2.

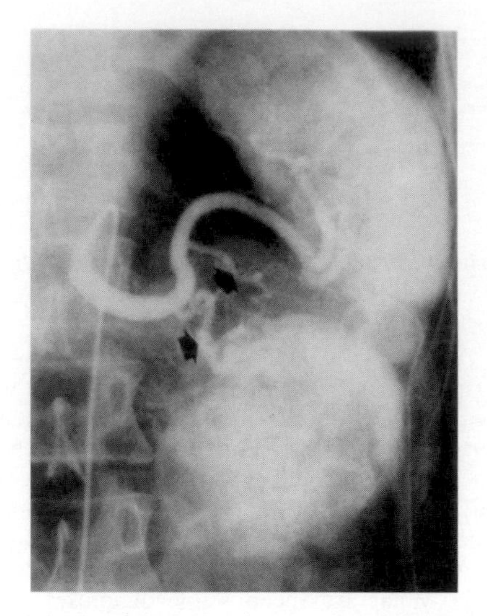

Figure 2. Selective splenic arteriogram showing feeding vessels (arrows) and a tumour blush.

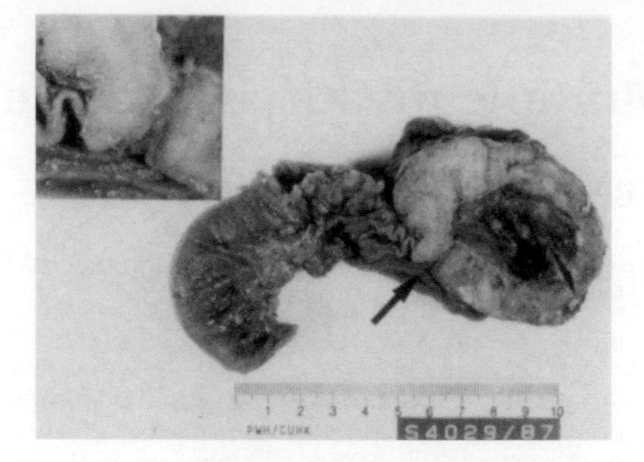

Figure 3. Resected specimen showing intramural site of the tumour and communication between the central cavity and the bowel lumen (arrow and inset).

The CT scan showed a well circumscribed, oval-shaped mass lying anterior to the left kidney. After iv contrast medium there was marked enhancement of a rim of soft tissue around a well defined central cavity which contained an air–fluid level. On these findings, the mass could be arising from the pancreatic tail, small bowel, colon or mesentery. The appearances of a thick-walled cavity indicate that a necrotic neoplasm, pancreatic pseudo-cyst or intraabdominal abscess would all be considered in the differential diagnosis.

Taken with the history of recurrent melaena, the signs on CT of a rounded, enhancing lesion with central cavitation should suggest the possibility of a smooth muscle tumour (leiomyoma or leiomyosarcoma) arising in the wall of the small bowel. The normal result of the follow-through examination would not be unusual since these tumours often grow outwards on the serosal surface of the bowel [1] and may therefore escape detection on conventional barium studies [2].

The diagnosis is often only established at angiography by the characteristic signs of a dense tumour blush and arteriovenous shunting [3]. In this patient, selective angiography showed the mass to be supplied mainly by two enlarged pancreatic branches of the splenic artery. There was a tumour blush (Figure 2) with early filling of a large vein. The inferior margin of the tumour was supplied by the left colic branch of the inferior mesenteric artery. The superior mesenteric angiogram was normal.

At operation, a lobulated tumour was found in the bowel wall just beyond the duodeno-jejunal flexure. Macroscopic inspection of the resected specimen showed a communication between the central cavity of the tumour and the bowel lumen (Figure 3). Histological examination confirmed a leiomyomatous tumour, with nuclear atypia but few mitoses. Local tumour infiltration was observed, the features overall suggesting a low grade leiomyosarcoma.

In the small bowel, leiomyomas account for almost 20% of primary benign neoplasms [1] and leiomyosarcoma is among the commonest small bowel malignancies. Cavitation, often with well defined areas of complete liquefaction, is seen on CT in most cases [4].

Our case illustrates that, in the correct clinical context, the characteristic features on CT of leiomyomatous tumours may suggest the diagnosis. CT has an inherent advantage over barium studies in demonstrating these tumours, which often do not project into the bowel lumen. It also illustrates the importance of performing comprehensive coeliac and mesenteric angiography in patients with recurrent melaena. Our patient went undiagnosed for 6 years, but was more fortunate than the case reported by Hanno and Mensch [5], which was diagnosed at post-mortem examination, 14 years after the first bleed.

References

1. Morson BC, Dawson IMP. Tumours of smooth muscles (leiomyomatous tumours). In: Gastrointestinal Pathology. Oxford: Blackwell Scientific, 1979:423–5.
2. Megibow AJ, Balthazar EJ, Hulnick DH, Naidich DP, Bosniak MA. CT evaluation of gastrointestinal leiomyomas and leiomyosarcomas. AJR 1985;144:727–31.
3. Forbes WSC, Nolan DJ, Fletcher EWL, Lee E. Small bowel melaena: two cases diagnosed by angiography. Br J Surg 1978;65:168–70.
4. McLeod AJ, Zornoza J, Shirkhoda A. Leiomyosarcoma: computed tomographic findings. Radiology 1984;152:133–6.
5. Hanno HA, Mensch M. Leiomyoma of the jejunum. Intermittent melanena of 14 years' duration and fatal haemorrhage. Ann Surg 1944;120:199–206.

Size is not important

[1]J S MILLAR and [2]M S CHOKSEY

Departments of [1]Radiology and [2]Neurosurgery, Royal London Hospital, Whitechapel, London E1 1BB, UK

A 14-year-old boy presented with a 4 day history of headache and vomiting. On the morning of admission he had developed left sided weakness and had become drowsy. 2 weeks previously he had suffered a "flu" like illness and had received a course of amoxycillin. He had recovered sufficiently to return to school prior to the presenting illness.

On examination he was pyrexial (38.2 °C), disorientated and had a left hemiparesis. CT was performed (Figure 1). What is the diagnosis and what course of action would you recommend?

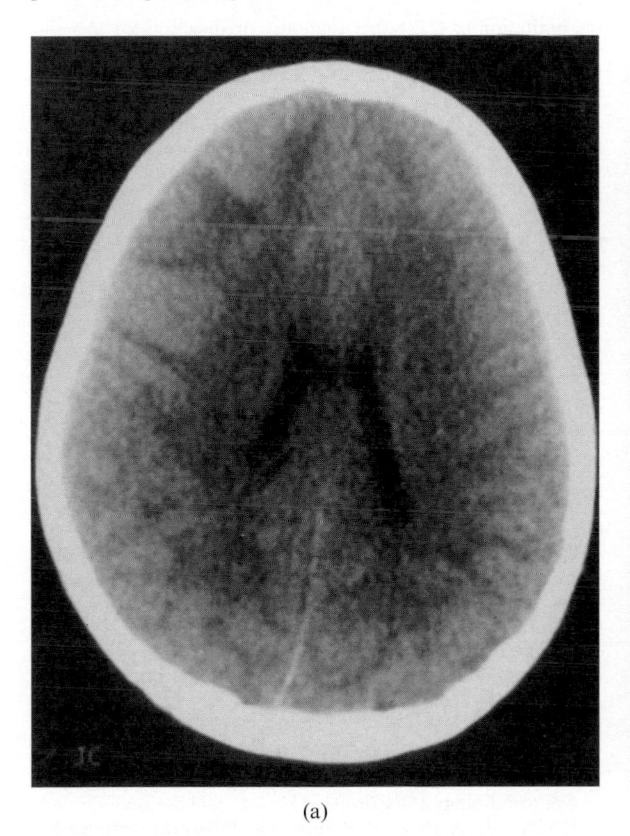

(a)

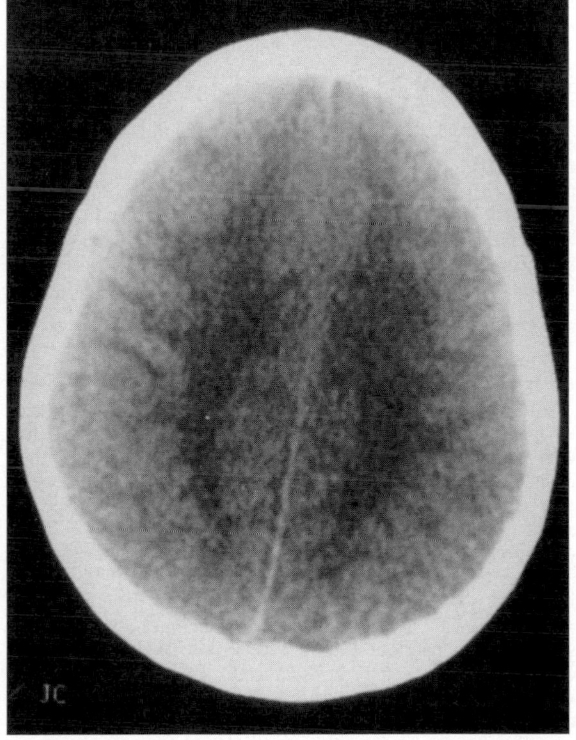

(b)

Figure 1. (a) and (b) CT scans at presentation.

Based on the case of the month originally published in Br J Radiol 1996;69:87–8.

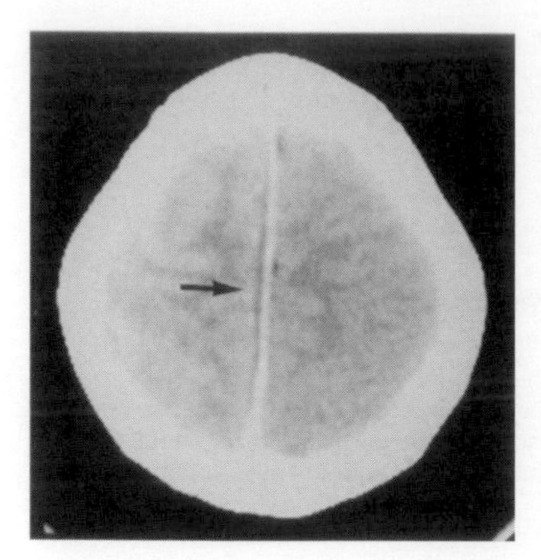

Figure 2. Contrast enhanced CT showing gyriform of enhancement over the right hemisphere and a small right parafalcine collection (arrow). The adjacent sulci are effaced indicating that this is in the subdural and not the subarachnoid space.

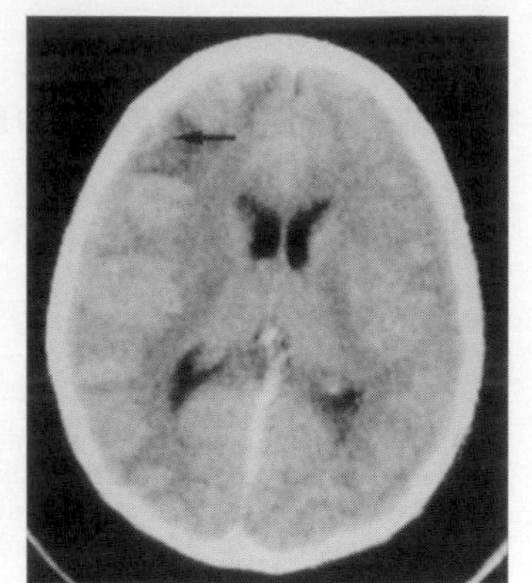

Figure 3. Contrast enhanced CT showing a small rim enhancing subdural locule over the right frontal lobe with low attenuation in the adjacent cortex and subcortical white matter (arrow).

The CT scan showed low attenuation in the right frontal lobe, mainly confined to the white matter consistent with vasogenic oedema. A contrast enhanced scan performed at that time showed no focal enhancement. The differential diagnosis was encephalitis or cerebritis and treatment with broad spectrum antibiotics and acyclovir was commenced.

The clue to the correct diagnosis is the small parafalcine collection seen just posterior to the splenium of the corpus callosum (Figure 1a) and more obviously on the higher slice (Figure 1b). The patient was re-scanned on transfer and the enhanced scan clearly shows the right parafalcine subdural empyema (Figure 2). Despite craniotomy and drainage of the subdural empyema the patient deteriorated rapidly and died 3 days after admission.

Subdural empyema (SDE) is an uncommon but often devastating form of intracranial sepsis. It usually occurs in adolescents as a result of paranasal sinus disease [1, 2]. Despite the proliferation of CT over the past 2 decades the diagnosis is often delayed or missed. There are several reasons why this might occur. The importance of performing a contrast enhanced scan and repeat scanning in the context of suspected intracranial sepsis needs to be emphasized. The often subtle findings of the condition must, however, be one of the foremost reasons.

The pattern of presentation is remarkably stereotyped. Severe headache, often frontal but becoming generalized is accompanied by fever, malaise and meningism in the early stages. A stable period of up to 2 weeks is followed by the rapid onset of altered level of consciousness, focal deficit and convulsions. Despite the strong association with sepsis in the paranasal sinuses this usually is not clinically apparent [2]. Trauma, previous surgery, ear disease and meningitis are other recognized causes but occasionally the source is never established [1].

The important early CT features of SDE include: (i) generalized unilateral hemispheric swelling; (ii) paranasal sinus disease; (iii) thin hypodense subdural collections and locules; (iv) enhancement of the capsule; (v) focal parenchymal abnormalities; (vi) gyral enhancement; and (vii) venous sinus thrombosis.

In the early stages of the condition the abnormalities are invariably asymmetric. The diagnosis should be suspected when diffuse unilateral hemispheric swelling is observed in the appropriate clinical setting [3]. Bone artefact on CT dictates that thin subdural collections are more easily appreciated at a parafalcine site than over the convexities. The emphasis in the literature placed on scrutinizing this area in suspected cases reflects the limitation of CT rather than any predilection for this site. The frequent association with paranasal sinus disease means that reviewing the scan on bone window settings is mandatory when intracranial sepsis is suspected.

The other diagnostic considerations in a febrile patient with hemispheric mass effect include cerebritis/abscess, herpes simplex encephalitis (HSE) and ischaemia/infarction due to an inflammatory vasculitis [4]. Subdural effusion or empyema is a recognized feature of pyogenic intracranial sepsis most notably meningitis in children due to *Haemophilus influenza* type B [5]. It is not a feature of encephalitis.

MRI is superior to CT in every respect, demonstrating the presence, nature and extent of an extraaxial empyema and the associated parenchymal abnormalities with greater accuracy [3]. Where available it would be the imaging modality of choice.

Conventional teaching considers early surgical treatment of subdural empyema to be an absolute requirement on the basis that even with appropriate chemotherapy there will not be adequate penetration of the subdural space. This view is challenged by some authors who document successful outcome with antibiotics alone [6]. It seems unlikely that earlier neurosurgical intervention in this case would have altered the outcome but nonetheless when SDE is diagnosed it must be considered a neurosurgical emergency. This requires a high index of suspicion on the part of the radiologist, and CT in suspected intracranial sepsis must be scrutinized for the often subtle signs of subdural empyema. If the clinical index of suspicion is high, exploratory burr holes are justified even if the scan appears normal.

References

1. Moseley IF, Kendall BE. Radiology of intracranial empyemas with special reference to computed tomography. Neuroradiology 1984;26:333–45.
2. Hodges J, Anslow P, Gillett G. Subdural empyema—continuing diagnostic problems in the CT scan era. Q J Med 1986;228:387–93.
3. Weingarten K, Zimmerman RD, Becker RD, et al. Subdural and epidural empyemas: MR imaging. AJR 1989;152:615–21.
4. Weisberg L. Subdural empyema. Clinical and computed tomographic correlations. Arch Neurol 1986;43:497–500.
5. Suchet I, Horowitz T, Kitay S, Cruz RM. The predictive value of computed tomography and *Haemophilus influenzae* capsular antigen in subdural effusion collections. Clin Radiol 1988;39:265–8.
6. Leys D, Destee A, Petit H, Warot P. Management of subdural intracranial empyemas should not always require surgery. J Neurol Neurosurg Psychiatr 1986;49:635–9.

Now you see it . . . now you don't

J S MILLAR

Department of Radiology, Coventry and Warwickshire Hospital, Stoney Stanton Road, Coventry CV1 4FH, UK

A 52-year-old female presented with a 6 month history of left iliac fossa pain and alteration of bowel habit. She was rather overweight but examination was otherwise unremarkable. She was anaemic with a haemoglobin level of 10.1 g dl^{-1}. A barium enema was requested.

The appearances shown in Figures 1 and 2 were unchanged by intravenous administration of Buscopan 20 mg (hyoscine butylbromide). What is your differential diagnosis?

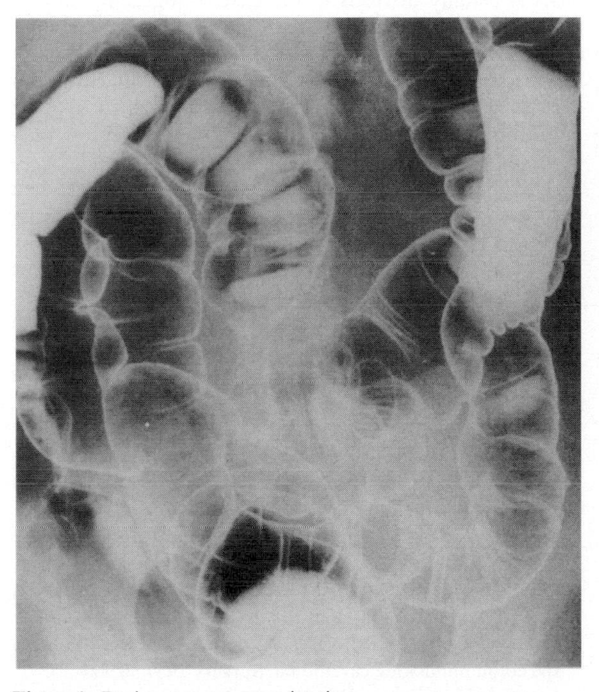

Figure 1. Barium enema examination.

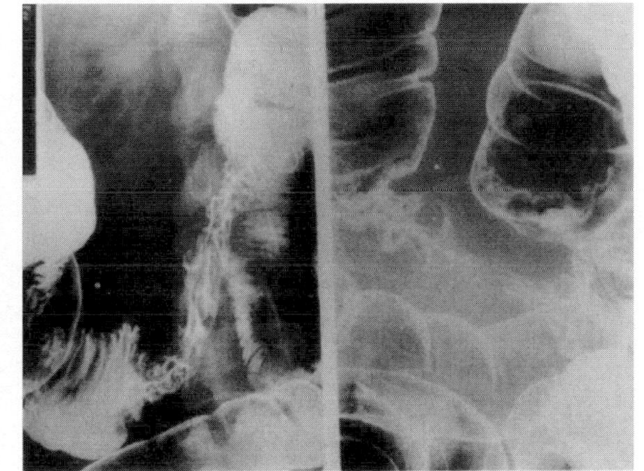

Figure 2. Spot views of the mid-transverse colon. Normal retrograde filling of the small bowel has occurred, accounting for opacification of the loop overlying the spine.

Based on the case of the month originally published in Br J Radiol 1992;65:183–4.

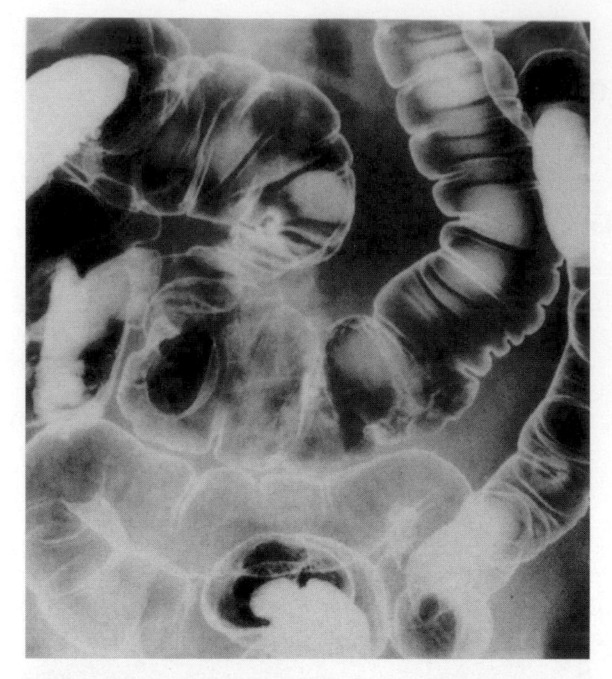

Figure 3. Film taken immediately after reduction of the patient's paraumbilical hernia. Allowing for the presence of some faecal residue and a twist in the proximal transverse colon one can see that the bowel is normally distended with a normal mucosal pattern.

There are long strictures affecting adjacent segments of an area of distorted bowel with an abrupt cut-off between normal and abnormal bowel. In some views there appears to be shouldering (Figure 2). The lumen is circumferentially narrowed and there is a normally distended segment of bowel between the strictures.

Primary colonic neoplasm can invade an adjacent segment of bowel and produce this appearance, as can Crohn's disease. However, there was no evidence of mucosal destruction. Serosal or intramural metastases and endometriosis can produce similar patterns to this, but it would be unusual for them to involve such long segments. The very rare linitis plastica type of primary colonic neoplasm can result in long segment stricturing with relative preservation of the mucosal pattern [1].

Local segmental spasm could produce these appearances [1], but, judging by the remainder of the large bowel, the Buscopan had been effective. Diverticular strictures can affect long segments of bowel with mucosal preservation. Although there are a few scattered diverticula there are none in the region of the stricture; this would be a very unusual site. Local spread from an adjacent primary tumour, primary, or secondary lymphoma would be associated with an extracolonic mass and destruction of mucosa.

A number of benign extrinsic processes can cause colonic strictures. These include pancreatic pseudocysts, colonic retroposition, congenital bands and adhesions [2]. There was no history of previous surgery in our patient but this is not essential for the formation of adhesions. Inflammation of omentum or the appendices epiploicae, which are particularly abundant in the transverse colon, are well recognized causes [3].

The possibility of a hernia should always be considered when faced with an atypical colonic stricture. The diagnosis is usually obvious in the case of inguinal, femoral or diaphragmatic hernia. In situations where there is no external mass there may be diagnostic confusion as in the case of obturator hernia and sometimes in Spigelian hernias [4]. Similarly ventral hernias such as the paraumbilical variety which rarely contain colon may be easily overlooked.

During air insufflation in this patient the abdomen became noticeably protuberant. On palpation an easily reducible paraumbilical hernia was found to be the cause. The aetiology of a midline "loop-type" stricture of the transverse colon in this patient was therefore obvious. The diagnosis was confirmed by a radiograph taken immediately after reduction of the hernia (Figure 3).

Considering the prevalence of ventral hernia in the adult population this complication is surprisingly rare. One other report [5] describes five cases. This is probably because the colon rarely enters the smaller defects while the larger ventral hernias cause little constriction of the bowel contained within them.

References

1. Thomas BM. In: Sutton D. A textbook of radiology and imaging. London: Churchill Livingstone, 1987:924–8.
2. Overton RC, Bolton BF, Usher FC. Extrinsic deformities of the colon mimicking carcinoma. Surgery 1954;36:906–15.
3. Kyaw MM, Koehler PR. Pseudotumours of colon due to adhesions. Radiology 1972;103:597–9.
4. Balthazar EJ, Subramanyam BR. Radiographic diagnosis of Spelian hernia. Am J Gastroenterol 1983;78:525–8.
5. Forrest JV, Stanley RJ. Transverse colon in adult umbilical hernia. AJR 1978;130:57–9.

"All's well that ends well"

[1]J BELL, [1]J KABALA and [2]M HORROCKS

Departments of [1]Radiodiagnosis and [2]Surgery, Bristol Royal Infirmary, Bristol BS2 8HW, UK

An 80-year-old man was admitted for repair of a right inguinal hernia. While on the ward, he complained of back pain in the lower thoracic and upper lumbar region, present for around 3 months, with some pain in the right groin. He was found to have reduced pin-prick sensation in the T12 to L2 dermatomes and a numb area on the lateral aspect of the right thigh.

Radiographs of his thoracolumbar spine are shown (Figure 1). CT was performed (Figure 2).

What does CT show, what is your differential diagnosis and how would you proceed?

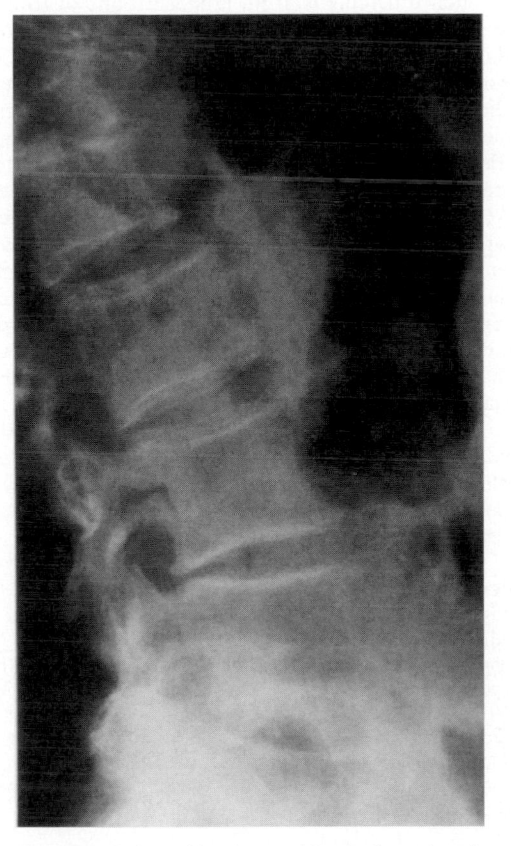

Figure 1. Lateral view of lumbar and lower thoracic spine.

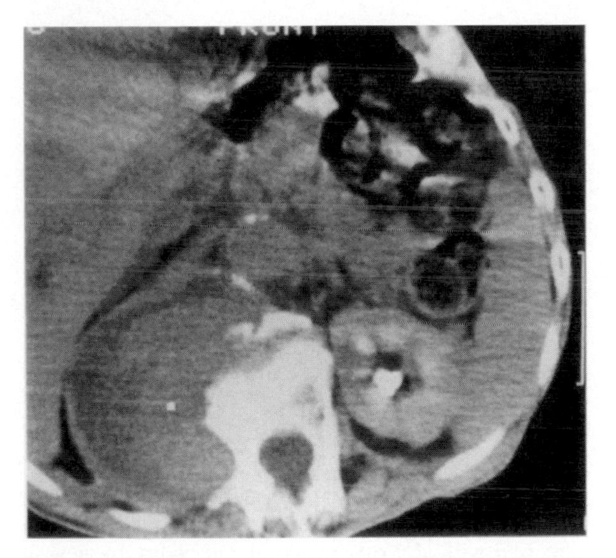

Figure 2. CT scan (window 350, centre 44) through upper abdomen at level of L1 (density measurement at site of white square to right of spine = 51).

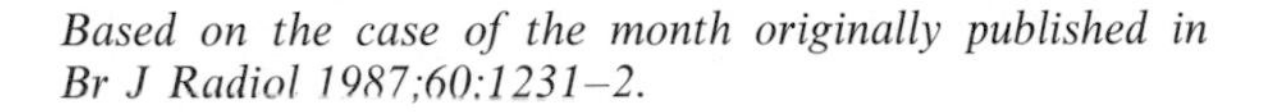

Based on the case of the month originally published in Br J Radiol 1987;60:1231–2.

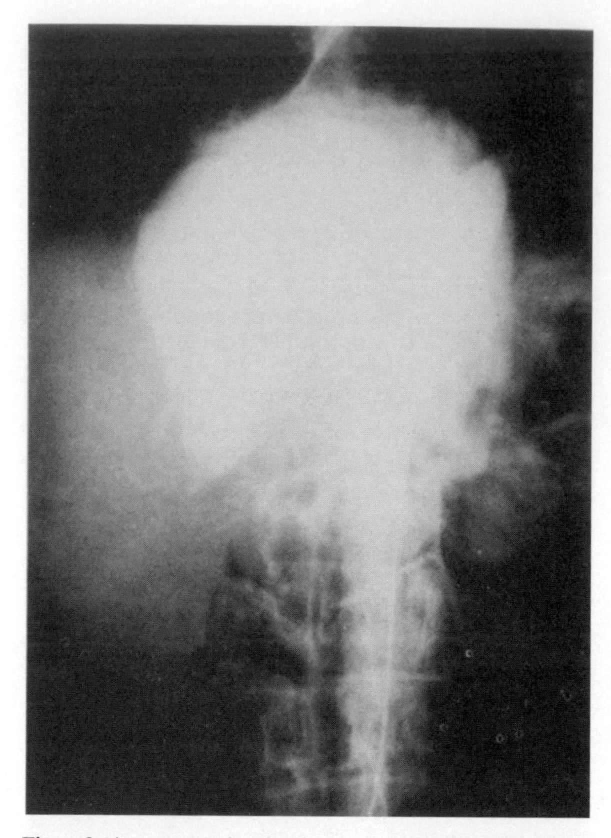

Figure 3. Aortogram showing large aneurysm lying anteriorly and mainly to the right of the aorta. Some contrast medium has passed inferiorly and to the right into the lumen of a false aneurysm.

The radiographs of the thoracolumbar spine showed anterior erosions and wedge collapse of the bodies of T12 and L1. The T11–12 and T12–L1 disc spaces were narrowed with sclerotic vertebral end-plates. In view of the associated disc space narrowing, an infective lesion was considered, although the patient was apyrexial with a normal white cell count.

CT showed a large soft tissue mass of mixed attenuation lying anteriorly and to the right of the upper lumbar vertebral bodies, which were eroded anteriorly. It apparently extended down the right psoas muscle. It was felt that this confirmed the presence of a large psoas abscess and a needle aspiration to identify the responsible organism was done. Only blood was aspirated, the flow being slightly pulsatile. Injection of contrast medium down the biopsy needle showed a large cavity connecting with the aorta. Aortography (Figure 3) confirmed the diagnosis of an aneurysm and demonstrated its full extent. A large aneurysm was shown anterior and to the right of the lower thoracic and upper lumbar vertebral bodies. Some contrast medium passed inferolaterally into the lumen of a false aneurysm. The findings were confirmed at operation when an aortic graft was successfully inserted.

There are many possible causes of anterior erosions of the vertebral bodies. While metastatic deposits are one of the commonest causes, myeloma, lymphoma and extrinsic compression from aneurysms, lymphadenopathy and abscesses can all produce similar appearances.

Paraspinal abscesses may occur with spread of infection, often tuberculous, from adjacent bone or from the disc space. In either instance, both the vertebral bodies and the intervening discs become involved, with narrowing of the disc space and erosion of the vertebral bodies [1]. Although new bone formation may cause some sclerosis, this is usually ill defined and not limited to the vertebral end-plates as in this case. The latter is more typically associated with degenerative disc disease.

Aortic aneurysms are well known to produce anterior erosion of the vertebral bodies. The bone margins are often well defined and the discs not involved. Such changes can be well shown by CT [2, 3]. In this case, anterior erosion has been extensive enough to produce some secondary collapse. This appearance, combined with coexistent degenerative changes, produced an initially misleading picture in this patient.

A dynamic scan with intravenous contrast medium would have clearly demonstrated the nature of the mass in this case. An ultrasound scan [*or MRI, ED*] of the upper abdomen would probably also have led to the correct diagnosis.

References

1. Epstein BS. In: The spine: a radiological text and atlas (4th edn). Philadelphia: Lea and Febiger, 1976:424.
2. Twigg HL, Axelbaum SP, Schellinger D. Computerised body tomography with the ACTA scanner. J Am Med Assoc 1975;234:314–7.
3. Godwin JD, Herfkens RL, Skiolderbrand CG, Federle MP, Lipton MJ. Evaluation of dissection and aneurysms of the thoracic aorta by conventional and dynamic CT scanning. Radiology 1980;136:125–33.

A pain in the pelvis

T M S GEAKE

Department of Radiology, Royal Adelaide Hospital, Australia

A 36-year-old woman, whose only relevant past history was of a right tubal pregnancy, presented with a 6-month history of lower abdominal discomfort. Pelvic examination showed a poorly defined mass in the right adnexal region, palpation of which induced paraesthesiae down the right leg.

Chest and abdominal radiographs were normal, as was an excretory urogram. Pelvic ultrasound was performed (Figure 1), followed by CT after oral contrast medium and intravenous contrast medium to outline the distal ureters and bladder base (Figures 2 and 3).

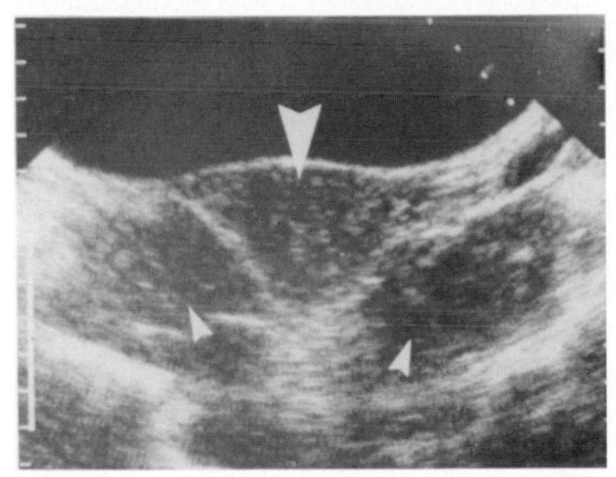

Figure 1. Transverse ultrasound scan above the pubic symphysis.

What abnormalities are shown and what is the diagnosis?

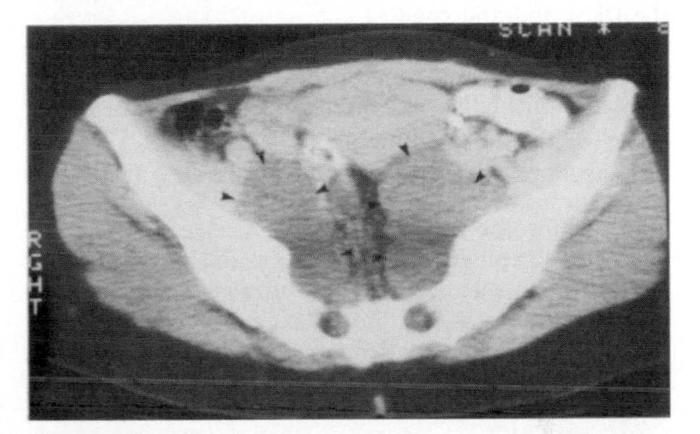

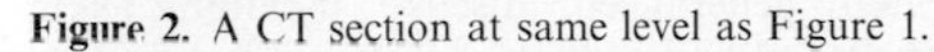

Figure 2. A CT section at same level as Figure 1.

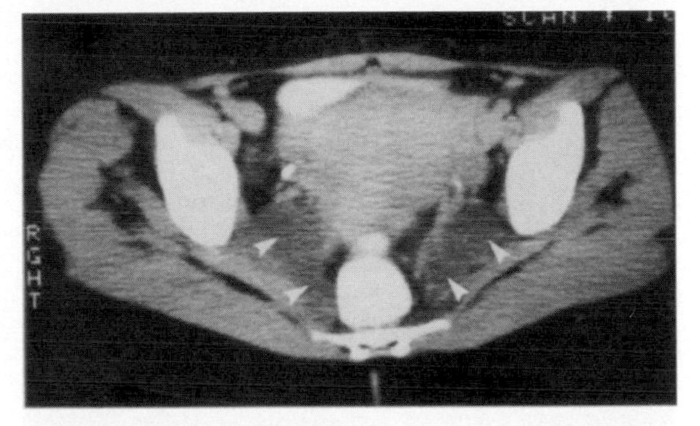

Figure 3. A CT section immediately above acetabulum.

Based on the case of the month originally published in Br J Radiol 1986;59:943–4.

Figure 1 shows two areas of reduced echogenicity lying behind and lateral to the bladder. A low density mass is seen at these sites in Figure 2, and the sacral foramina are large. Bilateral low density masses are seen posteriorly in Figure 3.

The appearances are those of plexiform neurofibromatosis, which is a form of generalized dysplasia of neuroectodermal and mesodermal tissue characterized by multiple nerve sheath tumours. Localized nervous tissue overgrowth may be fusiform and multiple in nature and form an intricate and communicating network, entrapping adjacent non-neural soft tissue. These lesions occur most commonly in the neck and limbs, and less often in the chest and abdomen [1].

After making the diagnosis radiologically, a single café-au-lait spot was found on the patient's back, and a localized thickening of a peripheral nerve could be felt in the right buttock (Figure 4).

Neurofibromatosis (von Recklinghausen's disease) has characteristic clinical manifestations and rarely presents a problem in diagnosis. Skin lesions may be absent in 10% of patients with a proven diagnosis of neurofibromatosis and 30% of patients have between one and six café-au-lait spots [2]. All, except one, previously reported cases of pelvic plexiform neurofibromatosis have exhibited generalized disease including skin stigmas. Our patient had a single skin lesion but on CT showed the characteristic features and distribution of pelvic plexiform neurofibromatosis as previously described [3, 4].

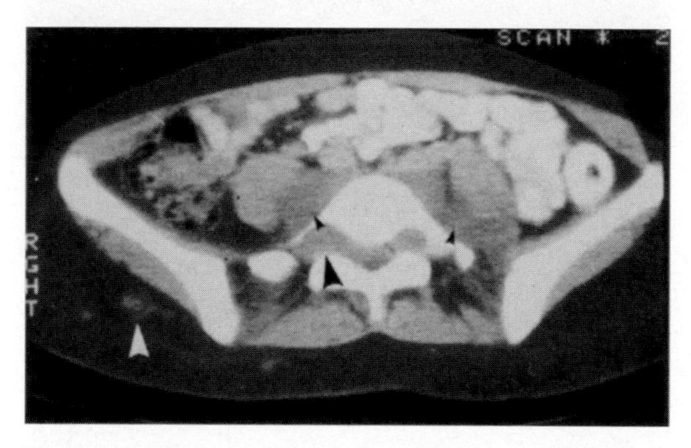

Figure 4. A CT scan at a level above Figure 2 shows displacement of the psoas muscles by lower density soft tissue (small arrowheads), enlarged sacral foramina (large black arrowheads) and an enlarged soft-tissue density in the fat posterior to the right ilium (white arrowhead).

The presence of pelvic side-wall masses of high echogenicity in the absence of acoustic shadowing on ultrasound should suggest a fat-containing tumour.

Simple and plexiform neurofibromas on CT have attenuation values of 20–30 HU and may enhance by 10 HU following contrast medium. When such lesions are homogeneous and have the distribution and configuration typical of neurofibromatosis, histological confirmation is unnecessary since it may be hazardous [3]. Low attenuation areas may result from haemorrhage or necrosis developing in areas of sarcomatous degeneration within the mass (17–30 HU) [5], a high content of lipid-rich Schwann cells within the tumour (5–17 HU) or fat incorporation within the tumour (−50–0 HU) [1]. In general, the higher the fat content of a mass (*i.e.* the lower the attenuation value), the less likely the mass is to be malignant.

In this patient, since large areas of the mass exhibited attenuation values of −20–0 HU with no evidence of associated bone destruction, it was considered to be benign and biopsy confirmation was not sought.

[*Neurofibromatosis (NF) is now separated into two definite groups: NF1 (von Recklinghausen disease) and NF2 (bilateral acoustic neurofibromatosis). NF1 has an abnormal chromosome 17 and NF2 has an abnormal long arm of chromosome 22. Lesions found in NF2 include optic pathway gliomas and other varieties of astrocytomas, spinal cord gliomas, osseous dysplasia, plexiform or peripheral nerve neurofibromas, café-au-lait spots, axillary linguinal freckling and pigmented hamartomas of the iris. NF2 includes bilateral acoustic neuromas, meningiomas of brain, spine and cranial nerve or spinal schwannomas, ED*]

References

1. Kumar AJ, Kuhajda FP, Martinez CR, Fishman EK, Jezic DV, Siegelman SS. Computed tomography of extracranial nerve sheath tumours with pathological correlation. JCAT 1983;7:857–65.
2. Crowe FW, Schull WJ. Diagnostic importance of café-au-lait spots in neurofibromatosis. Arch Intern Med 1953;91:758–66.
3. Paling MR. Plexiform neurofibroma of the pelvis in neurofibromatosis: CT findings. JCAT 1984;8:476–8.
4. Lanzieri CF, Hilal SK. Computed tomography of the sacral plexus and sciatic nerve in the greater sciatic foramen. AJR 1984;143:165–8.
5. Coleman BG, Arger PH, Dalinka MK, Obringer AC, Raney BR, Meadows AT. CT of sarcomatous degeneration in neurofibromatosis. AJR 1983;140:383–7.

The expanding infant

R J PECK

Department of Radiology, Prince of Wales Hospital, Shatin, Hong Kong

A 9-month-old child was seen with a history of diarrhoea of varying severity present for several months. The child had, in addition, developed ankle oedema and swelling around the eyes. On examination the abdomen was soft but distended. The major biochemical abnormality was a low serum albumin (19 $g\,l^{-1}$). Figure 1 is a plain radiograph of chest and abdomen.

Ultrasound showed a normal liver, gallbladder, pancreas and kidneys. Ascites was present. Figure 2 is a transverse scan of lower abdomen, and Figure 3 is an early radiograph from the barium follow-through.

What is your provisional diagnosis and how would you confirm it?

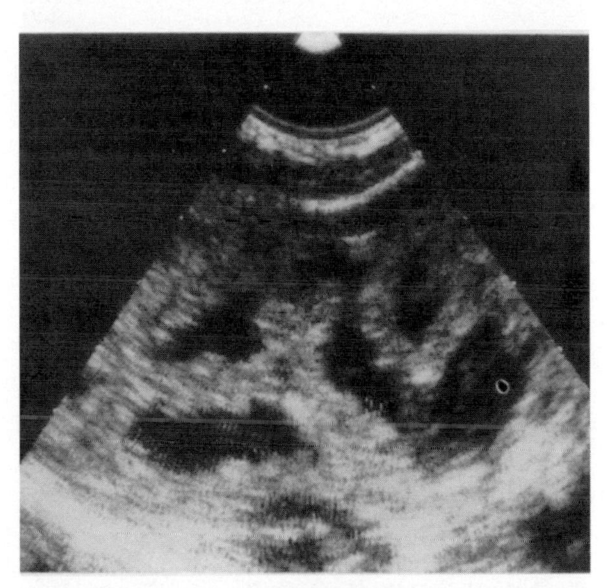

Figure 2. Ultrasound scan of lower abdomen.

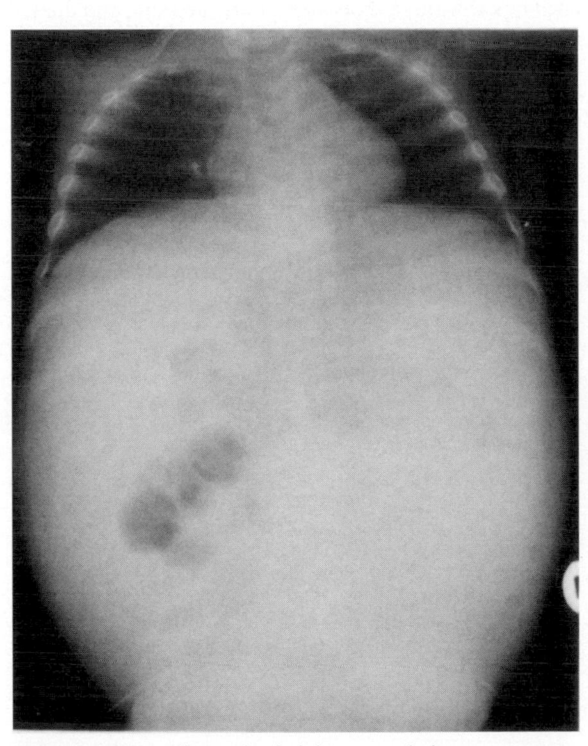

Figure 1. Plain radiograph of abdomen and chest.

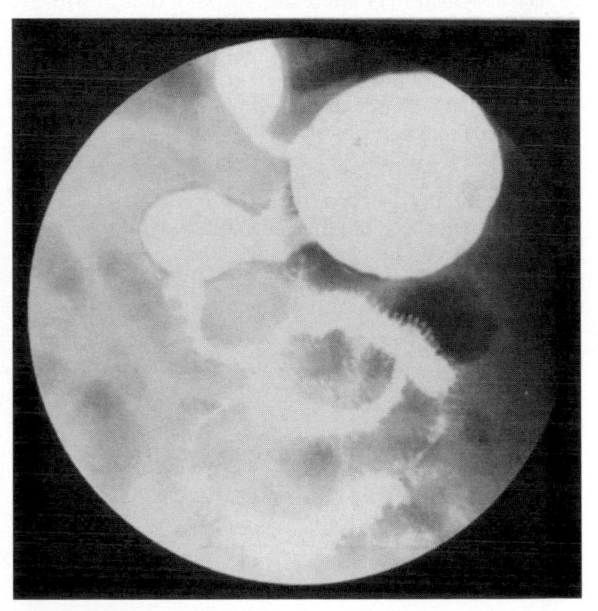

Figure 3. Barium follow-through examination.

Based on the case of the month originally published in Br J Radiol 1995;61:855–6.

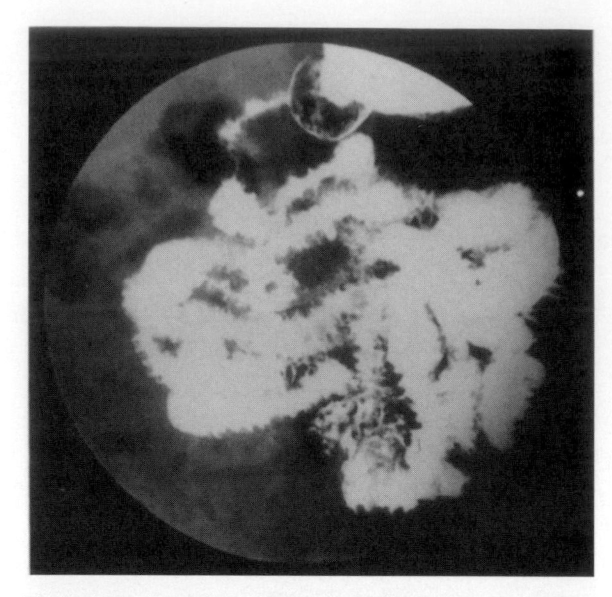

Figure 4. Barium follow-through examination.

The abdominal radiograph showed distension, an overall greyness, and centrally lying bowel loops, consistent with ascites. The ultrasound scan showed thick-walled, fluid-filled loops of small bowel. A later radiograph (Figure 4) from the barium series confirmed that the thickened valvulae conniventes were present throughout the small bowel.

The child presented with features of malabsorption. This is the clinical manifestation of many different disease processes which may affect the gut and alter absorptive or digestive functions, the commonest being coeliac disease. A wide variety of biochemical tests may show abnormal values but are unlikely to establish the precise diagnosis [1]. The thickened valvulae conniventes shown on the small bowel barium study can be due to the following causes.

(1) Inflammatory: Crohn's disease.
(2) Infiltratrive: eosinophilic enteritis, amyloidosis, mastocytosis, Whipple's disease.
(3) Neoplastic: lymphoma.
(4) Vascular: intramural haemorrhage, ischaemia.
(5) Infective: giardiasis, strongyloidiasis.
(6) Congenital: intestinal lymphangiectasia [2].

Small bowel biopsy is the definitive diagnostic test and, in this case, showed intestinal lymphangiectasia.

Intestinal lymphangiectasia is a generalized congenital disorder, thought to be due to hypoplasia of visceral lymphatic channels resulting in obstruction to lymph flow. Specimens of jejunal mucosa reveal dilated telangiectatic lymphatics in the lamina propria and submucosa. The villi may be club-shaped because of distortion from grossly dilated lymphatics, rather than because of partial villous atrophy such as is seen in coeliac disease. Clinical presentation is with diarrhoea, malabsorption, oedema, chylous ascites and hypoproteinaemia. The hypoproteinaemia and steatorrhea in lymphangiectasia are thought to be due to rupture of the dilated lymphatics with discharge of lymph into the bowel lumen.

The disease affects primarily children and young adults. The main biochemical abnormality is hypoproteinaemia with decreased serum levels of albumin, immunoglobulins G, A and M, transferrin and caeruloplasmin [1]. Lymphangiography may show hypoplastic peripheral and visceral lymphatics with absence of groups of retroperitoneal lymph nodes [3]. The ultrasound features of intestinal lymphangiectasia include diffuse, thickened bowel walls, ascites, mesenteric oedema, and dilated mesenteric lymphatics. Peristalsis appears reduced and pleural effusions may be seen. Recognition of these features is useful as ultrasound is frequently the first examination in children with abdominal disorders [4].

References

1. Braunwald E, Isselbacher KJ, Petersdorf RG, Wilson JD, Martin JB, Jauce AS. Harrison's Principles of Internal Medicine (11th edn). New York: McGraw-Hill, 1987:1276.
2. Nolan DJ. The small intestine. In: Grainger RG, Allison D, editors. Diagnostic Radiology. An Anglo-American Textbok of Imaging, Vol 2. Edinburgh: Churchill Livingstone. 1986:854.
3. Shimkin PM, Waldmann TA, Krugman RL. Intestinal lymphangiectasia. AJR 1970;110:827–41.
4. Dorne HL, Jecquier MD. Sonography of intestinal lymphangiectasia. J Ultrasound Med 1986;5:13–6.

Digging for a diagnosis

[1]H R JÄGER, [1]C O'DONNELL and [2]J SINHA

Departments of [1]Diagnostic Radiology and [2]Surgery, Hammersmith Hospital, Du Cane Road, London, UK

A 45-year-old man presented with a 1 week history of progressive painless jaundice. An ultrasound examination at the referring hospital indicated distal common bile duct (CBD) obstruction.

6 years previously he had noticed swelling around both mandibular angles and an orthopantomograph had shown two rounded radio-opaque masses in these areas (Figure 1). 1 year later, the patient had a colectomy with an ileorectal anastomosis.

On clinical examination, he was jaundiced, had multiple bony nodules in the region of the chin and forehead with two non-fluctuant, mobile lumps over the occiput and dorsum of the left foot. The liver was smoothly enlarged on palpation. A chest radiograph was normal. Endoscopic retrograde cholangiopancreatography (ERCP) (Figure 2) and a hypotonic duodenogram (Figure 3) are shown.

What is your diagnosis?

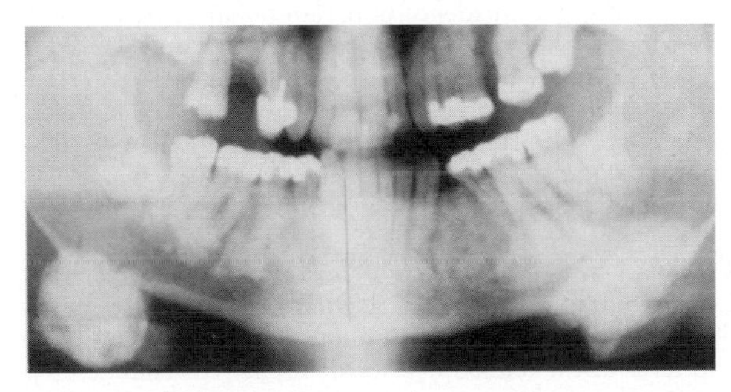

Figure 1. Orthopantomograph of the mandible.

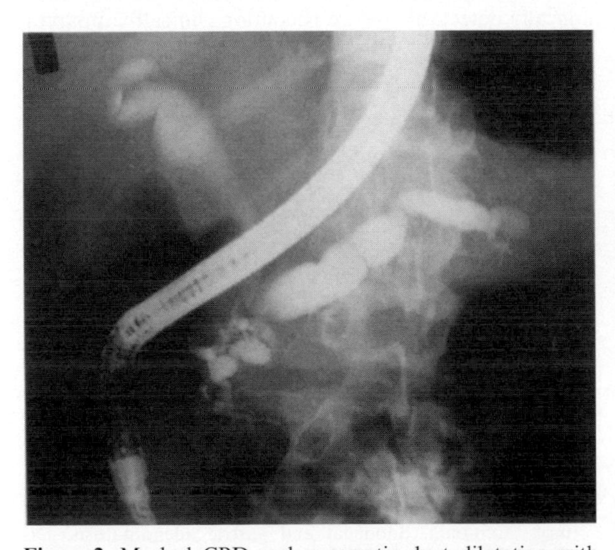

Figure 2. Marked CBD and pancreatic duct dilatation with preservation of pancreatic duct side branches shown by ERCP.

Based on the case of the month originally published in Br J Radiol 1990;63:143–4.

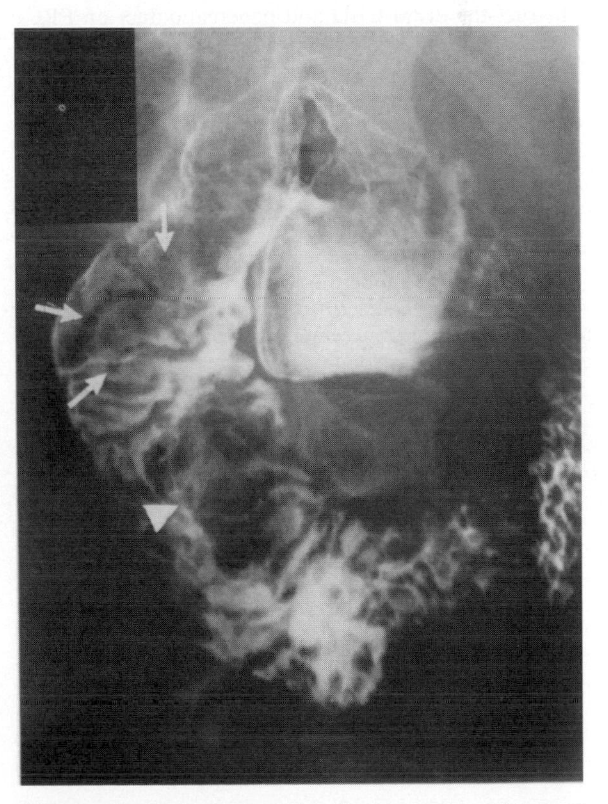

Figure 3. Hypotonic duodenogram demonstrates multiple small filling defects (arrows) and a larger mass in the region of the ampulla (arrowhead).

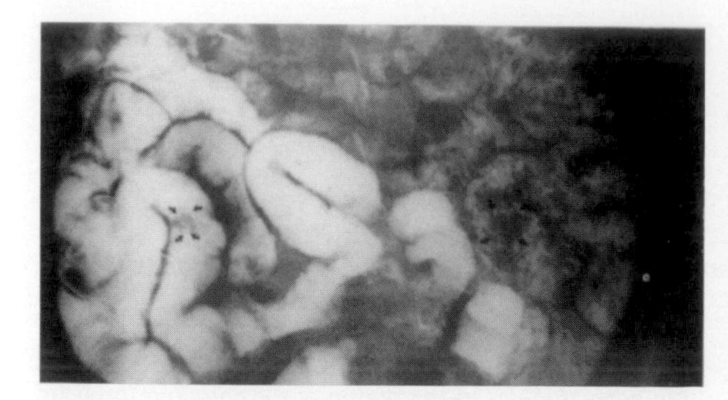

Figure 4. A small bowel follow-through demonstrates multiple polyps in jejenum and ileum (arrows).

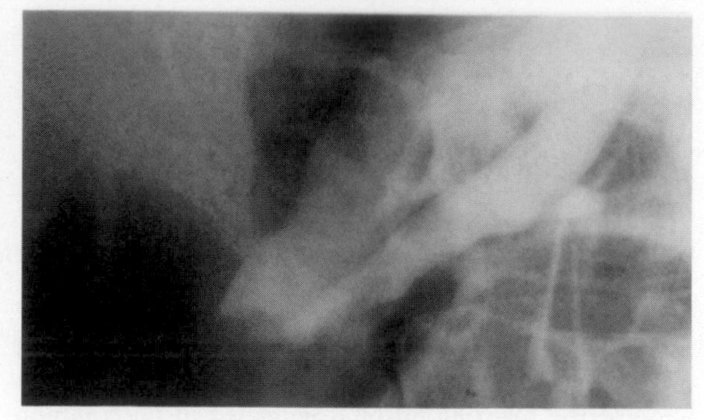

Figure 5. Close-up view of CBD and pancreatic duct confluence showing a mass lesion with irregular margin protruding into and obstructing both ducts.

The diagnosis is Gardner's syndrome, complicated by a periampullary carcinoma.

Our patient had initially presented with two large osteomas of the mandible (Figure 1). A subsequent barium enema had shown extensive colonic polyposis and led to the diagnosis of Gardner's syndrome. A colectomy had then been performed. Subsequent barium studies of the upper gastrointestinal (GI) tract demonstrated gastric polyps (sparing the antrum), polyps in the duodenum (small arrows, Figure 3) and polyps in the jejenum and ileum (Figure 4). The periampullary lesion seen on the duodenogram was shown to protrude into and obstruct the distal CBD and pancreatic duct on ERCP (Figure 5).

The patient had a proximal pancreaticoduodenectomy and histology revealed a villous adenoma with a small area of malignant invasion of the muscularis mucosa.

Gardner in 1953 described a syndrome of large bowel polyps with mandibular osteomas and epidermoid cysts as an autosomal dominant inherited disorder [1].

Subsequently, numerous other extracolonic manifestations have been described in the syndrome, including desmoid tumours, mesenteric fibromas, dental abnormalities, upper gastrointestinal and small bowel polyps. The most frequent extracolonic malignancy is periampullary carcinoma; other less common malignant tumours are papillary carcinoma of the thyroid, medulloblastoma, adrenal carcinoma and carcinoid of the small bowel [2]. There is increasing evidence that Gardner's syndrome and familial polyposis are one entity with the same underlying genetic defect but a variable phenotype [2, 3].

The polyps in the duodenum tend to be adenomatous (tubular or villous) and must be considered as a premalignant condition unlike gastric polyps, which are of the hyperplastic-fundus-cell type and usually follow a benign course. Duodenal polyps involve, most commonly, the second part of the duodenum and in particular the papilla of Vater. Adenomatous changes can even occur in a papilla that looks macroscopically normal [3], or can be confined to the distal CBD and then only be detectable as filling defects on ERCP examination [4].

The reported incidence of periampullary carcinoma in Gardner's syndrome varies between 2% and 12% [2, 3]. It seems to develop in a more advanced age group than colorectal carcinoma, the average age of manifestation being about 45 years [5]. Periampullary carcinoma is the most frequent cause of death in patients with Gardner's syndrome treated with colectomy and ileorectal anastomosis [2].

Small bowel polyps result histologically from either lymphoid hyperplasia in the terminal ileum or adenomatous polyps in the ileum and jejenum. They appear to have a low tendency towards malignant change [3].

Osteomas of the jaw are one of the originally described features of Gardner's syndrome. They may well occur before the appearance of colonic lesions and are radiologically detectable before becoming clinically apparent. Examination by orthopantomography has therefore been suggested as a useful screening test in children of polyposis coli families [2].

References

1. Gardner EJ, Richards RC. Multiple cutaneous and subcutaneous lesions occuring with hereditary polyposis and osteomatosis. Am J Hum Genet 1953;5:139–47.
2. Jagelman DG. Extracolonic manifestations of familial polyposis coli. Cancer Genet Cytogenet 1987;27:319–25.
3. Burt RW, Berenson MM, Lee RG, Tolman KG, Freston JW, Gardner EJ. Upper gastrointestinal polyps in Gardner's syndrome. Gastroenterology 1984;86:295–301.
4. Shemesh E, Bat L. A prospective evaluation of upper gastrointestinal tract and periampullary region in patients with Gardner's syndrome. Am J Gastroenterol 1985;80:825–7.
5. Sugihara K, Muto T, Kamiya J, Konishi F, Sawada T, Morjoka J. Gardner's syndrome associated with periampullary carcinoma, duodenal and gastric adenomatosis. Dis Colon Rectum 1982;25:767–71.

CT in the diagnosis of pyrexia of unknown origin

[1]R M J WILLIAMS, [2]R J MARSHALL and [3]J BRENNAN

[1]*Chiltern Wing, Sutton Hospital, Sutton, Surrey SM2 5NF,* [2]*Royal Cornwall Hospital (Treliske), Truro, Cornwall TR1 3LJ and* [3]*Royal Devon and Exeter Hospital (Wonford), Barrack Road, Exeter EX2 5DW, UK*

A 72-year-old Caucasian man presented to a medical clinic with a 6 month history of weight loss, epigastric discomfort, poor appetite, malaise and night sweats with low grade fever. In recent weeks he had become breathless and tired on minimal exertion, and had slight cough productive of yellow phlegm. He had complained of a peculiar sensation at the back of his mouth, but there was no visible lesion on ENT or dental examination.

During the Second World War he had served in Burma and India for 4 years where he had malaria. He had never since travelled outside Europe. He had had a left thoracoplasty for pulmonary tuberculosis in 1947. He had been a heavy smoker until he had suffered a myocardial infarct 15 years previously. Since then he had had an aortobifemoral bypass for peripheral vascular disease and a mild stroke from which he had made an excellent recovery. He was taking dipyrimadole, ranitidine and frusemide—this latter for a few days because his ankles had been swollen. He did not drink alcohol.

On examination he had clearly lost weight and had a temperature of 37.5 °C. The liver was felt 3 cm below the costal margin but there were no other remarkable findings. A chest radiograph showed no evidence of active disease. He had a normochromic normocytic anaemia (Hb 11.9 g dl^{-1}) with a normal white cell count and differential, a raised serum alkaline phosphatase at 218 IU l^{-1} (ref. 50–100) of hepatobiliary origin on isoenzyme analysis, a C-reactive protein of 47 mg l^{-1} (ref. <10) and an ESR of 22 mm h^{-1}. An upper gastrointestinal endoscopy showed gastritis associated with *Helicobacter pylorii*. Abdominal ultrasound revealed a thickened gall bladder only. Bone marrow aspiration and trephine were unremarkable, and a liver biopsy showed a granulomatous hepatitis. Cultures of sputum, urine and blood showed no mycobacterial or other growth. He was given a course of antituberculous therapy, and treatment for his gastritis. However, after 6 weeks he had deteriorated and had developed a troublesome itch. The antituberculous treatment was stopped. CT of the abdomen revealed bilateral adrenal enlargement (Figure 1).

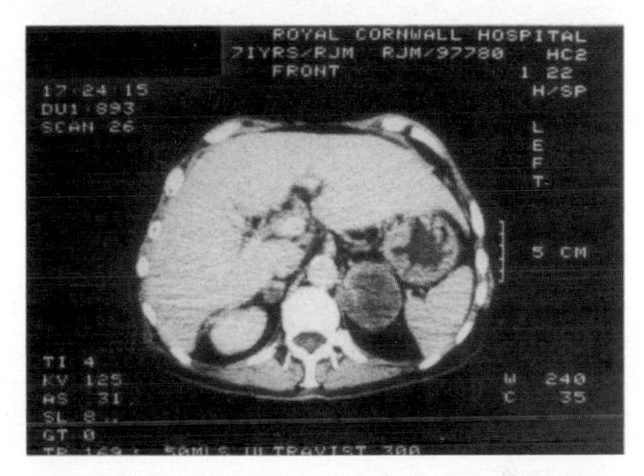

Figure 1. CT of the abdomen demonstrates enlarged adrenal glands.

What is your diagnosis?

Based on the case of the month originally published in Br J Radiol 1993;66:847–8.

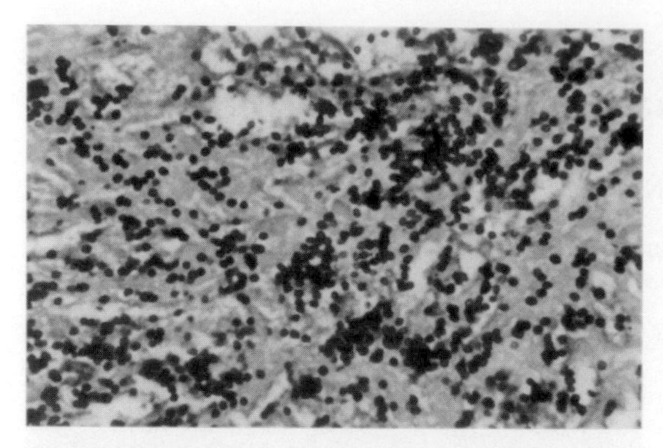

Figure 2. Numerous fungal spores are seen amongst necrotic material (Grocott methenamine—silver).

The diagnosis is chronic disseminated histoplasmosis with adrenal infiltration. A Trucut biopsy of the left adrenal showed necrotic material and a macrophage infiltrate, in both of which were numerous organisms consistent with *Histoplasma capsulatum* (Figure 2). On review of the liver biopsy no organisms were identified with special stains. The report of the specimen, on which in 1947 the diagnosis of tuberculosis was based, stated that acid-fast bacilli were seen with a Ziehl–Neelsen stain.

Histoplasmosis is caused by the dimorphic fungus *Histoplasma capsulatum.* The fungus grows in soil fertilized by bird excreta, particularly in humid river valleys, explaining the endemic distribution of histoplasmosis in parts of North and Latin America, and South East Asia [1]. Histoplasma skin test surveys suggest that the disease occurs much more widely. A single case has been contracted in the United Kingdom [2]. This may be explained by the existence of "microfoci" such as caves and bird roosts where favourably humid conditions occur.

In the vast majority of cases the disease is self-limiting causing either an influenza-like illness with patchy pneumonitis, or is asymptomatic. Chronic progressive pulmonary disease and acute or chronic disseminated histoplasmosis occur in less than 1% of cases, and are associated with pre-existing lung disease or defects in cell mediated immunity [1]. Dissemination occurs commonly via microphages in skin, brain and adrenal glands. However, only rarely (1 in 2000 cases) will this cause symptomatic disease [1]. Chronic disseminated disease tends to occur in the elderly, usually with a latent period of less than 2 years between exposure and onset of symptoms, at least with North American histoplasmosis [1]. St C Symmers, in 1972, [3] described a series of 48 cases of histoplasmosis in expatriates returning to the United Kingdom from South East Asia in whom the longest latent period was 33 years. Although histoplasmosis has occasionally been contracted in the United Kingdom [2], it seems fairly certain that this man originally contracted the disease in the Far East. The latent period of 44 years in our case is therefore the longest on record. In the series of St C Symmers in 1972 [3] all the cases had adrenal involvement and presented with oral, pharyngeal or genital ulceration, usually painful. In our case there was no such ulceration, although the patient had complained of abnormal sensations in the oropharynx.

The importance of considering treatable conditions such as histoplasmosis in the differential diagnosis of adrenal masses is well documented [4]. Other causes of bilateral adrenal masses include tuberculosis, blastomycosis and metastases (commonly from a bronchial primary). Phaeochromocytomas, adenomas and hyperplasia are primary adrenal conditions which may present as bilateral masses [5]. The diagnosis may be made by fine needle aspiration of the adrenal gland [4], or by large bore needle biopsy as in our case. Serological tests may be used as supportive evidence, although more specific tests are being developed [1]. Direct culture of the organism is successful in up to 90% of cases of chronic disseminated disease, the highest yield being from bone marrow [1]. In our case, the bone marrow specimen was sent for histology only.

This case exemplifies the importance of considering histoplasmosis in the differential diagnosis of bilateral adrenal masses, even when there is no history of recent exposure.

[*See also the review article by Conces [6], ED*]

References

1. Wheat LJ. Diagnosis and management of histoplasmosis. Eur J Microbiol Infect Dis 1989;8:480–90.
2. St C Symmers W. Histoplasmosis contracted in Britain. Br Med J 1956;ii:786–90.
3. St C Symmers W. Histoplasmosis in Southern and South Eastern Asia. Ann Soc Belg Med Trop 1972;52:435–52.
4. Valente PT, Calafati SA. Diagnosis and disseminated histoplasmosis by fine needle aspiration of the adrenal gland. Acta Cytol 1989;33:341–3.
5. Wilms GW, Baert AL, Kint EJ, et al. Computed tomographic findings in bilateral adrenal tuberculosis. Radiology 1983; 146:729–30.
6. Conces DJ. Histoplasmosis. Semin Roentgenol 1996;31: 14–20.

Another pain in the neck

[1]P M LOGAN, [2]K O'ROURKE and [1]R G GIBNEY

Departments of [1]Radiology and [2]Orthopaedic Surgery, St Vincent's Hospital, Dublin 4, Ireland

A 16-year-old male presented to the Accident and Emergency Department with an injury sustained by diving into a shallow swimming pool. He complained of pain in his neck and limitation of neck movements. Examination showed a marked torticollis and tenderness in the neck. Movement of the neck was limited to 15° on both flexion and extension and lateral rotation was limited to 30° bilaterally. The rest of the examination was unremarkable, in particular there was no neurological deficit.

Cervical spine radiographs were taken at the time of presentation (Figures 1 and 2), and he went on to have CT of the atlantoaxial area (Figure 3). What is your diagnosis? What other methods are employed to confirm the diagnosis?

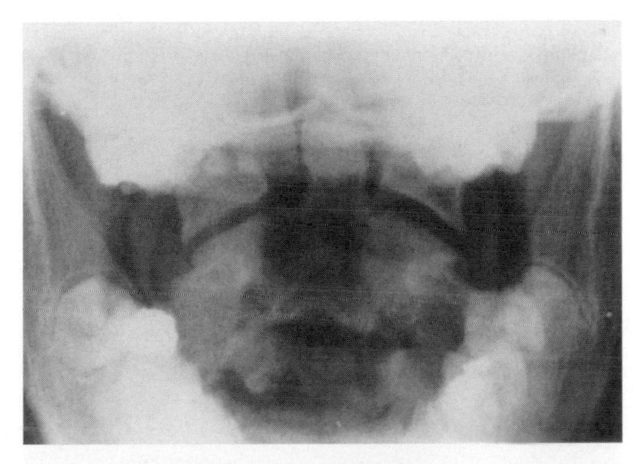

Figure 2. Open-mouth odontoid peg view.

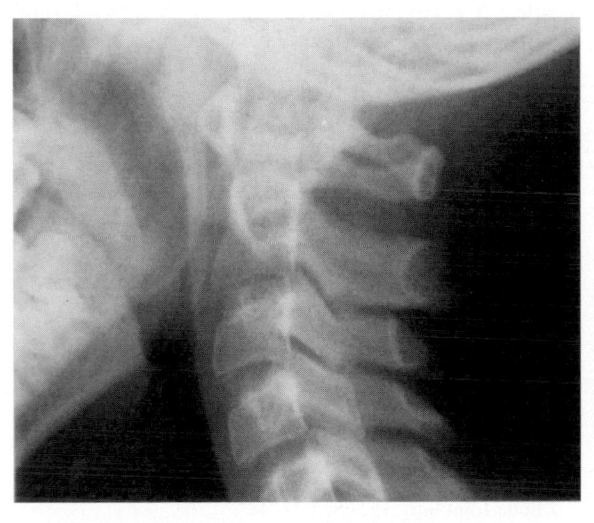

Figure 1. True lateral view of cervical spine.

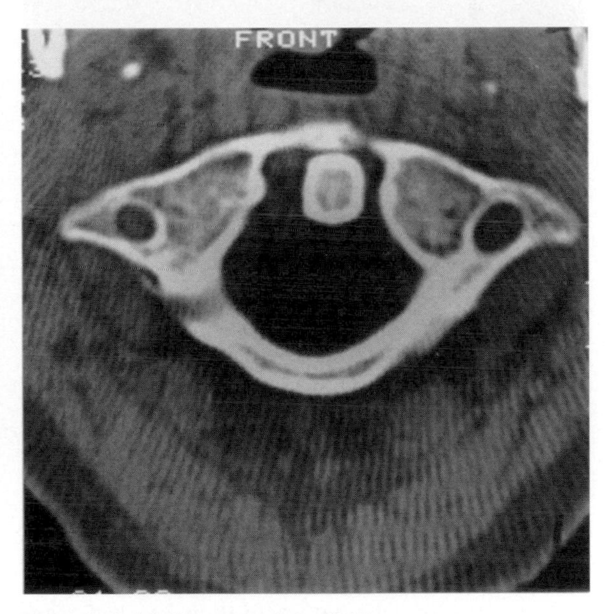

Figure 3. Axial CT section through C1.

Based on the case of the month originally published in Br J Radiol 1995;68:93–4.

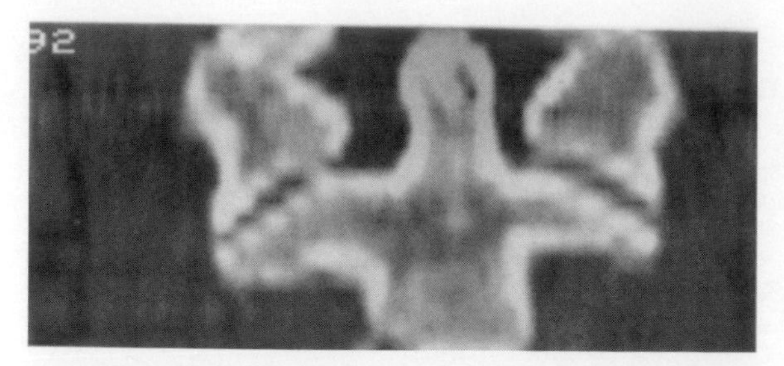

Figure 4. Coronal reconstruction of overlapping, thin section CT of the atlantoaxial level. The widened odontolateral mass distance on the right is demonstrated and the right atlantoaxial joint is narrowed due to the rotational subluxation.

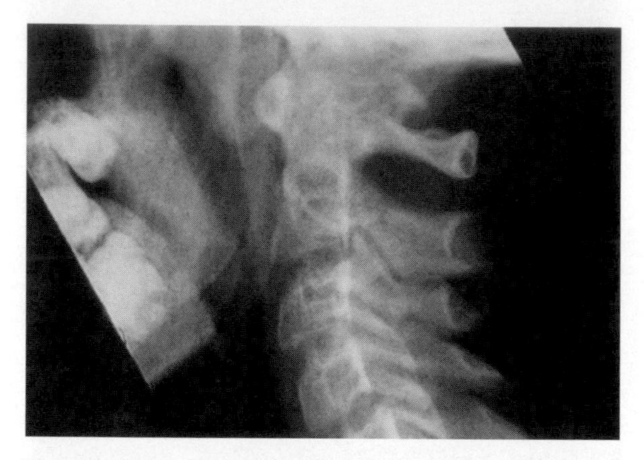

Figure 5. True lateral cervical spine radiograph on our patient post-reduction. The atlas is now in normal position.

The open-mouth odontoid peg view demonstrated widening of the right odontolateral mass interval. The lateral view of the cervical spine shows failure of superimposition of the two elements of the posterior arch of C1, despite it being a true lateral. This combination of signs strongly suggests the diagnosis of atlantoaxial rotatory fixation. This was confirmed by CT of the atlantoaxial region (Figures 3 and 4). The patient was placed on traction and anti-inflammatory and muscle relaxant agents were administered. After 5 days his condition had improved with no residual symptoms or signs. Repeat radiographs at this time were also normal (Figure 5). He was treated for a further 2 months in a soft collar and then discharged, suffering no long-term sequelae.

Since it was first described around the turn of the century, atlantoaxial rotatory fixation has had many names and there have been many reports of the condition, especially in children and young adults [1]. The aetiology can be either congenital or acquired. The commonest acquired cause is trauma, which is often surprisingly minimal, but other causes include local infection or surgery [2]. Despite the condition being well documented, its natural history remains unclear. Some cases spontaneously reduce with no lasting radiographic or symptomatic changes, some become asymptomatic (either spontaneously or as a result of skull traction) but may have persistent radiographic changes [1], and some need open reduction with atlantoaxial arthrodesis [3]. However, it is clear that early diagnosis is essential for optimal management of these patients [2, 4]. Untreated, the associated torticollis can become difficult to manage and occasionally rotation will progress, leading to at least one documented death due to spinal cord transection [3].

Less common in adults than children, atlantoaxial rotatory fixation appears to be more common in females and has recently been associated with fracture of the clavicle, especially in the young female subgroup [2].

The diagnosis should be considered on the plain film evidence, the classical findings being those already described in our patient. On an anteroposterior projection of the cervical spine the head may be seen to be turned to one side in the typical "cock-robin" deformity. Confirmation is achieved using either fluoroscopy or CT. On fluoroscopy the odontolateral mass widening is seen to remain unchanged when the head is turned from side to side. CT again demonstrates the so-called "wink sign" of asymmetrical odontolateral mass distance. It may also show rotation of the lateral mass of C1 over that of C2 on the affected side. However, some pitfalls have been identified using CT for the diagnosis of atlantoaxial rotatory fixation and a CT scan performed with the head turned in two different directions may be necessary [5]. MRI's ability to demonstrate soft tissue injury suggests that it may have a role in the early identification of those cases which are likely to need surgical intervention.

References

1. Wortzman G, Dewar FP. Rotary fixation of the atlantoaxial joint: rotational atlantoaxial sublaxation. Radiology 1968; 90:479–87.
2. Goddard NJ, Stabler J, Albert JS. Atlanto-axial rotatary fixation and fracture of the clavicle. J Bone Joint Surg 1990;72B:72–5.
3. Fielding JW, Hawkins RJ. Atlanto-axial rotatary fixation. J Bone Joint Surg 1977;59A:37–44.
4. Van Holsbeeck EMA, MacKay NNS. Diagnosis of acute atlanto-axial rotatory fixation. J Bone Joint Surg 1989; 71B:90–1.
5. Kowalski HM, Cohen WA, Cooper P, Wisoff JH. Pitfalls in the CT diagnosis of atlanto-axial rotary sublaxation. Am J Neuroradiol 1987;8:697–702.

Bleeding and cholangiographic filling defects—an unavoidable link

[1]W C G PEH, [2]E C S LAI and ^{1}H NGAN

Departments of [1]Diagnostic Radiology and [2]Surgery, The University of Hong Kong, Queen Mary Hospital, Hong Kong

A 61-year-old woman presented with repeated episodes of intermittent gastrointestinal bleeding. Haemoglobin level was 7.7 g dl^{-1}. On examination, she had telangiectasia of the tongue, lips and nasal cavities. Gastroscopy showed two small vascular malformations in the stomach, but no bleeding source was identified. Except for some altered blood, no lesion was detected on colonoscopy.

An ultrasound scan of the upper abdomen was performed (Figure 1). Based on these ultrasound findings, an endoscopic retrograde cholangiopancreatogram (ERCP) was attempted. During this procedure bleeding was seen from the ampulla of Vater, and so the cannulation for the cholangiogram was abandoned. Superior mesenteric and coeliac (Figure 2) angiograms were twice performed but no active bleeding point was identified. A technetium-99m red cell scan also failed to demonstrate a source of bleeding. The patient underwent laparotomy and a pylorus-preserving Whipple's operation was subsequently performed.

What do the liver ultrasound (Figure 1), coeliac angiogram (Figure 2) and T-tube cholangiogram (Figure 3) show? What produced the cholangiographic filling defects? Can all these radiological findings be correlated? What is the diagnosis?

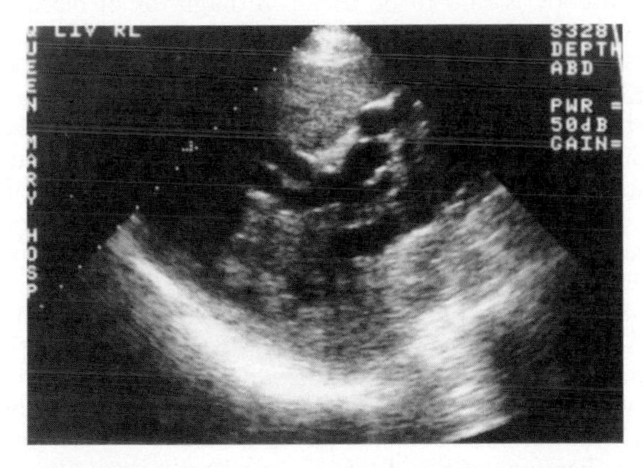

Figure 1. Ultrasound of liver.

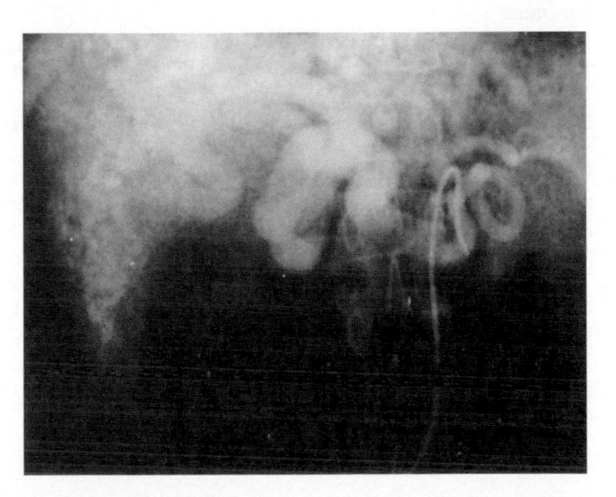

Figure 2. Coeliac angiogram.

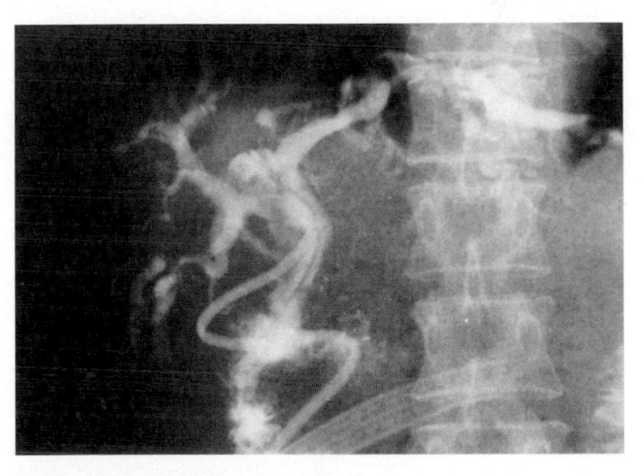

Figure 3. T-tube cholangiogram.

Based on the case of the month originally published in Br J Radiol 1996;69:281–2.

Ultrasound showed multiple hypoechoic tubular structures throughout the liver. These had a branching pattern and were thought to represent dilated intrahepatic ducts, hence the indication for the ERCP. The coeliac angiogram demonstrated gross ectasia of the hepatic artery and its branches. The multiple filling defects involving the intrahepatic ducts seen on cholangiography had smooth convex margins and formed obtuse angles with the adjacent unaffected ducts. Appearances of these filling defects were highly suggestive of lesions extrinsic to the biliary tree.

The tubular structures demonstrated sonographically represented ectatic hepatic arteries, which also produced the cholangiographic filling defects. Subsequent colour Doppler studies showed that all these tubular structures (Figure 4) were caused by grossly dilated intrahepatic arteries. A typical arterial waveform pattern was obtained from these vessels.

During surgery, pulsating vessels could be felt in the region of the head of the pancreas and there was uncertainty as to its exact pathology, hence the performance of a pylorus-preserving Whipple's operation. Pathological examination showed vascular ectasia in the mucosa and submucosa of the ampulla of Vater, with slight extension into the head of the pancreas, as the cause of the bleeding. The patient did not have any more bleeding episodes in the 7 months following surgery.

This patient had clinical and radiological features of Rendu–Osler–Weber syndrome (hereditary haemorrhagic telangiectasia).

Rendu–Osler–Weber syndrome is a familial disorder characterized by telangiectasia of the skin, mucous membranes or internal organs. There is no sex predominance. It usually manifests clinically as bleeding from rupture of telangiectatic vessels. The most frequently reported sites of internal lesions are the lungs, liver and gastrointestinal tract. Clinical presentation depends on the site involved [1].

Intestinal telangiectasia may appear as arteriovenous fistulas, localized arteriovenous malformations, and diffuse scattered lesions indicated by early filling of veins and phlebectasia. Gastrointestinal bleeding occurs in 13% of cases, 90% of which require blood transfusion. This bleeding tends to be more frequent and severe with increasing age. Identification of the source of bleeding remains a diagnostic and therapeutic problem. Angiography is required as the telangiectatic lesions are difficult to identify at surgery. If multiple lesions are seen at angiography and the patient is not actively bleeding at the time of examination, the current bleeding source cannot be accurately determined. Special angiographic techniques such as pharmacoangiography and magnification may be required to identify a small non-shunting lesion. Conversely, normal angiography does not exclude the presence of telangiectasia [1, 2]. Repeat endoscopy is said to be useful in diagnosis of bleeding from gastroduodenal vascular malformations [3].

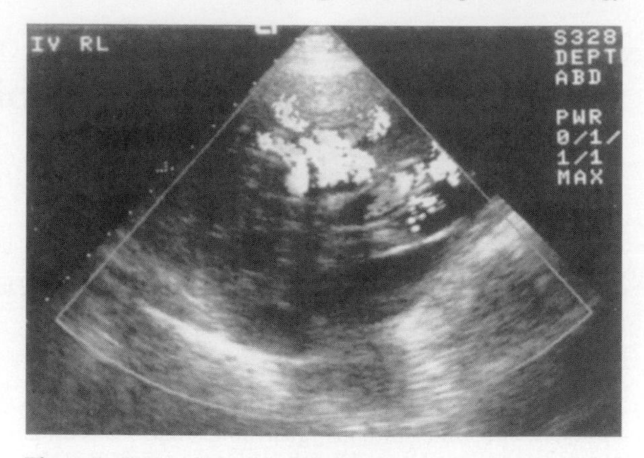

Figure 4. Colour Doppler ultrasound shows grossly dilated arteries throughout the liver.

The enormous size of the hepatic artery and its branches is an important diagnostic feature, as such arterial enlargement is now known to occur in any other condition [4]. As demonstrated in our case, the dilated intrahepatic arteries may be so large as to produce extrinsic filling defects on cholangiography. Other features not seen in our patient are early hepatic vein filling and venous pooling [1, 5].

Identification of one lesion should lead to an intensive search for other vascular lesions, especially if the initial findings are grossly ectatic hepatic arteries. This may save the patient from the potentially life-threatening gastrointestinal haemorrhage, pulmonary or cerebral complications of this disease.

References

1. Peery WH. Clinical spectrum of hereditary haemorrhagic telangiectasia (Osler–Weber–Rendu disease). Am J Med 1987;82:989–97.
2. Nyman U. Angiography in hereditary haemorrhagic telangiectasia. Acta Radiol Diagn 1977;18:581–92.
3. Quintero E, Piqué JM, Bombí JA, et al. Upper gastrointestinal bleeding caused by gastroduodenal vascular malformations. Incidence, diagnosis, and treatment. Digest Dis Sci 1986;31:897–905.
4. Thomas ML, Carty H. Hereditary haemorrhagic telangiectasia of the liver demonstrated angiographically. Acta Radiol Diagn 1974;15:433–8.
5. Lande A, Bedford A, Schechter LS. The spectrum of arteriographic findings in Osler–Weber–Rendu disease. Angiology 1976;27:223–40.

Not another case of aortic dissection!

J A SPENCER and S J GOLDING

The Regional Computed Tomography Unit, Churchill Hospital, Oxford OX3 7LJ, UK

A 70-year-old woman with a long history of ischaemic heart disease was admitted to hospital after a sudden onset of crushing central chest pain. 3 years previously a permanent transvenous pacemaker had been inserted following a bradycardic episode.

On examination there were signs of left heart failure. Peripheral pulses were normal and equal and she was normotensive. An electrocardiogram showed no features of acute myocardial infarction. A chest radiograph demonstrated cardiomegaly and widening of the superior mediastinum. The patient was referred for contrast CT examination of the chest (Figures 1 and 2) to exclude dissection of the thoracic aorta.

What abnormalities are present on the thoracic CT sections? What features might you expect to find on abdominal CT sections?

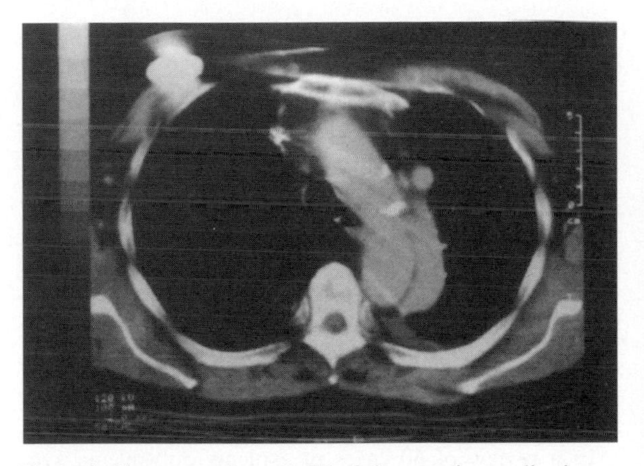

Figure 1. Contrast enhanced CT of the superior mediastinum.

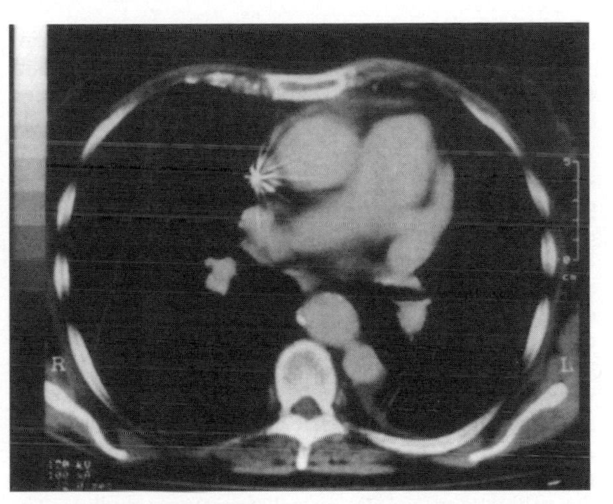

Figure 2. Contrast enhanced CT of the mediastinum at a more caudal level.

Based on the case of the month originally published in Br J Radiol 1993;66:565–6.

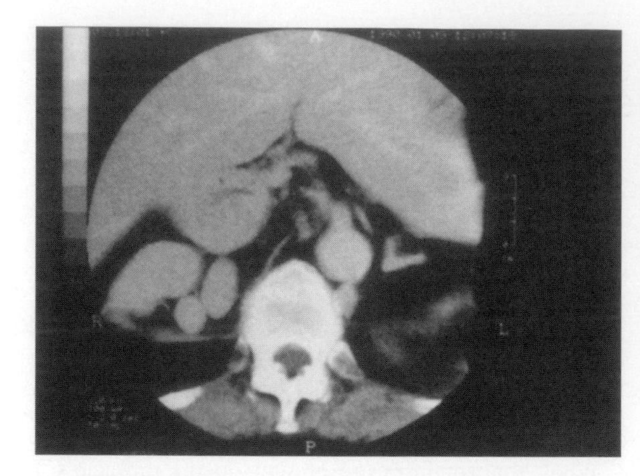

Figure 3. Detail of CT of the upper abdomen after enhancement shows a transverse liver, absence of the inferior vena cava and a right sided gastric fundus. Three right sided splenunculi are present on this section.

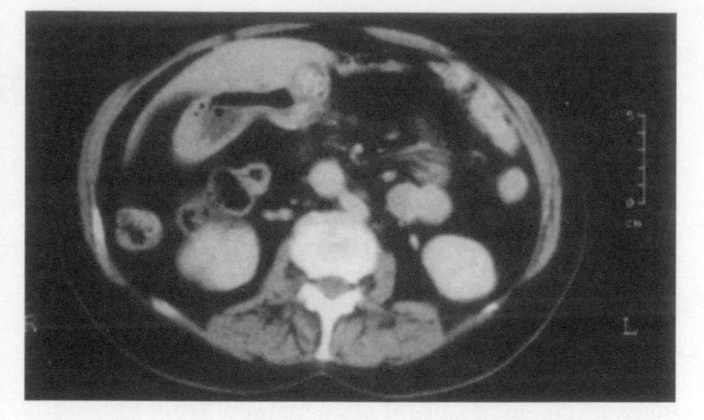

Figure 4. CT scan of the abdomen more caudally shows venous drainage via the left hemiazygos vein. A central gallbladder contains several gallstones and the stomach is again seen on the right of the abdomen.

The thoracic CT sections showed bilateral superior vena cavae; the right containing the pacemaker electrode, the left passing lateral to the aortic arch and draining inferiorly towards the coronary sinus (Figure 2). There was a large left hemiazygos vein draining lateral to the aortic arch into the left cava (Figure 1). There was no evidence of aortic dissection.

The superior mediastinal widening is therefore due to a left superior vena cava and a hemiazygos vein, both structures dilated from cardiac failure. The pleural thickening relates to a failed attempt to pass the pacemaker electrode into the right atrium from the left subclavian vein. The large left hemiazygos vein indicates anomalous venous drainage of the abdomen. The patient has hemiazygos continuation of a left inferior vena cava (IVC).

CT sections of the upper abdomen confirmed this pattern of venous drainage. The liver lay transverse and the gallbladder (containing gallstones) was midline. The gastric fundus was to the right of the midline with several splenunculi in the right upper quadrant (Figures 3 and 4). These are typical abdominal features of polysplenia.

A variety of venous anomalies are recognized in polysplenia and bilateral superior vena cavae are found in a third of cases [1]. There is a high incidence of intracardiac and other great vessel anomalies in association with the syndromes of asplenia and polysplenia, particularly with the former. An echocardiogram showed no intracardiac anomalies in our patient.

Pulmonary abnormalities may exist and more than 50% of cases have bilobed lungs bilaterally [1, 2]. This left thoracic isomerism may be found in isolation as part of the wide spectrum of manifestations of the heterotaxic syndromes [3]. Chest radiographs and CT in our patient suggested normal pulmonary anatomy.

Appearances in the abdomen were typical of polysplenia (Figures 3 and 4), the CT features of which have been reported previously [4]. CT has superseded visceral angiography and scintigraphy [5] as the definitive diagnostic study. A variety of other abdominal appearances have been described with polysplenia including partial and total forms of visceral situs inversus but an almost constant finding is of azygos drainage of the inferior vena cava with interruption of the suprarenal portion of the cava and direct drainage of the hepatic veins into the right atrium [1, 2] as in our patient. Our patient had a variant left sided configuration.

In a review of 60 cases of asplenia/polysplenia syndromes at the Hospital for Sick Children in Toronto, 79% of cases of asplenia died within the first year of life. Polysplenia cases were noted to be predominantly female and to survive longer [1]. Our experience of this septuagenarian accords with this finding.

References

1. Rose V, Izukawa T, Moes CAF. Syndromes of asplenia and polysplenia. Br Heart J 1975;37:840–52.
2. Vaughan TJ, Hawkins IF, Elliott LP. Diagnosis of the polysplenia syndrome. Radiology 1971;101:511–8.
3. Winer-Muram HT, Tonkin ILD. The spectrum of heterotaxic syndromes. Radiol Clin North Am 1989;27:1147–68.
4. Shadle CA, Scott ME, Ritchie DJ, Seliger G. Spontaneous splenic infarction in polysplenia syndrome. JCAT 1982; 6:177–9.
5. Baert AL, Myle J. Polysplenia. Br J Radiol 1975;48:496–8.

Smoke signals

M H S LOVE and K E BELL

Department of Neuroradiology, Royal Victoria Hospital, Grosvenor Road, Belfast BT12 6BA, UK

This male child had been well until the age of 8 years when he developed episodes of weakness and jerking of his right arm. He was felt to have partial seizures and treated with anticonvulsants. 4 years later he presented to hospital with a 5 day history of headaches and confusion associated with dysphasia. These symptoms gradually improved, but he was re-admitted the following month with left hemiplegia and a left homonymous hemianopia. CT (Figure 1) and cerebral arteriography (Figure 2) were performed. An anteroposterior view of the right common carotid injection is illustrated.

What is the diagnosis?

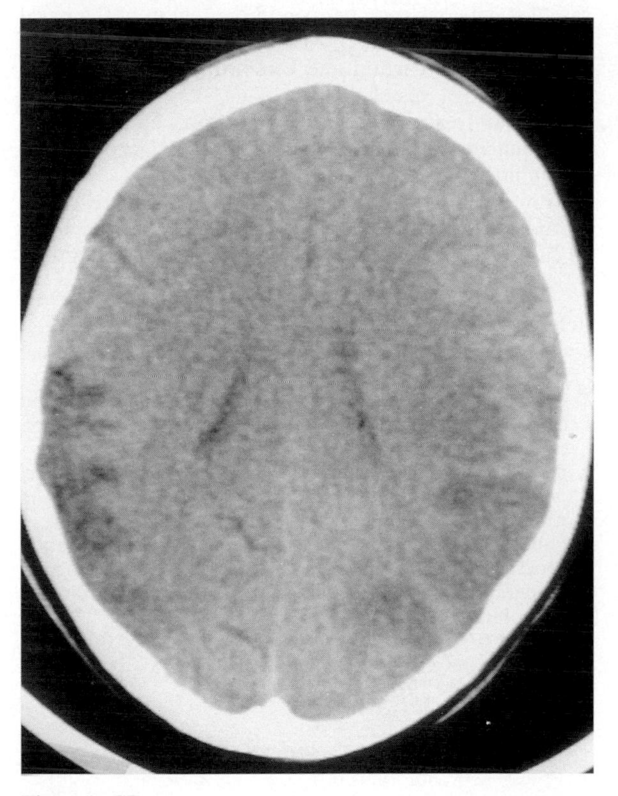

Figure 1. CT scan.

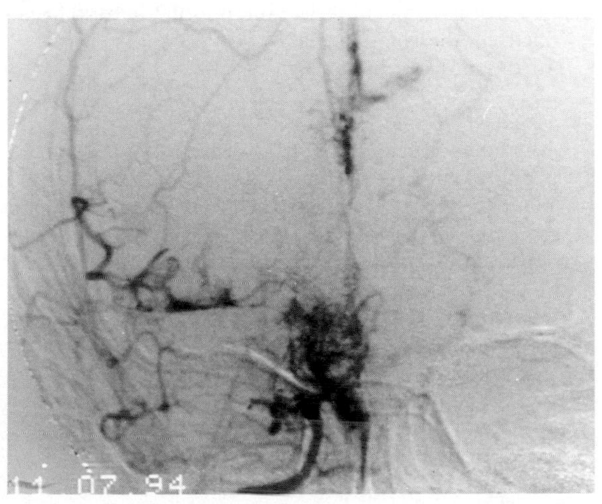

Figure 2. Cerebral arteriogram.

Based on the case of the month originally published in Br J Radiol 1997;70:427–8.

The CT scan showed widening of the cortical sulci in the left parietal region, consistent with focal atrophy due to an old cortical infarction. In the right parietal region an extensive zone of ill defined low density extending out to the cerebral cortex, associated with a slight mass effect, was consistent with a more recent evolving infarct.

The right carotid arteriogram showed occlusion of the internal carotid artery in the region of the carotid syphon. The artery terminated in a leash of tiny collaterals, probably meningohypophyseal vessels. The distal portions of the anterior and middle cerebral arteries filled via these collaterals.

The diagnosis is moyamoya disease.

Moyamoya disease was first described in Japan in 1957 by Takeuchi and Shimizu [1]. It is characterized by bilateral progressive occlusion of the intracerebral vessels, initially affecting the terminal parts of the internal carotid arteries and progressing to involve the anterior, middle and, in some cases, the posterior cerebral arteries. Simultaneously, a dense network of abnormal collateral vessels is formed at the base of the brain, angiographically resembling a puff of smoke, which is the meaning of the Japanese word "moyamoya".

The cause of moyamoya disease is unknown. It affects all races and has a female preponderance. There is an increased incidence in various unrelated conditions including Down's syndrome, neurofibromatosis, polycystic kidney disease, and following radiotherapy. Postmortem and angiographic studies sometimes show stenoses in extracranial arteries including the renal, pulmonary and external carotid arteries, suggesting that systemic factors may contribute to the pathogenesis. Histology of the affected arteries shows intimal thickening and medial thinning. Increased production of basic fibroblast growth factor (bFGF), a potent mitogen of vascular endothelial and smooth muscle cells, could be responsible. Raised levels of bFGF have been found in the superficial temporal arteries of patients with the disease [2].

The clinical presentation differs between adults and children. Children develop ischaemic events, including TIAs and strokes, as in this case. Seizures are common. The prognosis in this age group is better than in adults, who usually present with cerebral haemorrhage from the fragile, abnormal vessels. Additional cerebrovascular risk factors such as diabetes, hypertension and the oral contraceptive pill are likely to modify the natural history in adults.

The diagnosis of moyamoya disease is based primarily on the angiographic findings. Suzuki and Takaku noted six stages [3].

Stage 1. Suprasellar stenosis of carotid arteries.
Stage 2. Collateral "moyamoya" vessels develop at the base of the brain.
Stage 3. Major trunks of anterior circulation become severely stenosed or occluded.
Stage 4. All components of circle of Willis occluded.
Stage 5. "Moyamoya" vessels diminish and collaterals develop from the extracranial circulation.
Stage 6. "Moyamoya" vessels and cerebral arteries disappear. Cerebral hemispheres receive blood entirely from extracranial–intracranial anastamoses.

This case is considered to correspond to stage 3.

Laborde et al noted a good correlation between angiography and transcranial Doppler sonography and recommend this method in diagnosis, surgical planning and post-surgical follow-up [4].

The commonest CT finding is infarction, as in this case. Cerebral atrophy, haemorrhage or an abnormal vascular network may be seen in the region of the basal ganglia on CT and MRI. MR angiography will demonstrate occluded carotid and cerebral arteries as well as the moyamoya vessels [5].

Surgical treatment is aimed at revascularization of the ischaemic brain through extracranial–intracranial anastamosis.

Although moyamoya is a rare disease, it is increasingly recognized outside Japan and should be considered in all cases of childhood cerebral ischaemia and infarction.

References

1. Takeuchi K, Shimizu K. Hypogenesis of bilateral internal carotid arteries. No To Shinkei 1957;9:37–43.
2. Hoshimaru M, Kikuchi H. Involvement of external carotid arteries in moyamoya disease: neuroradiological evaluation of 66 patients. Neurosurgery 1992;31:398–400.
3. Suzuki J, Takaku A. Cerebrovascular "moyamoya" disease: disease showing abnormal net-like vessels in base of brain. Arch Neurol 1969;20:288–99.
4. Laborde G, Harders A, Klimek L, Hardenack M. Correlation between clinical, angiographic and transcranial Doppler sonographic findings in patients with moyamoya disease. Neurol Res 1993;15:87–92.
5. Trottier F, Dufour M, Grondin P, Bouchard G, et al. Magnetic resonance imaging in moyamoya disease. Can Assoc Radiol J 1994;45:137–9.

In what's my line?

[1]R ORME, [2]L HARPER and [1]J F C OLLIFF

Departments of [1]Radiology and [2]Nephrology, Queen Elizabeth Medical Centre, University Hospitals NHS Trust, Edgbaston, Birmingham B15 2TH, UK

A chest radiograph was performed on a man with renal failure following an apparently uneventful insertion of a double-lumen haemodialysis catheter from the left internal jugular vein (Figure 1). It was noted that although the initial puncture had been believed to be definitely venous, both lines yielded bright red and slightly pulsatile blood on aspiration.

Where is the catheter?

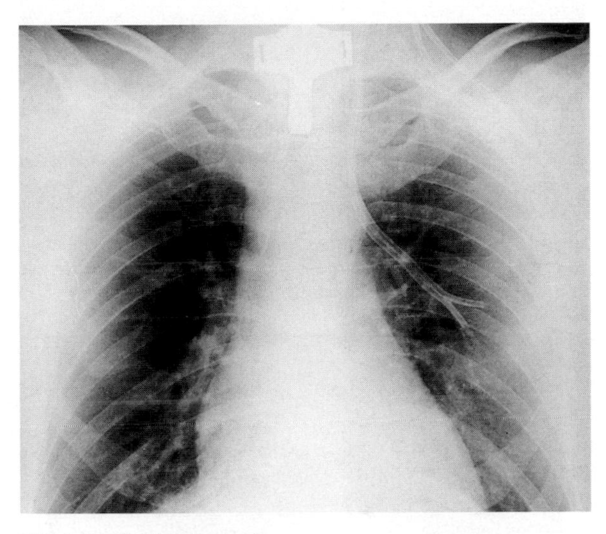

Figure 1. Chest radiograph.

Based on the case of the month originally published in Br J Radiol 1998;71:457–8.

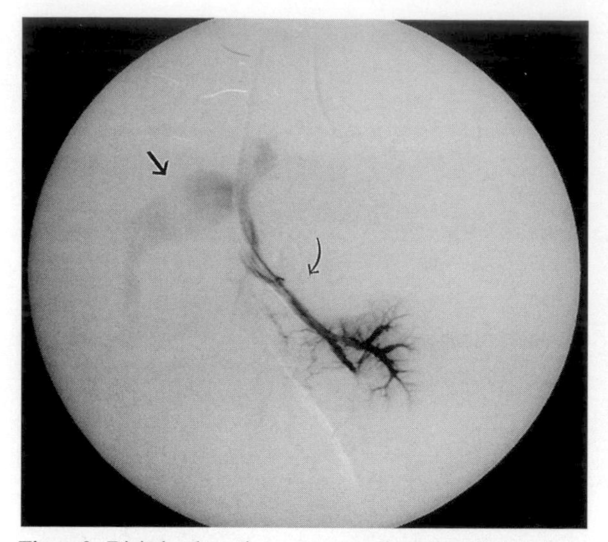

Figure 2. Digital subtraction venogram through catheter shows opacification of a large pulmonary vein (curved arrow) draining into the left innominate vein (straight arrow).

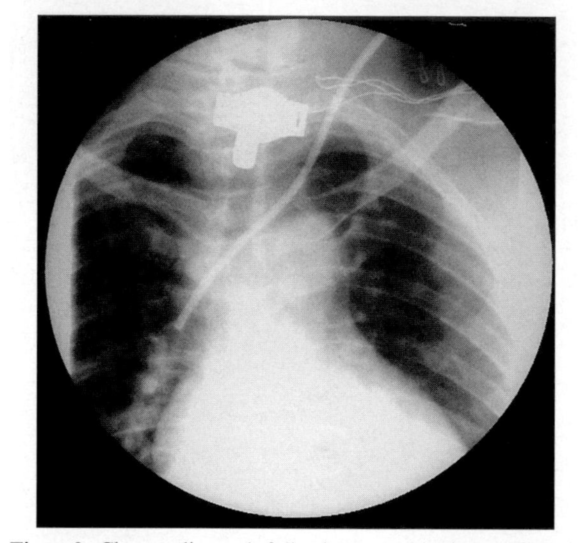

Figure 3. Chest radiograph following repositioning of dialysis catheter.

The catheter had entered an anomalous left superior pulmonary vein draining into the left innominate vein. This was confirmed at venography (Figure 2). Blood gas analyses were also performed, which showed an oxygen saturation of 100% with the catheter in its initial position, consistent with pulmonary venous blood, dropping to systemic venous oxygen saturation in the innominate vein.

Following guidewire manipulation, the catheter was uneventfully repositioned (Figure 3).

Radiological guidance has been advocated as a means of improving success rates and minimizing complications associated with the insertion of long-term central venous catheters [1]. A more reliable and safer initial puncture results from sonographic or fluoroscopic guidance, accurate final positioning of the catheter tip being all but ensured by fluoroscopic monitoring. Catheter tip malpositions are common with "blind" insertion of catheters, rates of 6–32% reported for insertion via the subclavian veins [2, 3]. Common aberrant sites are the contralateral innominate vein and the ipsilateral subclavian or internal jugular vein. Other tributaries of the major veins, such as the azygos, internal thoracic and left pericardiophrenic veins, are also potential sites for catheter malposition. Catheter tip position in smaller veins will usually manifest as a failure of normal catheter function, but malposition in larger veins may not be immediately apparent and is associated with an increased incidence of later complication from trauma to the vessel wall and pericatheter thrombosis [4]. The congenital anomaly of persistent left superior vena cava (SVC) may result in an abnormal appearance on chest radiography but with normal catheter function.

Partial anomalous pulmonary venous drainage of one or more lobes is present in approximately 0.4–0.7% of the "normal" adult population [5, 6]. A degree of left to right shunt is inevitably present but is usually asymptomatic. The anomaly commonly affects the upper lobes and is more frequent on the left, usually draining into the left innominate vein. Since it often causes no symptoms it may be discovered incidentally, for example during computed tomography performed for unrelated indications. Distinction from other venous anomalies, for example persistent SVC, can be made by careful tracing of the abnormal vein on sequential images from its systemic drainage to its tributaries in the pulmonary veins [7]. Three-dimensional reconstruction may be helpful while MRI has also been shown to be effective in evaluating anomalies of pulmonary venous return [8].

References

1. Adam A. Insertion of central venous catheters: time for a new look. Br Med J 1995;311:341–2.
2. Mansfield PF, Hohn DC, Fornage BD, et al. Complications and failures of subclavian catheterisation. N Engl J Med 1994;331:1735–8.
3. Conces DJ, Holden RW. Aberrant locations and complications in initial placement of subclavian vein catheters. Arch Surg 1984;119:293–5.
4. Horshal VL, Ause RG, Hoskins PA. Fibrin sleeve formation on indwelling subclavian central venous catheters. Arch Surg 1971;102:352–8.
5. Healey JE. An anatomic survey of anomalous pulmonary veins: their clinical significance. J Thorac Cardiovasc Surg 1952;23:433–44.
6. Adler SL, Silverman JF. Anomalous venous drainage of the left upper lobe. Radiology 1973;108:563–5.
7. Dillon EH, Camputaro C. Partial anomalous pulmonary venous drainage of the left upper lobe *vs* duplication of the superior vena cava: distinction based on CT findings. AJR 1993;160:375–9.
8. Masui T, Seelos KC, Kersting-Sommerhoff BA, Higgins CB. Abnormalities of the pulmonary veins: evaluation with MR imaging and comparison with cardiac angiography and echocardiography. Radiology 1991;181:645–9.

Contralateral thinking

S MEHTA and R WHITEHOUSE

Department of Diagnostic Radiology, University of Manchester, Stopford Building, Oxford Road, Manchester M13 9PT, UK

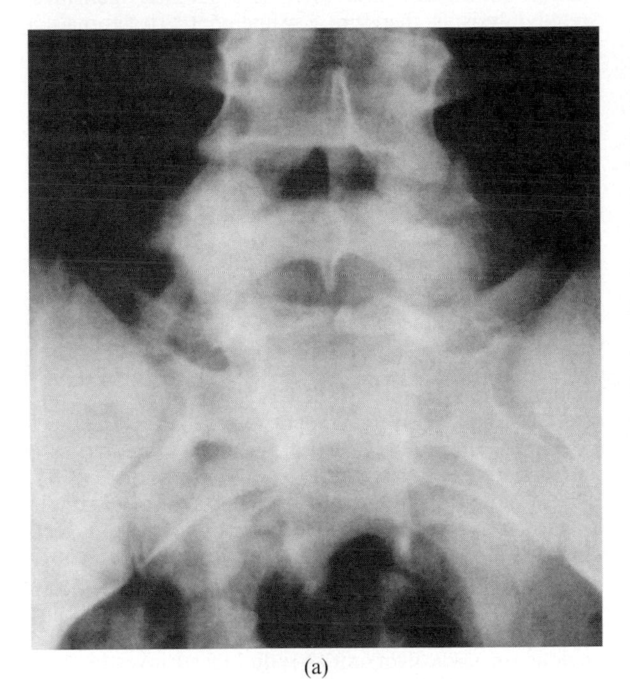

(a)

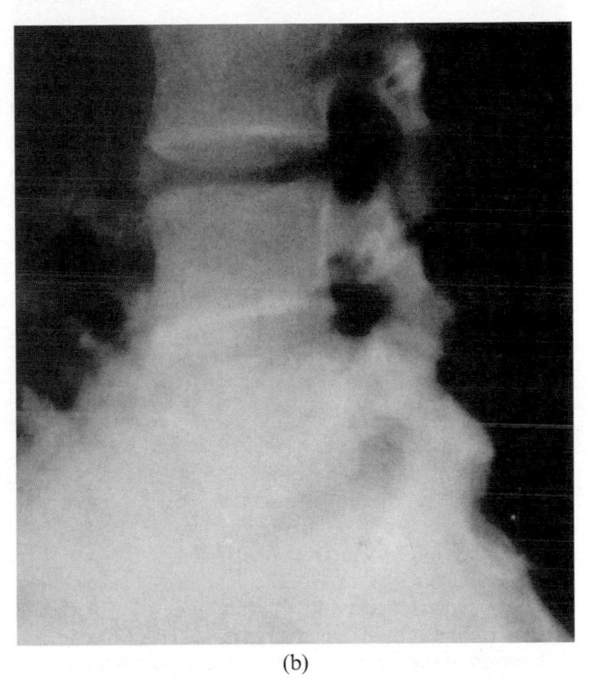

(b)

Figure 1. (a, b).

A 23-year-old man presented to a sports injury clinic with a 6 month history of exercise induced low back pain with radiation to his right buttock. 18 months previously he had been treated for osteomyelitis of the right medial malleolus. On examination there was no neurological deficit. Initial investigations consisted of anteroposterior (AP) and lateral lumbar spine films (Figure 1) and a $^{99}Tc^{m}$ HDP bone scan (Figure 2). Haematological and biochemical investigations were normal.

What is the differential diagnosis and what further investigations are appropriate?

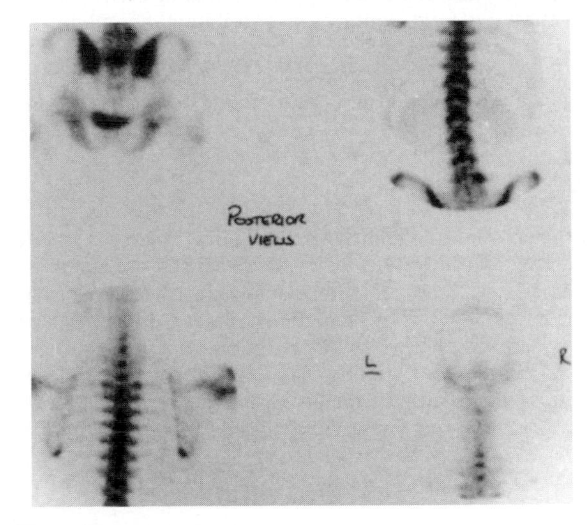

Figure 2.

Based on the case of the month originally published in Br J Radiol 1992;65:549–50.

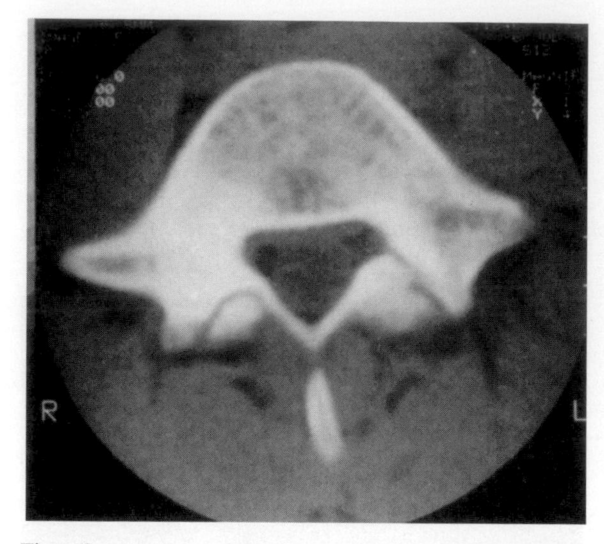

Figure 3.

The lumbar spine films showed a right sided localized area of sclerosis of the neural arch of the L5 vertebra and spina bifida occulta at S1. The bone scan confirmed increased uptake in the region of sclerosis but no other focal abnormality.

The patient was referred for CT with a differential diagnosis of an osteoid osteoma or possibly metastatic osteomyelitis. CT was performed with a GE 9800 scanner using contiguous 5 mm sections through the region of interest with the beam parallel to the end plate. Sclerosis of the pedicle and lamina on the right side of the L5 neural arch was confirmed. There was thickening and elongation of the lamina but no evidence of bone destruction, fracture or a nidus of an osteoid osteoma. On the left there was discontinuity of the neural arch anterior to the facet joint confirming a unilateral spondylolysis (Figure 3).

Sclerosis is a recognized change in the lamina and pedicle opposite a unilateral spondylolysis, reflecting increased stress [1]. Elongation of the lamina on CT has also been described [2].

Sclerosis of the pedicle in the lumbar spine has a wide differential diagnosis. Important causes are listed in Table 1. Yochum et al have comprehensively reviewed the causes [3]. These include the major differentials in this case: osteoid osteoma, infection and spondylolysis. The incidence of spondylolysis has been shown to be zero at birth with an increasing incidence as childhood progresses. Symptomatic spondylolysis often occurs in relation to exercise and there is a familial incidence. Spondylolysis is therefore considered to develop as a stress fracture in patients with a congenital predisposition. Standard AP and lateral plain films will miss up to 20% of cases. Oblique views are generally considered to be the most useful additional view, but a coned lateral view has been found to be the single most sensitive view, identifying 84% of defects. The lateralization, however, cannot be defined and the combination of standard AP, lateral and oblique views remains most sensitive identifying 96.5% of all defects visible on plain film [4].

Table 1. Sclerosis of the pedicle

Agenesis or hypoplasia of the contralateral neural arch
Ipsilateral or contralateral spondylolysis
Osteoid osteoma or osteoblastoma
Metastases, myeloma or lymphoma
Infection
Idiopathic

CT involves a higher radiation dose and defects obvious on plain films may not be easily visible as the pars defect merges with the adjacent facet joint. A CT examination may, however, prove necessary, as in this case, to exclude other pathology such as an osteoid osteoma, osteoblastoma or sclerotic metastases. Failure to detect a complete ring on any section has been suggested as a simple method for detection of spondylolysis on CT [5]. 13% of patients with spondylolysis or spondylolisthesis in one study were found to have a unilateral defect. There was often found to be contralateral sclerosis of the neural arch with elongation attributed to healing of microfractures [2].

In conclusion, unilateral spondylolysis may not be obvious on clinical or initial radiological investigation. The presence of unilateral sclerosis of the neural arch requires careful evaluation of the contralateral pars interarticularis.

References

1. Wilkinson RH, Hall JE. The sclerotic pedicle: tumour or pseudotumour? Radiology 1974;111:683–8.
2. Rothman SL, Glenn WV. CT: multiplanar reconstruction in 253 cases of lumbar spondylolysis. Am J Neuroradiol 1984; 5:81–90.
3. Yochum TR, Sellers LT, Oppennheimer DA, Peterson CK, Kirton DC, Dal Mas EC, et al. The sclerotic pedicle—how many causes are there? Skel Radiol 1990;19:411–7.
4. Amato M, Totty WG, Gilula LA. Spondylolysis of the lumbar spine: demonstration of defects and laminal fragmentation. Radiology 1984;153:627–9.
5. Langston JW, Gavant ML. "Incomplete ring" sign: a simple method for CT detection of spondylolysis. JCAT 1985;9: 728–9.

An unusual cause of abdominal pain

J WONG-YOU-CHEONG

Department of Diagnostic Radiology, Manchester Royal Infirmary, Oxford Road, Manchester M13 9WL, UK

A 57-year-old Asian woman presented with general malaise and intermittent pyrexia 3 months after a renal transplant. She was immunosuppressed with cyclosporin A. Examination showed low grade fever and tenderness in the upper abdomen. Chest and abdominal radiographs were unremarkable. An ultrasound scan showed a heterogeneous mass in the region of the head of the pancreas, displacing the superior mesenteric vein and compressing the inferior vena cava. There was no biliary dilatation. CT scans of the abdomen were then obtained with intravenous contrast enhancement (Figure 1), followed by endoscopic retrograde pancreatography (ERP) (Figure 2). What are the abnormalities and what is the differential diagnosis?

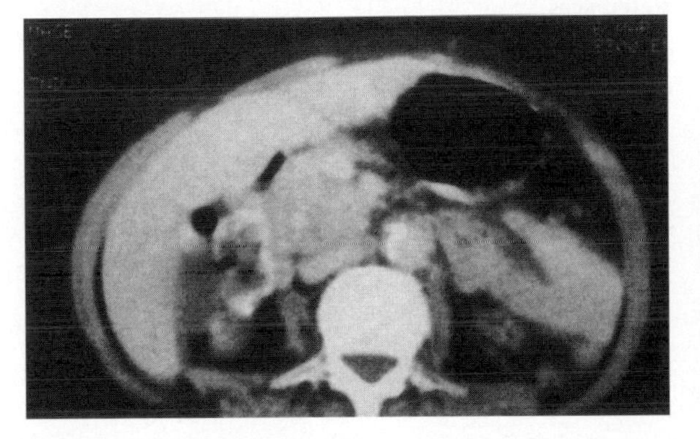

Figure 1. CT scan of upper abdomen with intravenous contrast enhancement.

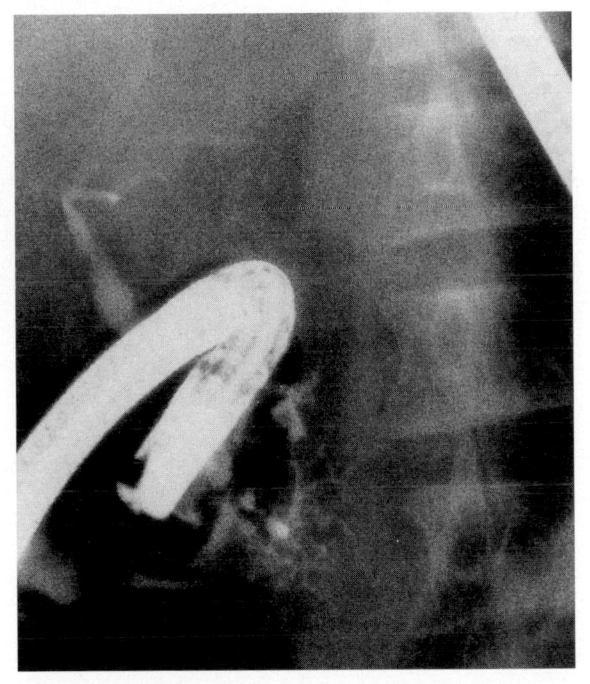

Figure 2. Endoscopic retrograde pancreatogram.

Based on the case of the month originally published in Br J Radiol 1990;63:981–2.

CT confirmed the presence of a heterogeneous, enhancing, hypodense mass in the head of the pancreas with displacement and compression of vessels as seen on ultrasound. On ERP the main pancreatic duct was occluded and the proximal side branches were disorganized with abnormal stenoses and beading. The main diagnoses were pancreatic carcinoma and chronic pancreatitis.

The patient underwent laparotomy where a hard mass was found in the pancreatic head, causing obstruction to the duodenum. The mass was inseparable from the superior mesenteric vein and was thought to be an inoperable pancreatic carcinoma. A gastrojejunostomy and two Tru-cut biopsies were performed.

There was no evidence of neoplasm in the biopsy samples but caseating granulomata were present, and a Ziehl–Neelsen stain was positive. The patient received antituberculous therapy and a follow-up ultrasound scan showed no evidence of a residual mass. The patient remained well on follow-up 4 years later.

Tuberculosis of the pancreas is rare, even in countries where tuberculosis is endemic. Involvement of the pancreas can occur as part of a generalized infection such as miliary tuberculosis. Focal involvement is rarer still. Tuberculosis may present as acute or chronic pancreatitis [1] and as a mass mimicking carcinoma [2]. It has been postulated that infection of the pancreas may occur by two different mechanisms: haematogenous dissemination or by penetration of the organ by adjacent lymph nodes. This patient had no other evidence of tuberculosis, but she had been immunosuppressed and she was of Asian origin.

Tuberculosis is well recognized in transplanted patients in whom the presentation is atypical and diagnosis is difficult. Infection is predominantly pulmonary [3] and responds well to antituberculous therapy.

The diagnosis of pancreatic tuberculosis is difficult. Clinical features may suggest the possibility, which should be investigated by CT and ERP. Confirmation, however, must be by histology.

References

1. Stock KP, Riemann JF, Stadler W, Rosch W. Tuberculosis of the pancreas. Endoscopy 1981;13:178–80.
2. Chandrasekhara KL, Iyer SK, Stanek AE, Herbstman H. Pancreatic tuberculosis mimicking carcinoma. Gastrointest Endosc 1985;31:386–8.
3. McWhinney N, Khan O, Williams G. Tuberculosis in patients undergoing maintenance haemodialysis and renal transplantation. Br J Surg 1981;68:408–11.

What is this breast mass?

M A RAMIREZ-ESCOBAR and I R SALMERÓN

Servicio de Radiodiagnóstico, Hospital Príncipe de Asturias, Alcalá de Henares, Madrid, Spain

A 63-year-old woman was referred for screening mammography. A nodular density was seen in the deep medial tissue of her right breast on the craniocaudal projection (Figure 1). No abnormality was seen on the lateral oblique projection. No palpable abnormality was noted on physical examination. An additional rotated craniocaudal view was performed (Figure 2). Ultrasound (US) of the breast showed no solid or cystic masses.

What does the mammogram show? What is the differential diagnosis of this radiological finding? What investigation would you carry out next?

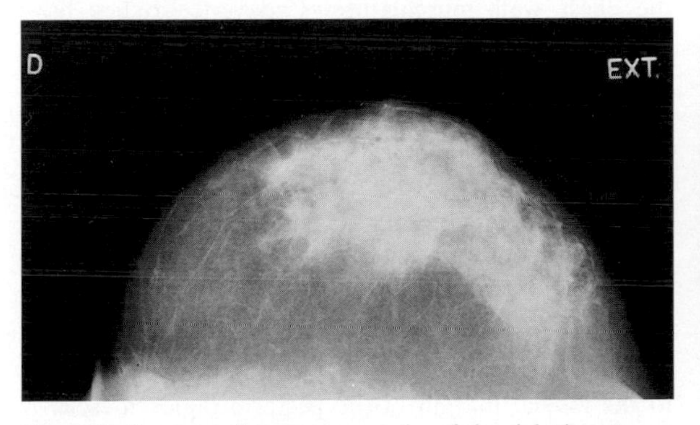

Figure 1. Craniocaudal mammography of the right breast.

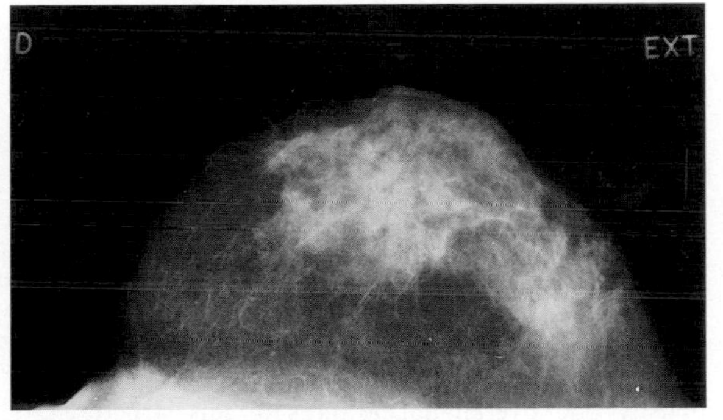

Figure 2. Rotated craniocaudal view.

Based on the case of the month originally published in Br J Radiol 1998;71:573–4.

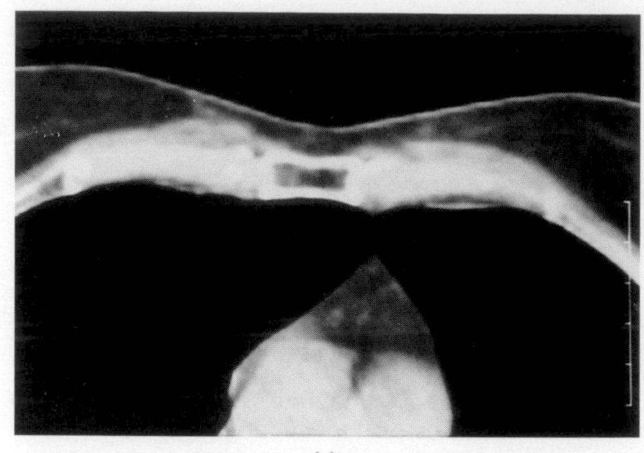
(a)

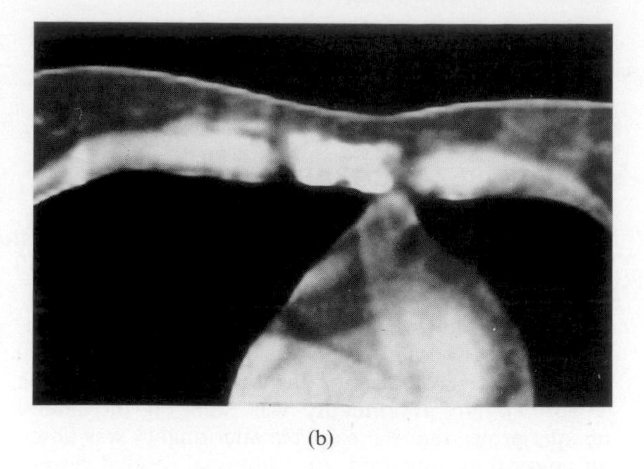
(b)

Figure 3. (a, b) Sequential axial CT scan of the chest wall.

The craniocaudal mammographic projection showed a mass, suspicious of carcinoma, in the medial aspect of the deep breast tissues. It had a rounded but irregular shape and was almost completely surrounded by fat (Figure 1). On a rotated craniocaudal projection, the density was in continuity with the pectoral muscle (Figure 2). This appearance is highly suggestive of a chest wall structure but breast cancer infiltrating the pectoralis muscle cannot be excluded. On CT images (Figure 3) there was a bandlike structure, 2 cm wide and 4 cm long, lying anterior to the medial margin of the pectoralis major muscle. A thin layer of fatty tissue lay between the sternalis and the pectoral major muscle. The density and overall appearances of this structure are consistent with a muscle running longitudinally along the border of the sternum: the sternalis muscle. The patient was re-examined 6 months later and no change was seen in the mammographic appearance of the density.

Improved mammographic positioning allows better imaging of deep breast tissues. When the craniocaudal view is properly performed, the pectoralis muscle is visualized in 30–40% of patients [1, 2]. This muscle is usually shown as a convex density along the posterior edge of the image. Occasionally, a small focal density is visible in the medial aspect of the breast, on the craniocaudal projection only, which cannot be explained as the pectoralis muscle. Bradley et al have shown that this unusual structure is the sternalis muscle [3]. They established the diagnosis by exploratory surgery in one case and with CT or MR in five other cases. The sternalis (or pre-sternalis) muscle is an unusual anatomical variant of the chest wall musculature. Cadaveric studies have shown that the sternalis muscle is present in 5–8% of males and females, and is more often unilateral than bilateral [4]. The sternalis muscle has a superficial parasternal location and runs from the infraclavicular region to the inferior aspect of the sternum, overlying the pectoralis major muscle. Its mammographic appearance is that of an irregular rounded soft tissue density at the sternal edge of the craniocaudal projection, almost completely surrounded by fat [3]. In general, it cannot be identified on the mediolateral oblique projection. On supine CT scans the sternalis muscle assumes a bandlike shape and is seen as a flattened structure lying anterior to the medial margin of the pectoral major muscle. A band of fat tissue is usually interposed between the sternalis and the pectoralis muscle. Familiarity with the mammographic appearance of the sternalis muscle on the craniocaudal projection is necessary to avoid confusion with a breast cancer. The correct diagnosis is suggested by the location and by the absence of an abnormality on the mediolateral oblique projection and on physical examination. CT, as in this particular case, or MRI will confirm the presence of the muscle and prevent unnecessary biopsy.

References

1. Eklund GW, Cardenosa G. The art of mammographic positioning. Radiol Clin North Am 1992;30:21–53.
2. Bassett LW. Clinical image evaluation. Radiol Clin North Am 1995;33:1027–39.
3. Bradley FM, Hoover HC Jr, Hulka CA, et al. The sternalis muscle: an unusual finding seen on mammography. AJR 1996;166:33–6.
4. Testut L, Latarget A. Músculos del tórax. In: Salvat, editor. Anatomía humana. Barcelona, 1985:895–920.

Castles in the air?

A J BRADLEY, N B THOMAS and S A SUKUMAR

Department of Radiology, North Manchester General Hospital, Delaneys Road, Manchester M8 6RL, UK

A 22-year-old Asian woman presented with a 2 year history of unproductive cough, which had not resolved with simple measures. Clinical examination and routine blood tests were normal. A chest radiograph was taken (Figure 1) and had not changed since a previous radiograph, taken 4 years earlier. Pre- and post-contrast CT examination was performed (Figure 2). What abnormality is shown on the chest radiograph and CT? Suggest a possible diagnosis.

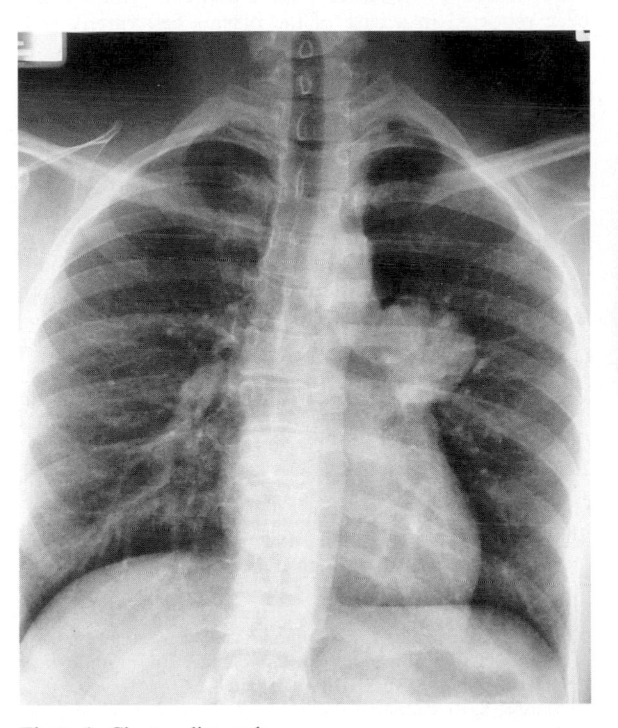

Figure 1. Chest radiograph.

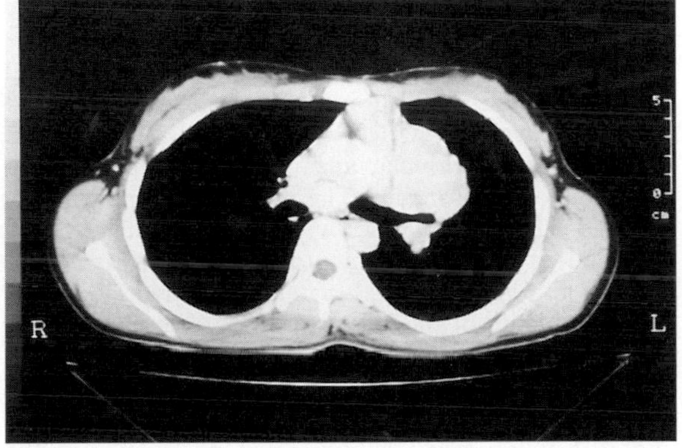

Figure 2. Post-contrast CT.

Based on the case of the month originally published in Br J Radiol 1997;70:767–8

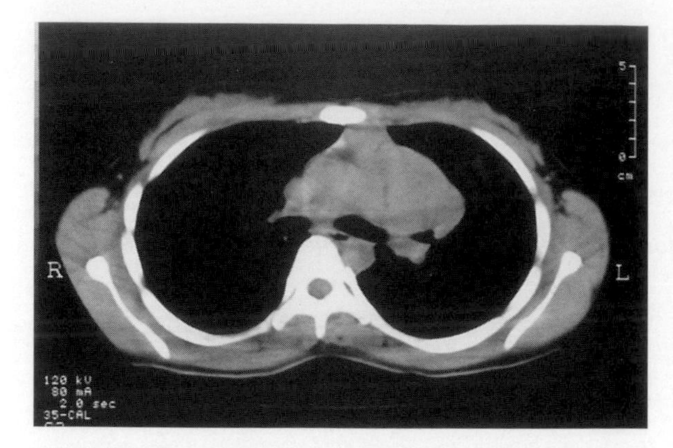

Figure 3. Follow-up CT scan demonstrating no change in the mass.

The chest radiograph showed a left sided mediastinal mass. The CT scan demonstrated a solitary lobulated soft tissue mass in the left anterior mediastinum. This mass was highly vascular and intimately related to the thymus and left bronchus. The mass was homogeneous, and had a smooth interface with the adjacent lung.

A limited anterior thoracotomy was performed. At operation, a vascular mass was found, surrounding the major branches of the left pulmonary artery, thus rendering it inoperable. Biopsy revealed typical features of hyaline vascular angiofollicular lymphoid hyperplasia (Castleman's disease). Follow-up CT (Figure 3), 2 years after the initial scan, demonstrated no change in the appearance, size or enhancement characteristics of the mass; and there was no change in symptoms.

Giant lymph node hyperplasia occurring in the mediastinum was initially described by Castleman in 1954 [1]. Since that time, over 200 cases have been reported in the literature. The hyaline-vascular type of angiofollicular lymphoid hyperplasia (AFLH) accounts for 90% of cases. The other 10% constitute the plasma cell group, characterized by large follicles surrounded by sheets of plasma cells [2]. The aetiology remains unknown [3] although, in the plasma cell type, altered immune parameters such as anergy or the absence of suppressor T cells have been described [4]. It is uncertain whether the plasma cell and hyaline vascular types represent different entities, or whether they arise from differences in host response to the same process [2]. 70% of cases in the literature occur in the chest; of these 85% are mediastinal, and the remainder intrapulmonary [5]. Thoracic cases are usually of the hyaline-vascular type, and present as an incidental finding in over 50% of cases. The commonest extrathoracic sites are in the lymph nodes of the retroperitoneum, mesentery, axilla and neck. Extralymphatic sites include muscles, parotid gland and pancreas.

The characteristic findings on a chest radiograph are of smooth mediastinal or hilar mass, with no central necrosis or cystic change. CT may show multiple discrete nodes, giving a lobulated appearance. Calcification was initially documented in 4% of mediastinal lesions, but has been found more frequently with the increasing use of CT. Marked enhancement with intravenous contrast is due to the vascular nature of these lesions. Digital subtraction angiography may show a marked capillary blush, and can be useful for excluding abnormality of a major vascular structure [3]. Uptake of gallium has been reported in a case of the plasma cell variety [6]. MRI demonstrates homogeneous low signal on T_1 weighted sequences, with marked contrast enhancement. Lesions are of high signal on T_2 weighted images [7]. MRI features are not specific and CT guided or operative biopsy are usually required for confirmation. The vascular nature can make biopsy or surgery hazardous, but pre-operative embolization has been successfully employed to reduce intraoperative haemorrhage [8].

Castleman's disease, although relatively rare, should be considered in the differential diagnosis of a smooth mediastinal or hilar mass in a young patient.

References

1. Castleman B. Case records of the Massachusetts General Hospital. Weekly clinicopathological exercise case No. 40011. New Engl J Med 1954;250:26–30.
2. Keller AR, Hochmolzer L, Castleman B. Hyaline vascular and plasma cell types of giant lymph node hyperplasia of the mediastinum and other locations. Cancer 1972;29:670–83.
3. Samuels TH, Hamilton PA, Ngan B. Mediastinal Castleman's disease: Demonstration with computed tomography and angiography. Can Assoc Radiol J 1990;41: 380–3.
4. Serour F, Liberman Y, Rosenman J, et al. Castleman's disease of the mediastinum, misleading clinical and radiological characteristics. Resp Med 1989; 83:509–12.
5. Meissel S, Rosenman J, Yellin A, et al. Castleman's disease: An uncommon computed tomographic feature. Chest 1988;6:1306–7.
6. Stansby G, Milson A, Hamilton G. Gallium scintigraphy in the diagnosis and management of multifocal Castleman's disease. Br J Radiol 1991;64:165–7.
7. Moon WK, Im JG, Han MC. Castleman's disease of the mediastinum: MR imaging features. Clin Radiol 1994; 49:466–8.
8. Walters JF, Tottenberg RW, Cannon WB, et al. Giant mediastinal lymph node hyperplasia (Castleman's disease): Angiographic and clinical features. AJR 1978;130:447–50.

A painful scoliosis

P G PRESTON

Department of Radiology, Edinburgh Royal Infirmary, Edinburgh, UK

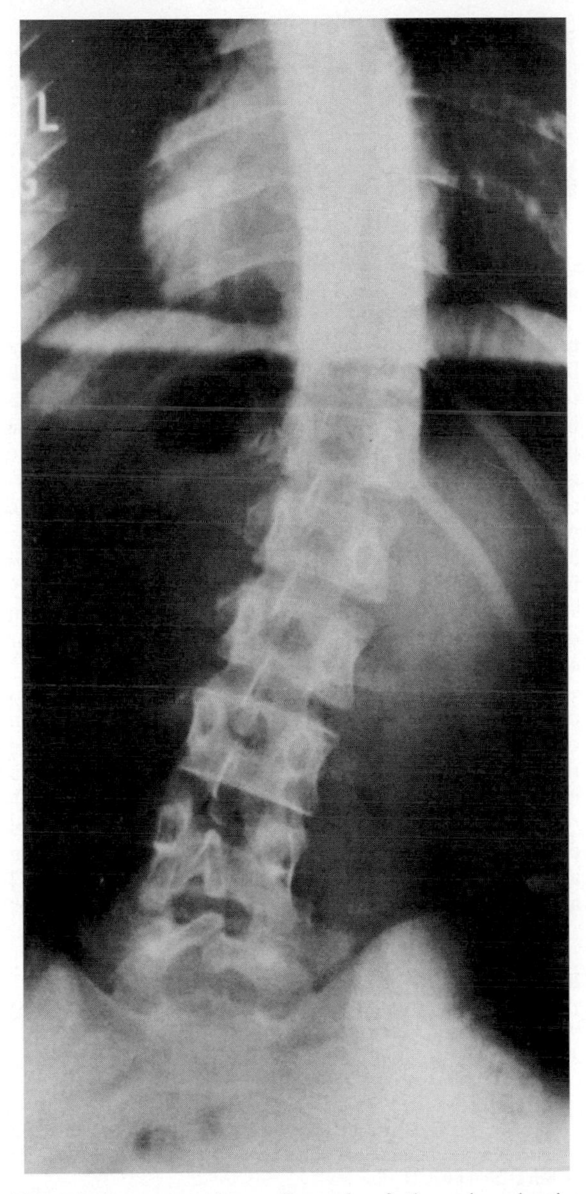

Figure 1. Posteroanterior radiograph of the spine showing scoliosis and an unfused neural arch at L5, but no other abnormality.

Based on the case of the month originally published in Br J Radiol 1986;59:1233–5.

A 14-year-old girl presented with a 2-year history of continuous pain in the lumbar region. The pain was worse at night, exacerbated by movement and partially relieved by analgesics. On initial examination she had a thoracolumbar scoliosis with severe restriction of all movements of the lumbar spine. Plain radiography of the spine (Figure 1) demonstrated a thoracolumbar scoliosis, extending from T7 to L3, concave to the left with a Cobb angle of 31° and no other abnormality.

An isotope bone scan was then performed (Figure 2).

What is the differential diagnosis and what other investigation would be helpful?

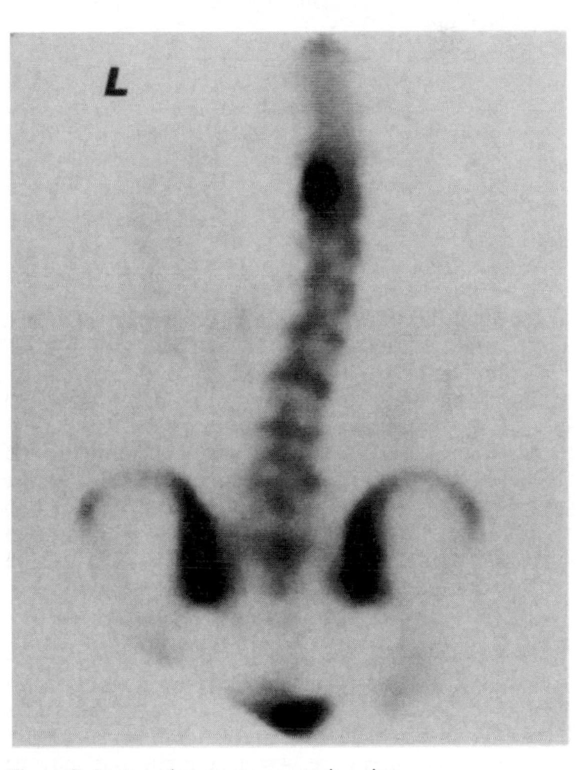

Figure 2. Isotope bone scan, posterior view.

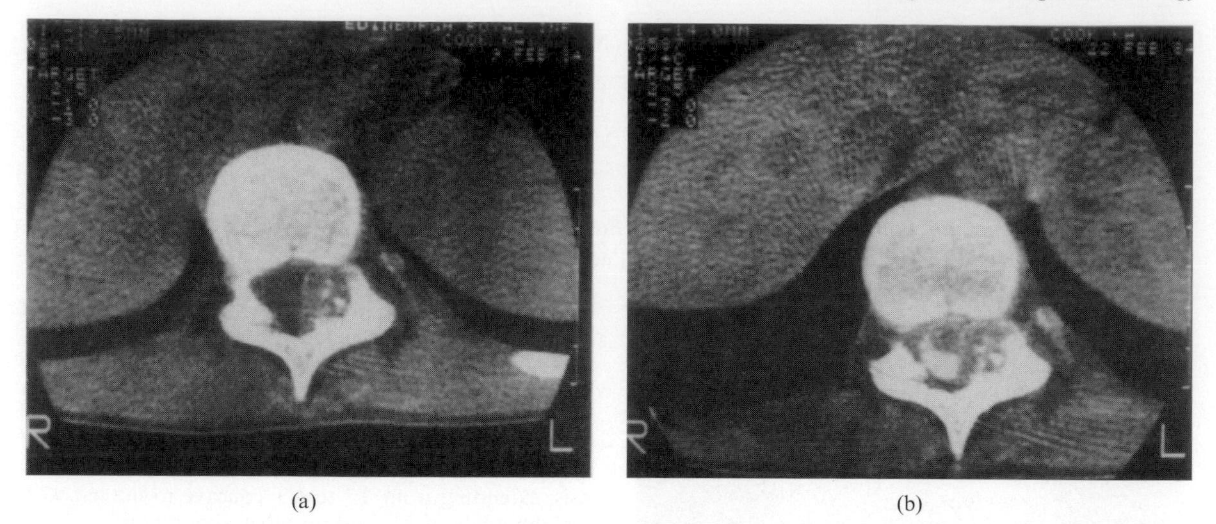

(a) (b)

Figure 3. CT of the spine at T11, (a) without and (b) with intrathecal contrast medium (L + 100, W 500). A soft tissue mass with calcified areas is extending into the canal from the left side of the neural arch and displacing the theca to the right.

Adolescent scoliosis may be seen at this age, but is not painful, and the history of pain should raise the possibility of underlying pathology. Night pain and relief by analgesics is seen in osteoid osteomas and in osteoblastoma.

The bone scan (Figure 2) showed a solitary area of increased uptake in the left side of T11, at the apex of the concavity of the scoliosis. CT was also performed at this level (Figure 3) and showed a mass arising from the left pedicle of T11 and extending into the spinal canal, with displacement of the thecal sac to the right. The mass was of mixed attenuation, having calcification and soft tissue densities within it.

At operation, a soft, red, lobulated tumour was found arising from the pedicle of T11 and extending into the spinal canal. The tumour was removed and an interfacet: intertransverse fusion was performed from T10 to T12. The tumour measured 3.2 cm × 1.5 cm × 1 cm. Histological examination showed immature woven bone and osteoid trabeculae within richly vascular connective tissue. There was little evidence of organization around a central nidus. Her pain disappeared within 24 h of the operation. Her scoliosis progressively resolved and 6 months after surgery the angle of the scoliosis had decreased from 31° to 15°. After 12 months the Cobb angle measured 6°.

There is considerable difficulty clinically, radiologically and histologically in distinguishing osteoblastoma and osteoid osteoma when they occur in the spine. Clinically, an osteoid osteoma is often associated with more pain, which can be worse at night and may be relieved by aspirin. Radiologically, the major differentiation can be based on size and degree of reactive sclerosis. Osteoid osteomas have a limited growth potential, whereas osteoblastomas enlarge progressively and have dimensions usually greater than 1.5 cm. A tumour which grows and expands into the spinal canal is much more likely to be an osteoblastoma. The location of both tumours in the spine is similar, usually in the neural arch in the region of the pedicle or base of the transverse process. Characteristically, osteoid osteomas cause more reactive sclerosis. CT usually shows this sclerosis surrounding a central nidus but in some cases only the reactive sclerosis is visible. Calcification and new bone formation within the tumour is more often seen in osteoblastomas [1]. Histologically, an osteoid osteoma may show organization around a central nidus, whilst an osteoblastoma shows mineralization and large vascular spaces [2].

A spinal bone tumour should be suspected if there is a painful scoliosis [3]. In a growing child, progression of the scoliosis with vertebral rotation may occur during this delay and subsequent surgical excision of the lesion may not result in complete resolution of the scoliosis [4].

Plain radiography is positive in less than 50% of patients [3]. An isotope bone scan will be positive in almost 100% of patients with an osteoid osteoma [5] and CT can then be performed at the appropriate level.

References

1. McLeod RA, Dahlin DC, Beabout JW. The spectrum of osteoblastoma. AJR 1976;126:321–35.
2. Marsh BW, Bonfiglio M, Brady LP, Enneking WF. Benign osteoblastoma: range of manifestations. J Bone Joint Surg 1975;57A:1–9.
3. Kirwan EO'G, Hutton PAN, Pozo JL, Ransford AO. Osteoid osteoma and benign osteoblastoma of the spine. J Bone Joint Surg 1984;66B:21–6.
4. Ransford AO, Pozo JL, Hutton PAN, Kirwan EO'G. The behaviour pattern of the scoliosis associated with osteoid osteoma or osteoblastoma of the spine. J Bone Joint Surg 1984;66B:16–20.
5. Lisbona R, Rosenthall L. Role of radionuclide imaging in osteoid osteoma. AJR 1979;132:77–80.

A colonic double bubble

[1]A HARRISON, [2]L MACHIN and [3]A GRUNDY

Departments of [1]Surgery, [2]Pathology and [3]Radiology, St George's Hospital, London SW17 0QT, UK

A 62-year-old woman presented with a 3-month history of two large abdominal swellings. There were no associated gastrointestinal or urinary symptoms and no history of previous abdominal surgery. On clinical examination, two 10 cm diameter, firm, mobile and non-tender masses were present in the left side of the abdomen. They were thought clinically to be arising within the abdominal wall. Clinical examination was otherwise unremarkable.

A supine abdominal radiograph (Figure 1) was taken. Subsequently, a double-contrast barium enema was performed (Figure 2). What is the most likely diagnosis?

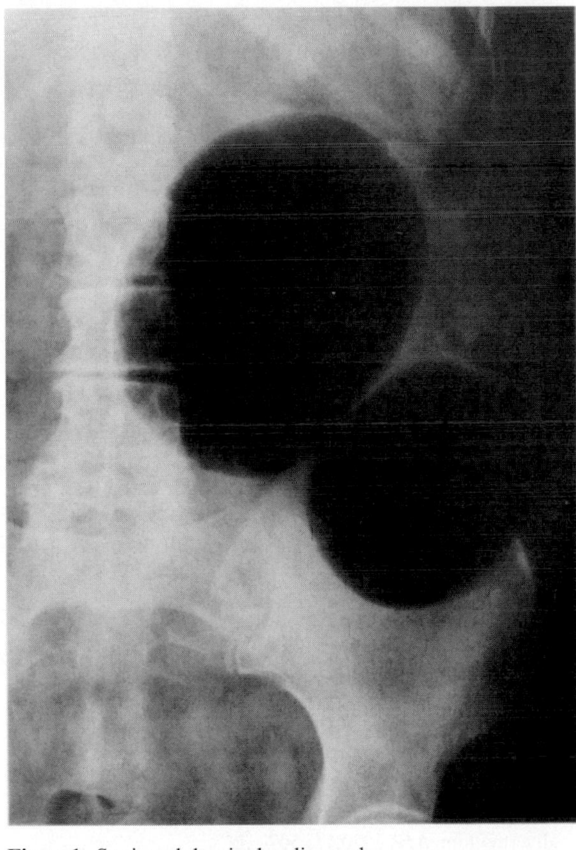

Figure 1. Supine abdominal radiograph.

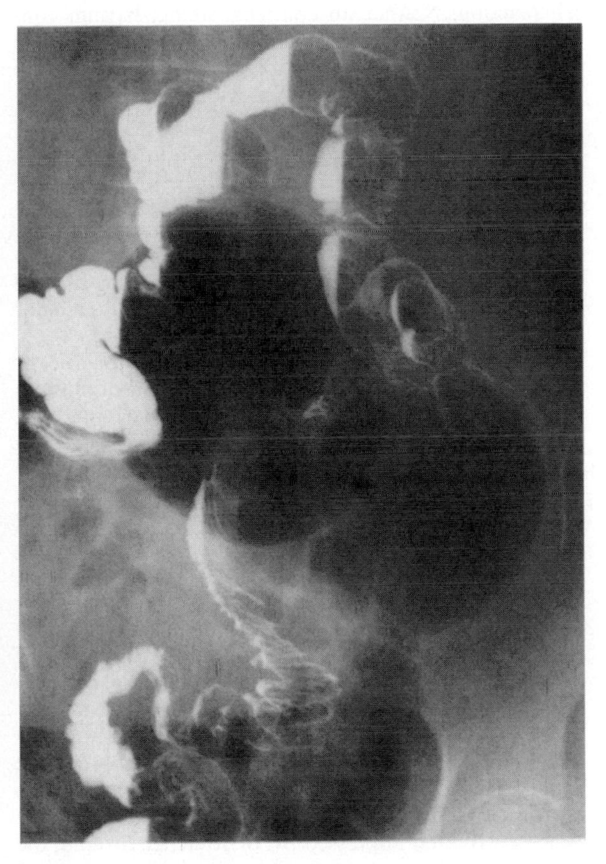

Figure 2. Double-contrast barium enema.

Based on the case of the month originally published in Br J Radiol 1989;62:85–6.

The plain abdominal radiograph showed two well circumscribed, oval, air-containing collections in the left side of the abdomen. The bowel gas pattern was otherwise unremarkable. The barium enema showed the sigmoid colon stretched around the two air-filled structures which did not fill with barium. There was diverticulosis in the adjacent sigmoid colon.

The patient underwent laparotomy at which two air-filled structures were identified attached to the sigmoid colon and communicating with each other. A segment of small bowel was adherent to the colon at this site. The involved segment of sigmoid colon was resected along with the segment of the adjacent small bowel (Figure 3). The patient made an uneventful post-operative recovery.

Histological examination of the resected specimen showed two communicating fibrous-walled cysts within the serosa of the sigmoid colon. There was faecal debris in their walls which had elicited both acute and chronic granulomatous inflammation and a foreign body giant cell reaction. Neither an epithelial lining, barium contents nor communication with the bowel lumen were demonstrated, although the presence of faecal debris within the cysts implied some previous communication.

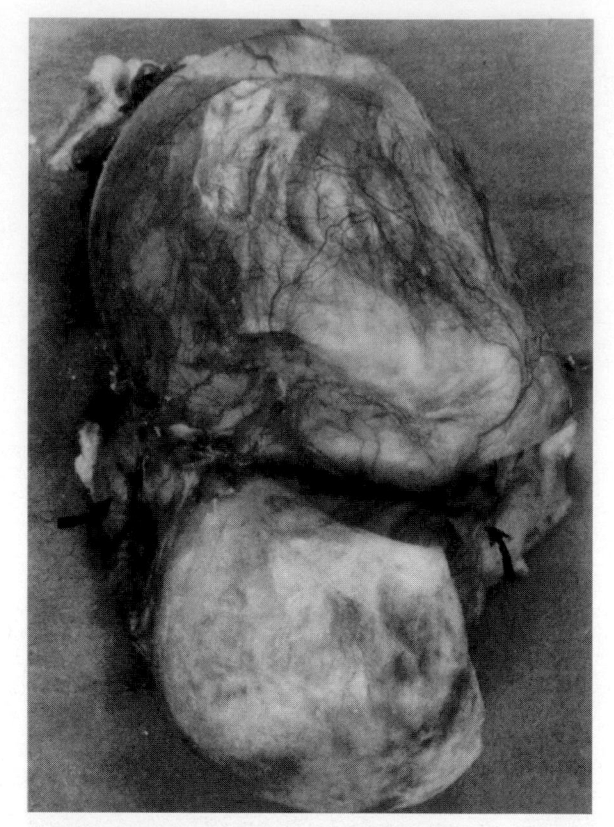

Figure 3. Resected specimen. Two giant sigmoid diverticula measuring 15 cm × 11 cm and 10 cm × 8 cm arising from and lying either side of the sigmoid colon (arrows).

Giant colonic diverticula or giant air-cysts of the colon may present as an unusual gas collection arising from the large bowel. In the majority of cases they arise from the sigmoid colon [1]. They are usually solitary, multiplicity having been described in only a small number of cases [2]. There is almost always evidence of diverticular disease elsewhere in the colon.

Giant colonic diverticula may be asymptomatic or may present with pain, vomiting, abdominal distension, malaena or more acute symptoms of diverticulitis [1], including perforation or, rarely, as a palpable abdominal mass.

Giant colonic diverticula can be detected on plain radiographs as rounded or elliptical, well circumscribed air collections, usually in the left side of the abdomen [3]. Such collections may exceed 20 cm in diameter. Differential diagnosis includes other causes of large air collections such as abscesses, which are usually less well circumscribed, or diverticula arising from other parts of the gastrointestinal tract, such as giant duodenal diverticula or a dilated air-containing Meckel's diverticulum.

On barium enema, these diverticula do not always fill with barium and a communication with the colonic lumen may be found in only 60% of cases [1]. They are invariably in close proximity to the sigmoid colon and the colon is often impressed by, or stretched around, the diverticula.

On histological examination the wall of a giant colonic diverticulum is often composed of acute and chronically inflamed tissue. Mucosal and muscular remnants may not be found. It is unusual not to find a communication with the colon [4]. In this case a communication was not visible on pathological examination although the presence of faecal debris within the lumen of the diverticula implies that a communication had existed.

Three mechanisms for the development of giant sigmoid diverticula have been proposed. Inflammation at the neck of a pre-existing diverticulum may lead to a ball-valve mechanism resulting in a massively enlarged pseudodiverticulum of mucosa and submucosa protruding through the wall of the colon. Alternatively, perforation of a diverticulum may occur, leading to a progressively enlarging pseudocyst, secondary to a ball-valve mechanism. The other suggested mechanism is that the neck of a diverticulum is occluded and the diverticulum becomes distended by gas-forming organisms.

References

1. Kricun R, Stasik JJ, Reither RD, Dex WJ. Giant colonic diverticulum. AJR 1980;135:507–12.
2. Gallagher JJ, Welch JP. Giant diverticula of the sigmoid colon: a review of differential diagnosis and operative treatment. Arch Surg 1979;114:1079–83.
3. Rosenberg RF, Naidich JB. Plain film recognition of giant colonic diverticula. Am J Gastroenterol 1981;76:59–69.
4. Muhletaler CA, Berger JL, Robinette CL. Pathogenesis of giant colonic diverticula. Gastrointest Radiol 1981;6:217–22.

A fit in a young woman

[1]A VALI, [1]C S McKINSTRY and [2]D DICK

Departments of [1]Neuroradiology and [2]Neurology, Regional Neurological Centre, Newcastle General Hospital, Westgate Road, Newcastle upon Tyne NE4 6BE, UK

A 33-year-old woman was admitted to hospital with a 4-day history of nausea and headache exacerbated by bending or coughing. On the day of admission she had a major seizure and two further major fits in the following 24 h. 3 weeks previously she had given birth to a normal child by a spontaneous vertex delivery. She had a past history of recurrent pulmonary emboli and at the time of admission was receiving prophylactic subcutaneous heparin 5000 units twice daily, which had been commenced during her pregnancy.

Physical examination on admission showed left-sided visual inattention with parietal sensory disturbance in the left hand. Reflexes were generally brisk but otherwise the power, tone and co-ordination in her limbs were normal. She was in sinus rhythm, normotensive with normal heart sounds and no abnormal pulses or bruits were detected.

Examination of the cerebrospinal fluid at the referring hospital showed 41 red blood cells mm^{-3}, 9 white blood cells mm^{-3} and an elevated protein concentration of $0.72\ g\,l^{-1}$.

CT of the head was obtained on an EMI 1010 scanner and this was repeated the following day on a GE 9800 machine following intravenous contrast enhancement (Figure 1).

What abnormalities are present? What is the diagnosis and how might this be confirmed?

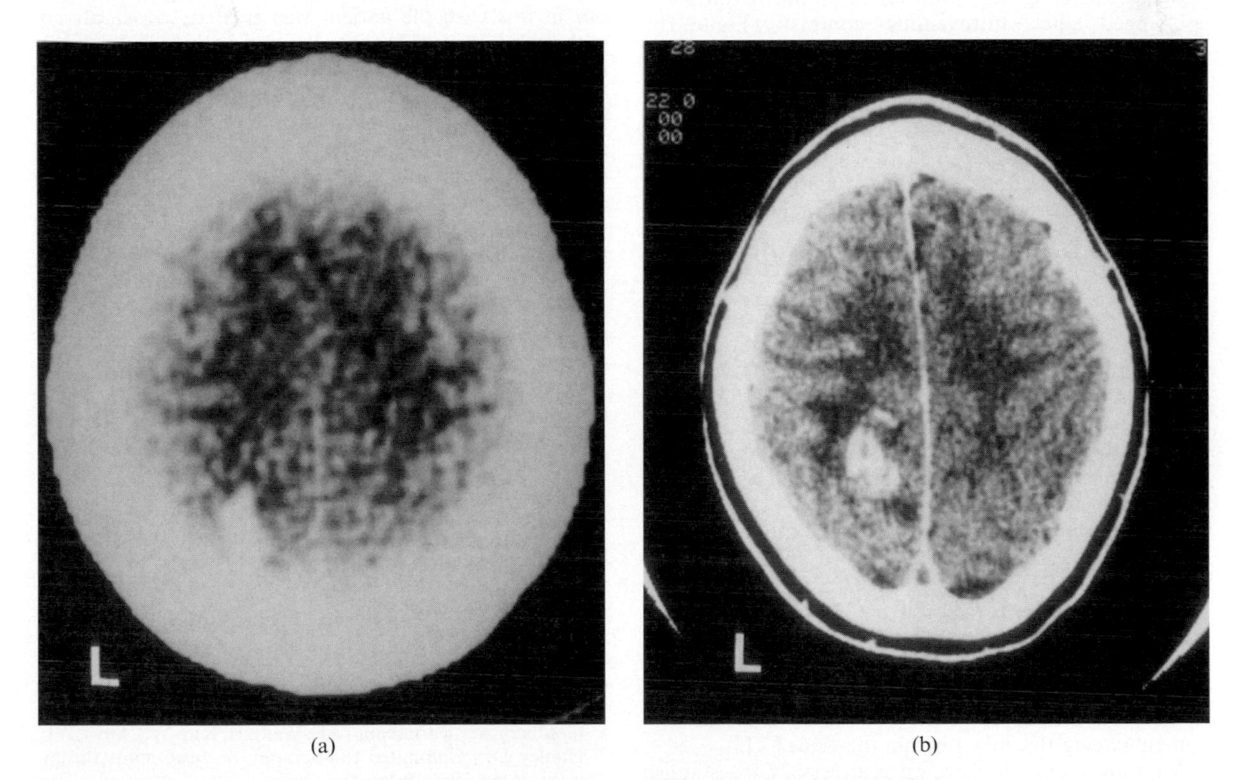

(a) (b)

Figure 1. (a) Unenhanced CT on admission. (b) Contrast enhanced CT on the day after admission.

Based on the case of the month originally published in Br J Radiol 1988;61:335–6.

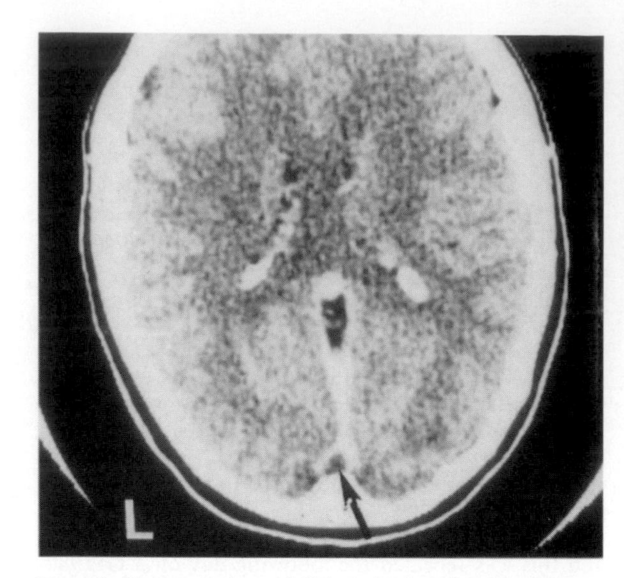

Figure 2. Contrast enhanced CT on the day after admission, at the level of the bodies of the lateral ventricles. Note an apparent filling defect within the posterior superior sagittal sinus (arrow).

Figure 1a showed a hyperdense area deep in the left parietal lobe consistent with an acute haematoma and unchanged after intravenous contrast (Figure 1b). Haemorrhage from an arteriovenous malformation or possibly an embolic infarction were considered as diagnoses in this case. However, Figure 1b showed an obvious triangular-shaped low density area with an enhanced rim in the region of the superior sagittal sinus (SSS). This was present on contiguous sections (Figure 2) and is an example of the so-called "empty triangle" or "empty delta" sign of SSS thrombosis.

Apart from pregnancy and the puerperium, other possible causes of SSS thrombosis include dehydration, steroids (including oral contraceptives), haematological disorders, neoplasms compressing the sinus and rarely arteriovenous malformations.

The empty triangle sign was first described in 1978 [1] and is considered to be pathognomonic of SSS thrombosis. A review of the literature listed 54 cases of SSS thrombosis out of a total of 76 cases of intracranial sinovenous occlusive disease in which the CT appearances had been reported [2]. The two most frequently observed signs were the empty delta sign (28.6%) and haemorrhagic venous infarction (22%). The origin of the empty delta sign is uncertain, although there is evidence that it may arise from congestion of dural vascular collateral channels in the leaves of the SSS which contrast with non-enhancing thrombus within the sinus [2].

A strong index of suspicion is necessary to establish the diagnosis and viewing of scans at wide window settings is essential [3]. The normal SSS usually enhances

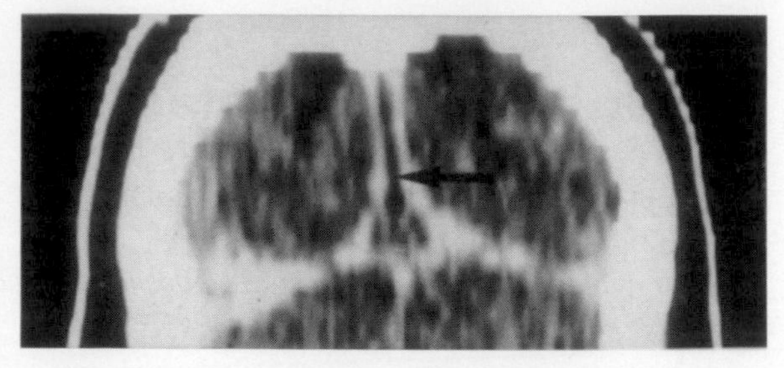

Figure 3. Coronal reformatted image through torcula and superior sagittal sinus confirms the presence of an extensive filling defect (arrow).

homogeneously and, although low density areas may be seen, these are usually limited to one section only and do not involve the full surface of the sinus [4].

Confirmation of the diagnosis may be achieved by angiography. The use of thin serial CT sections allows multiplanar reconstruction to provide sufficiently precise demonstration of the thrombus [5]. Contiguous 3 mm thick cuts through the torcula and SSS in this patient allowed coronal reformatting and demonstration of the abnormality extending into the SSS and transverse sinuses (Figure 3).

The presence of both an empty delta sign and haemorrhage has been reported to imply a worse prognosis [2] but in this case the patient was treated conservatively with withdrawal of heparin therapy and made an excellent clinical recovery. A follow-up scan 3 weeks later showed resolution of the haematoma and some reduction in the sinus lesion; complete resolution of the empty delta sign may take 1.5–2 months [3]. Use of the correct technique and a high index of suspicion will enable this rare diagnosis to be made.

[*Beware of false positives—when there is a delay between contrast injection and CT scanning (20–50 min), dural enhancement in wall of sinus will simulate a delta sign of SSS thrombus [6]. MRI demonstrates sagittal sinus thrombosis well, the normal flow void being lost. As with CT, the delta sign may be seen, ED*]

References

1. Buonanno FS, Moody DM, Ball MR, Laster DW. Computed cranial tomographic findings in cerebral sinovenous occlusion. JCAT 1978;2:281–90.
2. Virapongse C, Cazanave C, Quisling R, Sarwar M, Hunter S. The empty delta sign: frequency and significance in 76 cases of dural sinus thrombosis. Radiology 1987;162:779–85.
3. Brant-Zawadzki M, Chang GY, McCarty GE. Computed tomography in dural sinus thrombosis. Arch Neurol 1982; 39:446–7.
4. Zilkha A, Stenzler SA, Lin JH. Computed tomography of the normal and abnormal superior sagittal sinus. Clin Radiol 1982;33:415–25.
5. Goldberg AL, Rosenbaum AE, Wang H, Kim WS, Lewis VL, Hanley DF. Computed tomography of dural sinus thrombosis. JCAT 1986;10:16–20.
6. Ulmer JL, Elster AD. Physiologic mechanisms underlying the delayed delta sign. Am J Neuroradiol 1991;12:647–50.

A calcified brain

[1]J D GRAHAM, [2]C OWENS and [1]J N GODLEE

[1]*Department of Radiotherapy and Oncology, University College Hospital, Gower Street, London WC1E 6AU, and* [2]*Department of Radiology, The Hospital for Sick Children, Great Ormond Street, London WC1N, UK*

A 13-year-old boy complained of increasing headaches over a 3 month period. At the age of 7 years he had undergone craniotomy and complete resection of a medulloblastoma of the cerebellum. No metastases were detected and post-operative radiotherapy was given to the whole brain and spinal cord to a dose of 30 Gy in 20 fractions over 4 weeks, followed by a boost to the posterior fossa, which received a total dose of 50 Gy in 40 fractions over 8 weeks. CT 1 year after treatment showed no evidence of disease. Following treatment he required growth hormone replacement and there were behavioural problems that required medication. Incoordination of the right side had been present since cranial surgery but there had been no recent neurological deterioration. CT was performed (Figures 1 and 2). What does it show? What is the diagnosis and aetiology?

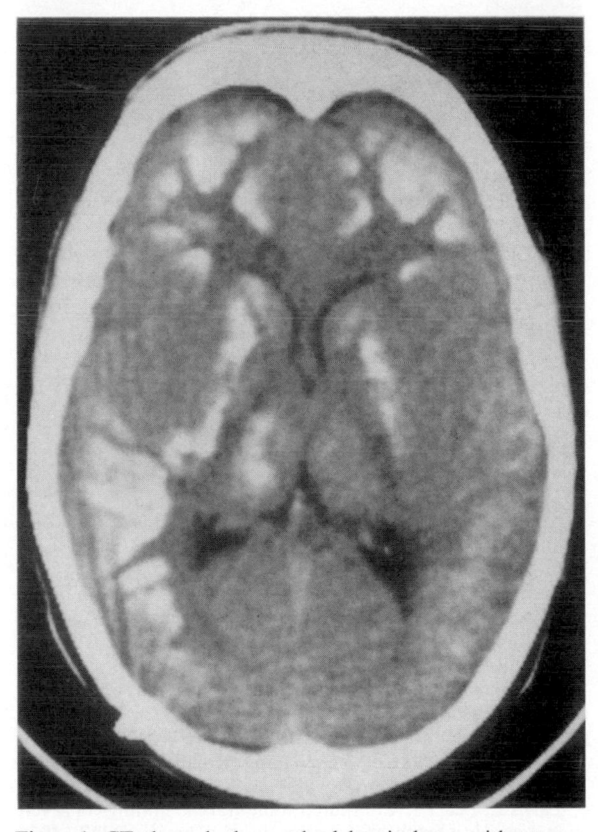

Figure 1. CT through the cerebral hemispheres without contrast enhancement.

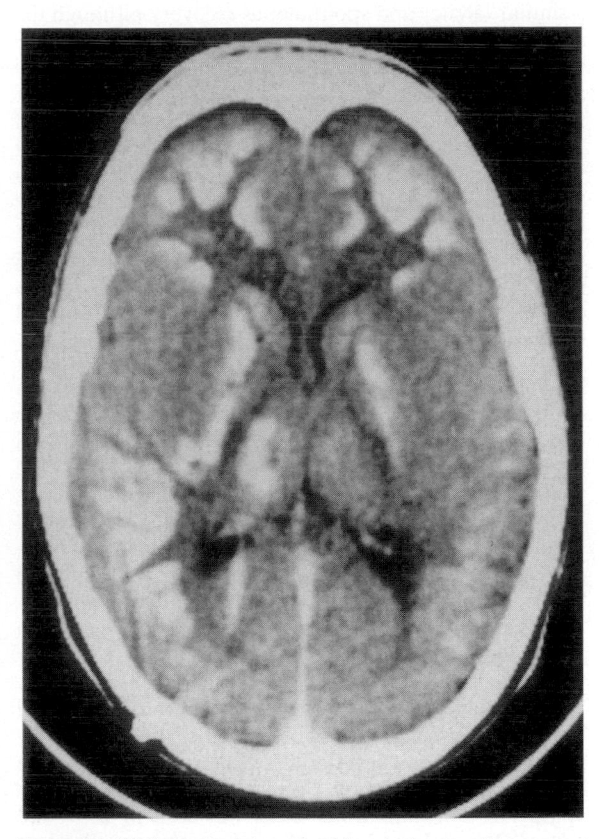

Figure 2. CT through the cerebral hemispheres with contrast enhancement.

Based on the case of the month originally published in Br J Radiol 1993;66:1065–6.

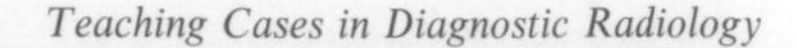

The CT scan showed extensive serrated calcification at the corticomedullary junction and within the basal ganglia. There was no evidence of tumour recurrence and the cerebellum showed relative sparing from the florid calcification (Figure 3). These are the classic features of mineralizing microangiopathy, a late effect of cranial irradiation. In the more acute stages bilateral leucoencephalopathy occurs with bifrontal low density within the white matter progressing to atrophy.

The effects of radiation on the brain may be classified as acute, early delayed and late reactions [1]. Acute reactions are seen during or immediately after treatment and are thought to be the result of increased oedema. Corticosteroid medication often gives rapid relief of symptoms.

The early delayed reaction occurs 6 to 8 weeks after irradiation as a transient deterioration seldom lasting more than 14 days. A more persistent course virtually always indicates progressive disease. There is some evidence that transient demyelination is the causative factor [2]. The somnolence syndrome, seen in children after whole brain irradiation with doses as low as 24 Gy, has a similar latency and spontaneous recovery although the underlying lesion remains obscure.

Late radiation damage occurs from about 4 months and while most lesions appear within 2 to 3 years, latent periods up to 7 years have been reported. The principal factor is vascular damage. Focal radionecrosis results when an end arteriole is occluded and is rare at doses below 60 Gy and at fraction sizes of 2 Gy or less. The lesion is indistinguishable from tumour recurrence both on CT and MR. Cerebral atherosclerosis is more common following irradiation and moya moya disease, a rare vasculitis of the circle of Willis, has also been reported.

The development of widespread vascular changes following lower dose irradiation was described in an autopsy series on the brains of leukaemic children who had received prophylactic cranial irradiation [3]. All cases occurred in children less than 10 years old and the mean radiation dose was 24 Gy. The term mineralizing microangiopathy was used to describe lesions around small blood vessels which contained calcium and mucopolysaccharides. In arteries the deposits were confined to the intima but in veins the entire wall was affected. The basal ganglia were uniformly involved with additional involvement of the cortical and cerebellar vessels.

The incidence of CT changes following cranial irradiation in children has been studied retrospectively [4] and the commonest finding was atrophy and volume loss (51%). Calcification from mineralizing microangiopathy in non-tumourous areas was seen in 28% and appeared as early as 3 months after treatment with doses from 35–50 Gy. The incidence was similar whether or

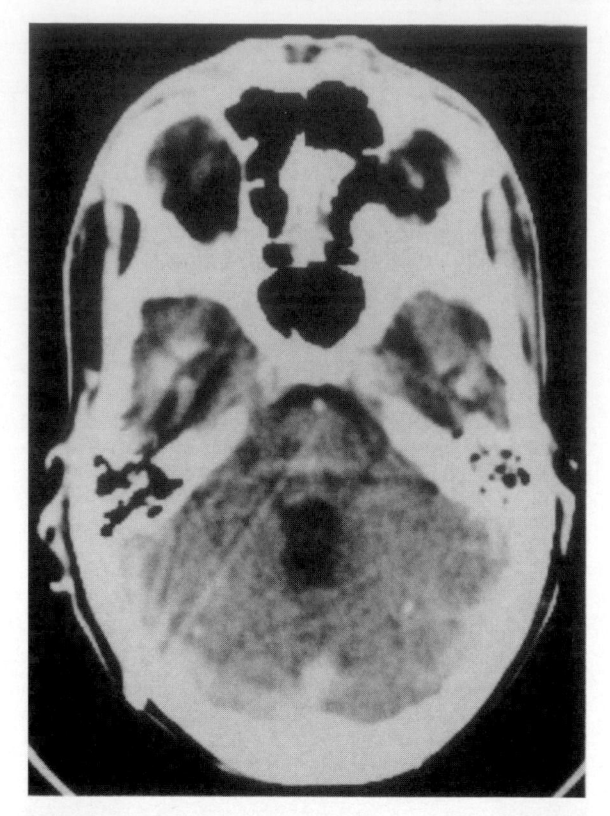

Figure 3. CT through the cerebellum with contrast enhancement.

not chemotherapy was given, suggesting that radiotherapy was the aetiological factor. The changes were more frequent and more severe in children irradiated before 3 years of age. In most children the appearances of mineralizing microangiopathy have been an incidental finding; however, they have been associated with the development of focal epilepsy, abnormal EEG tracings, focal neurological signs and headaches [4, 5].

References

1. Sheline GE, Wara WM, Smith V. Therapeutic irradiation and brain injury. Int J Radiat Oncol Biol Phys 1980; 6:1215–28.
2. Lampert PW, Davis RL. Delayed effects of radiation on the human central nervous system. "Early" and "late" delayed reactions. Neurology 1964;14:912–7.
3. Price RA, Birdwell DA. The central nervous system in childhood leukaemia. III. Mineralizing microangiopathy and dystrophic calcification. Cancer, 1978;42:717–28.
4. Davis PC, Hoffman JC, Pearl GS, Braun IF. CT evaluation of effects of cranial irradiation in children. AJR 1986; 147:587–92.
5. Lewis E, Lee YY. Computed tomographic findings of severe mineralising microangiopathy in the brain. JCAT 1986; 10:357–64.

Pseudo-pseudo-obstruction

[1]S C CHAKRAVERTY, [2]K H SIDDIQUI and [2]S M GRIFFIN

Departments of [1]Radiology and [2]Surgery, Newcastle General Hospital, Westgate Road, Newcastle-upon-Tyne NE4 6BE, UK

A 63-year-old man had recently undergone subtotal oesophagectomy for squamous carcinoma of the oesophagus. He had undergone a Heller's myotomy for achalasia of the oesophagus 30 years previously. A barium study was performed to evaluate post-operative swallowing and regurgitation problems. Unusual appearances were noted in the abdomen during screening. Radiographs were taken after completion of the upper gastrointestinal study (Figure 1) and 2 days later (Figure 2).

What abnormality is shown? What additional findings may there be on history and examination?

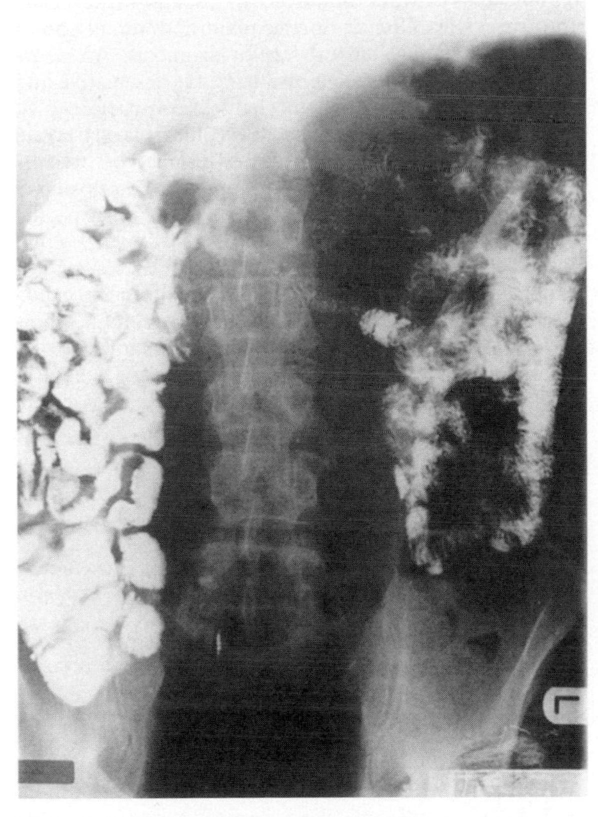

Figure 1. Radiograph taken after completion of the upper gastrointestinal study.

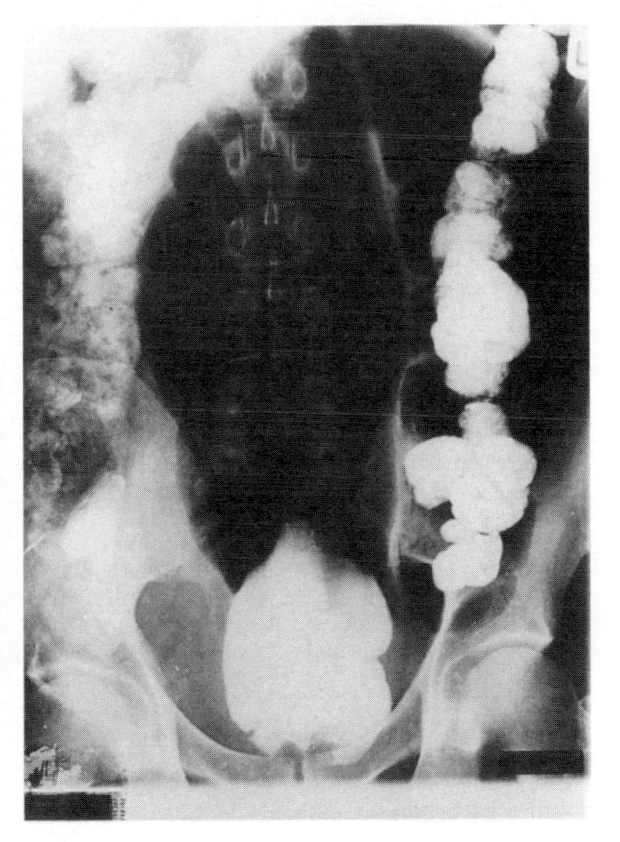

Figure 2. Radiograph taken 2 days after the upper gastrointestinal study.

Based on the case of the month originally published in Br J Radiol 1995;68:329–30.

The rectum and sigmoid colon were hugely dilated and extended well up into the upper abdomen, displacing barium-filled loops of small bowel to either side. The dilatation extended down as far as the anal margin. There was no obstruction to the passage of barium. The features of gaseous distension, with gas visible in the rectum and with no cut-off point of bowel gas are suggestive of intestinal pseudo-obstruction. The patient's swallowing difficulties were referrable to his recent surgery and he had no other symptoms at that stage. Rectal examination was not performed. He was well enough to be allowed home.

The patient was re-admitted a short while later with nausea, vomiting and watery diarrhoea that was associated with severe proctalgia. The plain abdominal film taken on admission is shown (Figure 3). Examination findings included a tight anal stenosis and further digital rectal examination was impossible. Examination under general anaesthesia confirmed the anal stenosis as well as disclosing a large anal fissure. Sigmoidoscopy revealed large amounts of fluid and solid faeces. Deep rectal biopsy showed normal acetylcholinesterase activity. An anal stretch to three fingers was performed. Post-operative treatment was continued with laxatives and anal dilators for use at home. This led to complete resolution of his symptoms and improvement in the radiographic appearances.

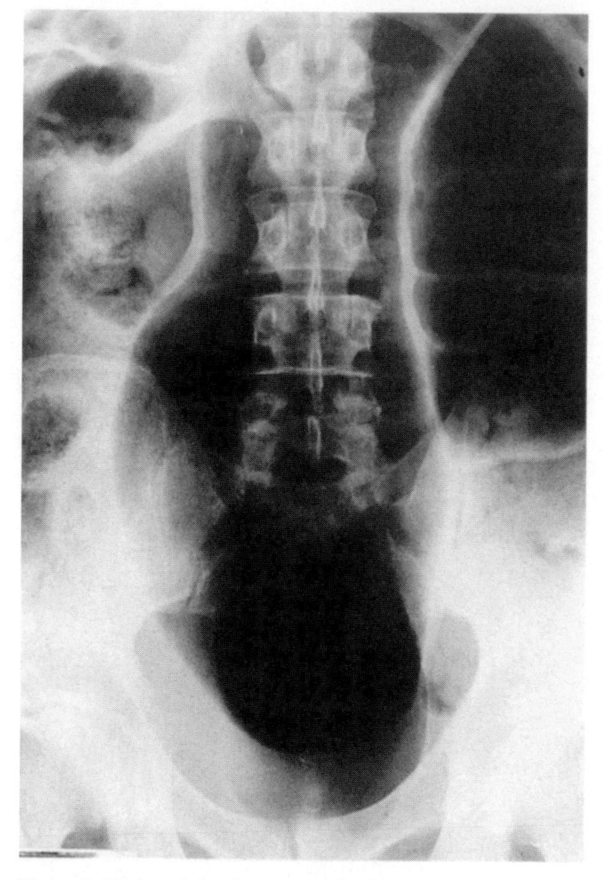

Figure 3. Plain abdominal radiograph taken on patient's readmission to hospital.

Mechanical large bowel obstruction and intestinal pseudo-obstruction can be difficult to differentiate as the clinical symptoms and signs can be identical. The context of presentation may be helpful. The patient with pseudo-obstruction is usually elderly with some other illness or injury [1]. On the plain abdominal radiograph, the appearances of gaseous distension of the colon extending into the rectum with no cut-off point are generally held to represent features of intestinal pseudo-obstruction. However, over-reliance on the plain abdominal radiograph may lead to an erroneous diagnosis. An acute contrast enema has been shown to be more sensitive and more specific in excluding mechanical obstruction [2]. Its use in the circumstances of clinical large bowel obstruction will save a substantial number of patients from unnecessary laparotomy, as well as disclosing a mechanical cause in a smaller number of unsuspected cases [3].

Anal stenosis can mimic exactly the classical radiographic appearances of intestinal pseudo-obstruction [4] as in this case. Misdiagnosis is avoided by careful examination of the rectum and anus. Outside of Chagas' disease endemic areas, there is no association of achalasia and megacolon, although a single case has been reported [5].

References

1. Dudley HAF, Paterson-Brown S. Pseudo-obstruction. Br Med J 1986;292:1157–8.
2. Chapman AH, McNamara M, Porter G. The acute contrast enema in suspected large bowel obstruction: value and technique. Clin Radiol 1992;46:273–8.
3. Koruth NM, Koruth A, Matheson NA. The place of the contrast enema in the management of large bowel obstruction. J Roy Coll Surg Edinburgh 1985;30:258–60.
4. Sagar PM, Wedgwood KR. Anal canal stenosis and pseudo-obstruction. Br J Clin Pract 1990;44:786–9.
5. Okamoto S, Ohno H, Sakai Y, et al. A case of achalasia with megacolon. Nippon Shokak Gakkai Zasshi 1989;86:916–20.

Puerperal right iliac fossa pain

[1]J P HENEGHAN, [1]D COLL, [2]J J MURPHY and [1]R G GIBNEY

Departments of [1]Diagnostic Imaging and [2]Surgery, University College Dublin and St Vincent's Hospital, Dublin 4, Ireland

A 32-year-old woman presented with gradual onset of right iliac fossa pain 10 days after an uncomplicated vaginal delivery of twins. Physical examination showed a pyrexia of 38 °C and right iliac fossa tenderness. No mass was palpable. A leucocytosis of 36×10^9 was present and *E. coli* was isolated from blood cultures. A clinical diagnosis of acute appendicitis was initially made, but the presence of a severe toxic illness associated with only mild localized signs prompted further investigation.

Ultrasound (US) of the pelvis demonstrated a 5.5 cm complex right adnexal mass, the superior aspect of which appeared tubular and extended cephalad to the right side of the inferior vena cava (IVC) (Figure 1). Colour Doppler US demonstrated no flow within the mass, but normal flow within the IVC. Fluid was present within the endometrial cavity. Sagittal and coronal T_1 weighted magnetic resonance images of the abdomen and pelvis were obtained (Figure 2, overleaf).

What is the diagnosis?

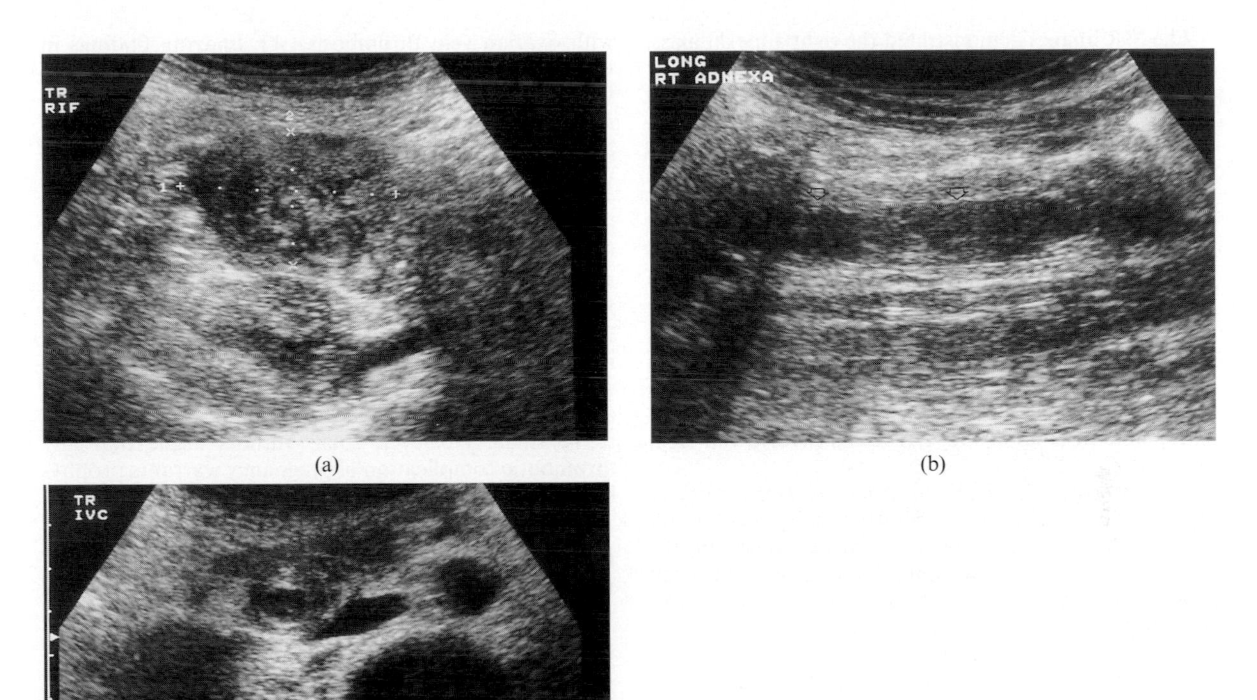

(a) (b) (c)

Figure 1. (a) Transverse image of right adnexal mass. (b) Longitudinal image of the tubular superior aspect of the mass (arrows) extending superomedially towards the IVC. (c) Transverse image of the aorta and IVC below the level of the renal vessels.

Based on the case of the month originally published in Br J Radiol 1997;70:967–8.

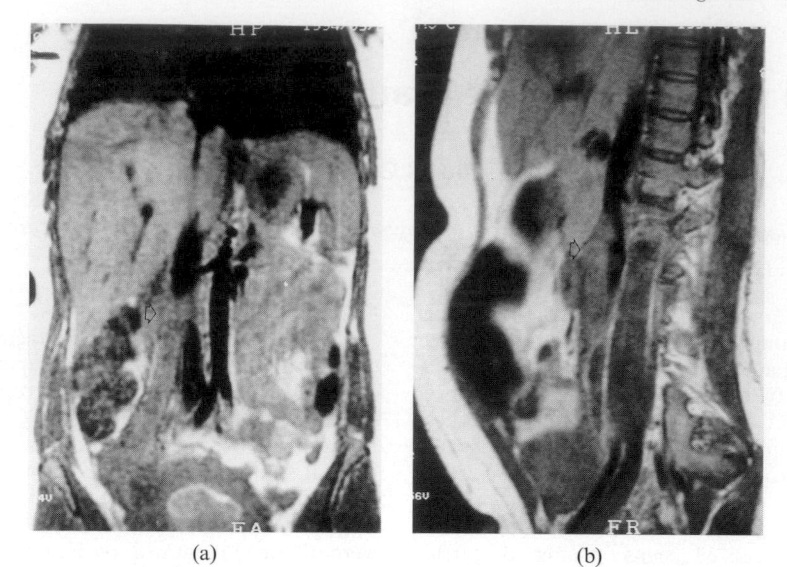

(a) (b)

Figure 2. (a) Coronal and (b) sagittal T_1 weighted (TR 520, TE 25) images of the abdomen and pelvis.

The MR images demonstrated the right adnexal mass, which was of homogeneous intermediate signal intensity and represented an oedematous right ovary. A well defined tubular structure (arrows) extended superomedially from the ovary to enter the normal IVC. This represented a thrombosed right ovarian vein.

Post-partum ovarian vein thrombosis is an uncommon entity, complicating approximately one in 2000 deliveries and abortions [1]. The majority of cases occur within 1 week of delivery, although later cases have been reported up to 70 days after delivery [2]. Ovarian vein thrombosis has also been reported in association with uterine leiomyomata, pelvic inflammatory disease, malignancy and trauma. 80–90% of cases involve the right ovarian vein [3].

The pathogenesis of this disorder involves a number of factors. An infectious thrombophlebitis may result from the combination of post-partum stasis in the ovarian vein, endothelial injury from bacterial invasion (usually endometritis), and the general hypercoagulable state of pregnancy and the puerperium.

The usual clinical presentation consists of right iliac fossa pain, typically accompanied by nausea and fever. A tender mass is often palpable in the right lower quadrant. The clinical diagnosis is difficult, particularly if a mass is not palpable. A wide differential diagnosis must be considered, including acute appendicitis, tubo-ovarian abscess and complicated ovarian cyst. Imaging has an important role to play in these cases.

In addition to US and MR evaluation, CT may be helpful in both the diagnosis and follow-up of patients with ovarian vein thrombosis [4]. Imaging findings in this condition may include an adnexal mass, an enlarged fluid-filled uterus and ovarian vein thrombus, as demonstrated in this case. Thrombus may extend into the IVC and pulmonary embolism may develop. Right hydroureter has also been described.

Ovarian vein thrombosis is treated with anticoagulation and broad spectrum antibiotics. Interruption of the inferior vena cava or ligation of the ovarian vein is recommended only if medical treatment fails [2]. Symptoms, particularly fever, generally subside within 72 h. Treatment with Warfarin is continued for several months. Our patient made an uncomplicated recovery with US and MRI at 3 months demonstrating normal appearances. The risk to future pregnancies is considered to be small. However, some authors argue that any thrombotic complication of pregnancy warrants prophylaxis in the puerperium of future pregnancies [5].

References

1. Dunnihoo DR, Gallaspy JW, Wise RB, Otterson WN. Post-partum ovarian vein thrombophlebitis: a review. Obstet Gynecol Surv 1991;46:415–27.
2. Musnick RA, Gillanders LA. A review of the syndrome of puerperal ovarian vein thrombophlebitis. Obstet Gynecol Surv 1981;36:57–66.
3. Simons GR, Piwnica-Worms DR, Goldhaber SZ. Ovarian vein thrombosis. Am Heart J 1993;126:641–7.
4. Savader SJ, Otero RR, Savader BL. Puerperal ovarian vein thrombosis: evaluation with CT, US, and MR imaging. Radiology 1988;167:637–9.
5. Rutherford SE, Phelan JP. Deep venous thrombosis and pulmonary embolism in pregnancy. Obstet Gynecol Clin N Am 1991;18:345–70.

An unusual cause of baldness

[1]D A COLLIE, [1]A J M STEVENSON and [2]A M LESSELLS

Departments of [1]Radiology and [2]Histopathology, Western General Hospital, Crewe Road North, Edinburgh EH4 2XU, UK

A previously well 85-year-old man initially presented with a 6 month history of anorexia and weight loss, together with a 1 month history of vomiting. A barium meal was performed (Figure 1). An abdominal ultrasound showed a normal liver and biliary tree but diffuse thickening of the stomach wall consistent with infiltration. Endoscopic biopsies of the gastric antrum and duodenum demonstrated non-specific inflammatory changes and mucosal oedema only.

He was managed conservatively with H_2-antagonists for 1 month but represented with steatorrhoea and rectal bleeding. At this time, in addition to the development of pitting oedema to the level of the umbilicus, he was noted to have scalp alopecia and dystrophic nail changes. A barium enema was performed (Figure 2).

What abnormalities are seen and what is the diagnosis?

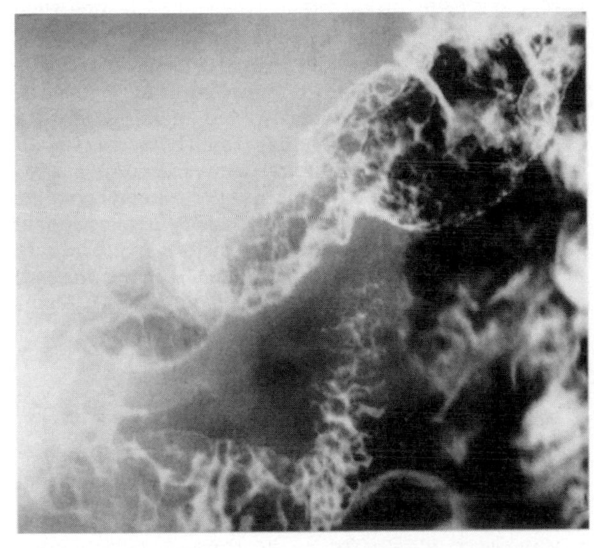

Figure 1. Spot view from barium meal series of gastric antrum and duodenum.

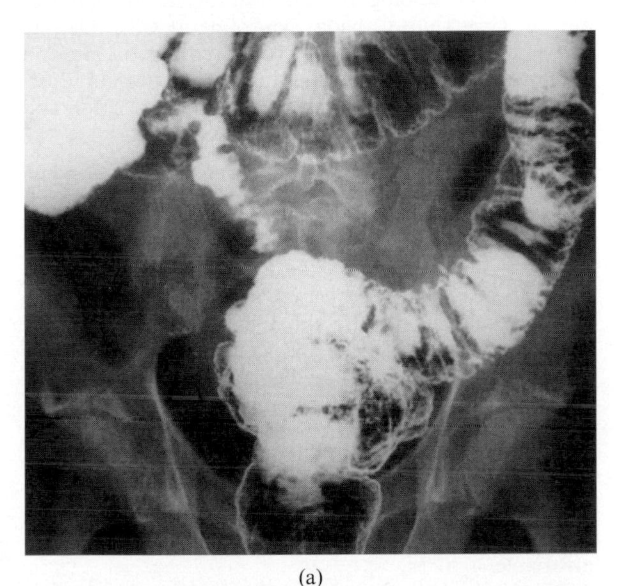

(a)

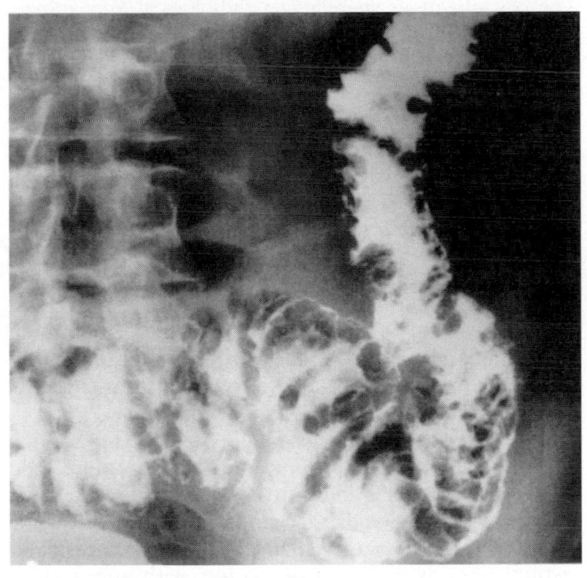

(b)

Figure 2. Barium enema: (a) supine film and (b) spot view of sigmoid colon.

Based on the case of the month originally published in Br J Radiol 1995;68:773–4.

The spot view of the barium meal series showed a diffuse nodularity and thickening of the rugal folds with a "whiskered" mucosal pattern affecting the antrum. No frank ulceration was demonstrated. The barium enema showed innumerable polypoid filling defects and although under-distended, the terminal ileum appeared similarly affected.

Biopsy of the colonic mucosa demonstrated a mild inflammatory infiltrate disease (Figure 3). The features were distinct from those of ulcerative colitis and Crohn's disease. The radiological and histological appearances are of Cronkhite–Canada syndrome (CCS). Despite active treatment, the disease progressed inexorably, and the patient died 4 months after initial presentation. Post-mortem confirmed polyposis in the stomach, colon and terminal 12 cm of ileum.

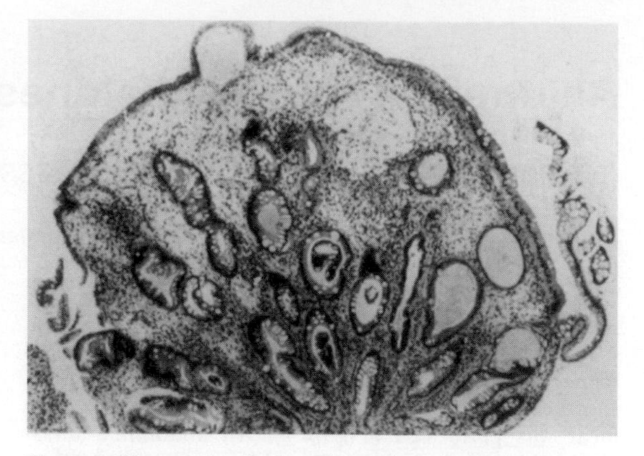

Figure 3. Biopsy of colonic polyp. There is cystic glandular dilatation with a mild inflammatory infiltrate and oedematous thickening of the lamina propria. Note the preservation of mucosal integrity and goblet cells.

Cronkhite–Canada syndrome, originally described in 1955 [1], is a rare, acquired, generalized gastrointestinal polyposis syndrome associated with ectodermal changes. It has a peak incidence between 50 and 70 years. The aetiology remains obscure although a defect in immunity is thought to play a part, and associations with erosive arthritis, systemic lupus erythematosis, hypothyroidism and myeloma have been documented. The commonest presenting symptoms are non-specific: nausea, vomiting, abdominal pain, weight loss, diarrhoea, steatorrhoea and oedema. The ectodermal changes include patchy hair loss and hyperpigmentation and can occur anywhere, including the pubic areas. Nail dystrophy and onycholysis are invariable.

Polyps may occur in the stomach, small bowel and colon. The oesophagus is spared. The radiological appearances have been well described previously [2]. The number of polyps may vary from a few scattered lesions to a confluent carpet, their size varying from 1–2 mm to 1 cm in diameter. In the stomach they are found particularly in the body and antrum, and are associated with thickened rugal folds and "whiskering"; a fine irregularity of the mucosa when seen in profile due to coarse area gastricae pattern [3] (Figure 1). Small bowel barium studies are not often performed but appearances indicating malabsorption, including dilution, flocculation and segmentation of contrast may be seen. Post-mortem studies have revealed small bowel polyps in 90% of fatal cases, particularly in the duodenum and terminal ileum [4]. In the colon the appearances are more patchy and match the severity of the gastric disease. The underlying haustral pattern is retained.

Histologically, the mucosa is polypoidal owing to the oedema of the lamina propria and there is only a mild inflammatory cell infiltrate, associated with the occasional cystic glands. The clue to the diagnosis is the presence of inflammatory changes in the upper gastrointestinal tract as well as in the colon, with appearances similar to those seen in juvenile polyposis [5].

The response to treatment and the prognosis are variable. Supportive therapy with parenteral nutrition together with high dose steroids may control disease. Approximately 50% recover, but the rest succumb to unabating malabsorption. Relative youth and male sex are good prognostic factors [2].

The diagnosis is often delayed, and malignancy suspected on the basis of the relentless clinical course. The differential diagnosis of the appearance in the stomach are of lymphoma and Menetrier's disease. Although the polyps do not have unique radiological features, differentiation of CCS from the other causes of gastrointestinal polyposis (familial polyposis, Gardner's syndrome, Peutz–Jegher's syndrome and Turcot's syndrome) can be made on the basis of age. Colonic appearances may be mistaken both colonoscopically and radiologically for inflammatory bowel disease, particularly ulcerative colitis with pseudopolyp formation. The presence of gastrointestinal polyps with diarrhoea and ectodermal changes presenting *de novo* in a relatively elderly patient should alert the radiologist to the diagnosis of CCS. The case presented here also serves as a reminder that the presence of polyps at one end of the gastrointestinal tract warrants examination of the remainder.

References

1. Cronkhite LW, Canada WJ. Generalised gastrointestinal polyposis. An unusual syndrome of polyposis, pigmentation, alopecia and onychotrophia. N Engl J Med 1955;252:1011–5.
2. Dachman AH, Buck JL, Burke AP, Sobin LH. Cronkhite–Canada syndrome: radiological features. Gastrointest Radiol 1989;14:285–90.
3. Kilcheski T, Kressel HY, Laufer I, Rogers D. The radiographic appearance of the stomach in Cronkhite–Canada syndrome. Radiology 1981;141:57–60.
4. Daniel ES, Ludwig SL, Lewin KJ, et al. The Cronkhite–Canada syndrome: an analysis of the clinical and pathological features and therapy in 55 cases. Medicine 1982;61:293–309.
5. Burke AP, Sobin LH. The pathology of Cronkhite–Canada syndrome: a comparison with juvenile polyposis. Am J Surg Pathol 1989;13:940–6.

The third dimension

A D KING and A L HINE

Department of Radiology, Central Middlesex Hospital, Acton Lane, London NW10 7NS, UK

A 31-year-old Indian woman presented with a 6 month history of pain in the neck and 2 months of swelling below the right ear. She had an 8 year history of rheumatoid arthritis, treatment for which included prednisolone 5 mg twice a day and monthly gold injections. There was no history of trauma. Physical examination showed a marked torticollis, pyrexia and a fluctuant mass below the right ear, but no neurological signs. Plain radiographs were difficult to assess because of the torticollis and, therefore, CT of the neck with bone windows and three-dimensional (3D) reconstruction was performed.

What abnormalities are demonstrated and what are the two most likely causes of the appearance at the atlas and axis in this patient?

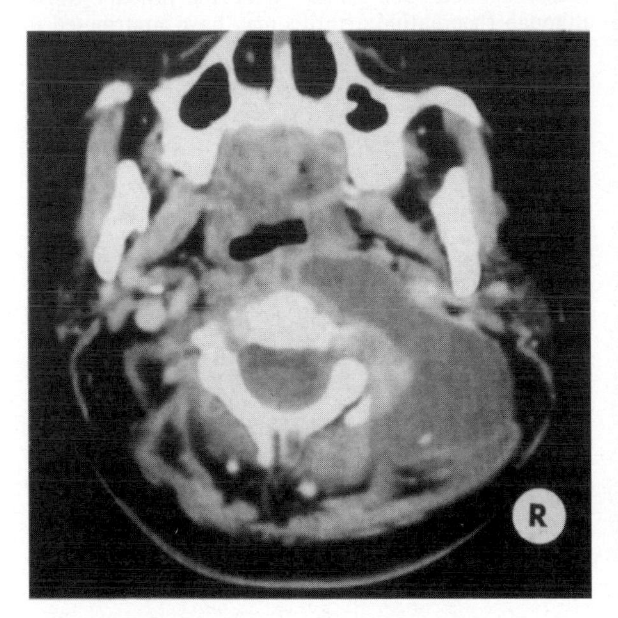

Figure 1. Axial CT section at level of C2 vertebra.

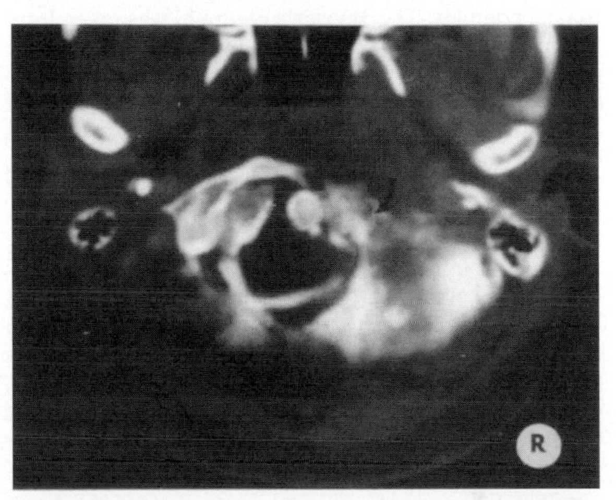

Figure 2. Axial CT bone window section of the atlantoaxial complex.

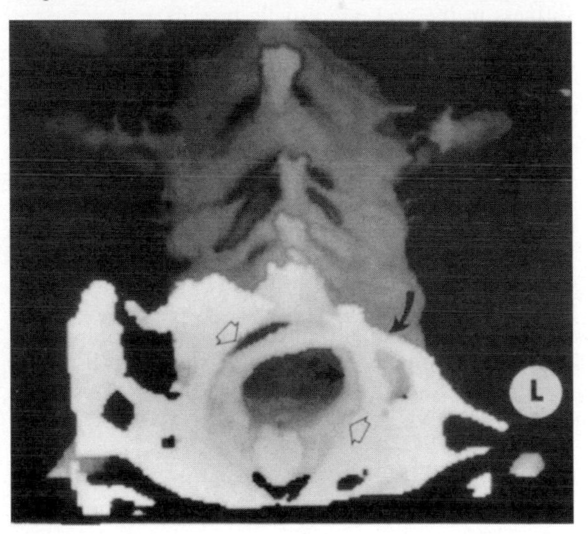

Figure 3. 3D CT reconstruction looking down the cervical spine from the rim of the foramen magnum (open arrows).

Based on the case of the month originally published in Br J Radiol 1992;65:871–2.

CT (Figure 1) demonstrated an extensive retropharyngeal fluid collection which extended posteriorly on the right to involve the atlas. The bone windows (Figure 2) showed destruction of the right lateral mass of the atlas which was associated with lateral movement of the atlas (curved arrow) to the left and dislocation of the left facet joints. There was also some rotation about the atlantoaxial joint, but no significant anterior subluxation. 3D reconstruction was found to be useful in demonstrating the relationship of the foramen magnum to the atlantoaxial complex. The 3D view (Figure 3) was taken from the foramen magnum looking down the cervical spine and it demonstrated lateral dislocation of the atlas (curved arrow) to the left with the foramen magnum and remainder of the cervical spine remaining aligned (smaller arrow = axis).

Acid fast bacilli were identified from aspiration of the retropharyngeal abscess and mycobacterium tuberculosis was later cultured. The chest radiograph was normal. Treatment initially involved bed rest, antituberculous chemotherapy and a stiff collar, the latter two being continued for 18 months. Follow-up examination after 1 year demonstrated resolution of the retropharyngeal abscess and normal neurological examination but no change in the degree of bone destruction or subluxation.

Tuberculosis of the atlantoaxial joint producing subluxation is rare but well documented [1–4]. Pain and stiffness in the neck are usually present and may occur before there are any radiographic changes [5]. Constitutional symptoms, dysphagia and a retropharyngeal abscess are also common. Neurological findings range from normal to tetraparesis. Torticollis is well recognized, particularly in atlantoaxial rotation where the head is held in the "cock robin" position [6].

Tuberculous involvement may be direct from a retropharyngeal abscess or from haematogenous spread. Usually, the pathological process at the atlantoaxial complex initially involves ligaments and bone erosions, particularly around the odontoid. This may lead to subluxation which is usually anterior. Rotatory subluxation, as seen to a minor degree in this case, has also been reported in tuberculosis [2], although it is more commonly seen following upper respiratory tract infections, trauma and rheumatoid arthritis [5]. More extensive destruction of bone occurs in the later stages of tuberculosis. At the axis this tends to involve the body and the odontoid; the latter may either fracture just above the base or be completely destroyed. The atlas is usually eroded at the anterior arch or the lateral masses. This is demonstrated in the present case and has resulted in not only rotatory subluxation around an intact odontoid, but also lateral subluxation of the atlas as clearly seen on the 3D scan. This had caused considerable narrowing of the right side of the spinal canal.

Atlantoaxial disease may be caused by other pyogenic infections, trauma, malignancy or the arthritides. The major differential diagnosis of atlantoaxial disease in this patient is rheumatoid arthritis. This most commonly causes anterior subluxation as a result of erosions of the odontoid and may occur with an intact transverse ligament. The synovial process can also involve the lateral facet joints [7] producing lateral subluxation, lateral mass collapse and rotatory subluxation. However, in this patient the large tuberculous retropharyngeal abscess adjacent to the extensively destroyed lateral mass of the atlas suggested tuberculosis to be the primary cause, although rheumatoid arthritis may have contributed to the severity of the subluxation.

References

1. Wang LX. Peroral focal debridement for treatment of tuberculosis of the atlas and axis. Ch J Orthopaed 1981;1:207–9.
2. Fang D, Leong JCY, Fang HSY. Tuberculosis of the upper cervical spine. J Bone Joint Surg 1983;65(B):47–50.
3. Dowd CF, Sartoris DJ, Haghighi P, Resnick D. Case report 344. Skel Radiol 1986;15:65–8.
4. Lifeso R. Atlanto-axial tuberculosis in adults. J Bone Joint Surg 1987;69(B):183–7.
5. Shi-Dy. Early diagnosis of atlanto-axial tuberculosis. Chung-Hua-Wai-Ko-Tsa-Chih 1989;27:78–9, 124.
6. Fielding JW, Hawkins RJ. Atlanto-axial rotary fixation. J Bone Joint Surg 1977;59(A):37–44.
7. Halla JT, Hardin JG, Vitek J, Alarcon GS. Involvement of the cervical spine in rheumatoid arthritis. Arthr Rheum 1989;32:652–9.

Just another case of varicose veins?

[1]R C TRAVIS, [2]D M ROWAN and [1]J MILLER

Departments of [1]Radiology and [2]Dermatology, Middlemore Hospital, Otahuhu, Auckland, New Zealand

A 49-year-old Maori woman was referred to the Surgical Outpatients Department because of increasing discomfort and disability in the left leg. She had had varicose vein surgery as a child, and the veins later recurred. Views from her left lower limb venogram and bilateral aortofemoral angiogram are shown. What is the diagnosis?

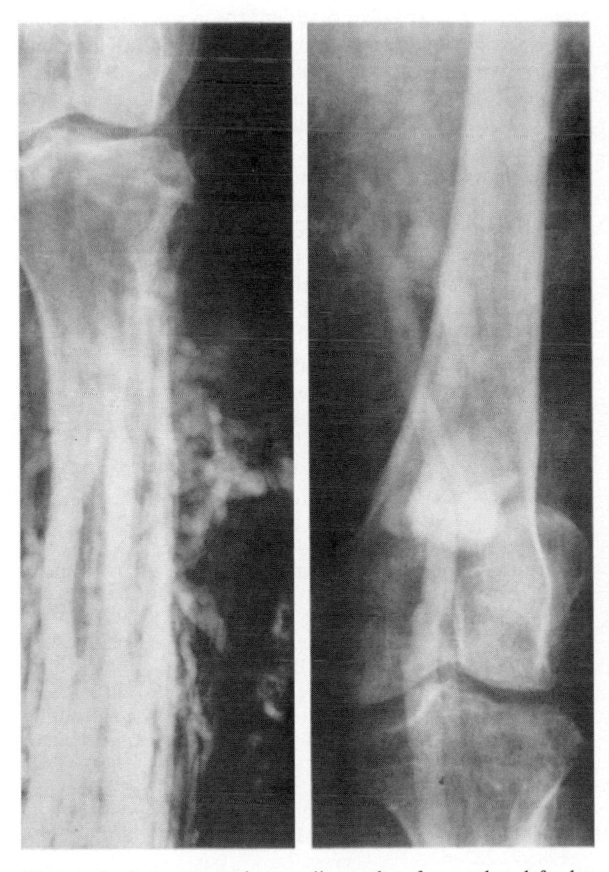

Figure 1. Anteroposterior radiographs from the left leg venogram.

Based on the case of the month originally published in Br J Radiol 1990;63:581–2.

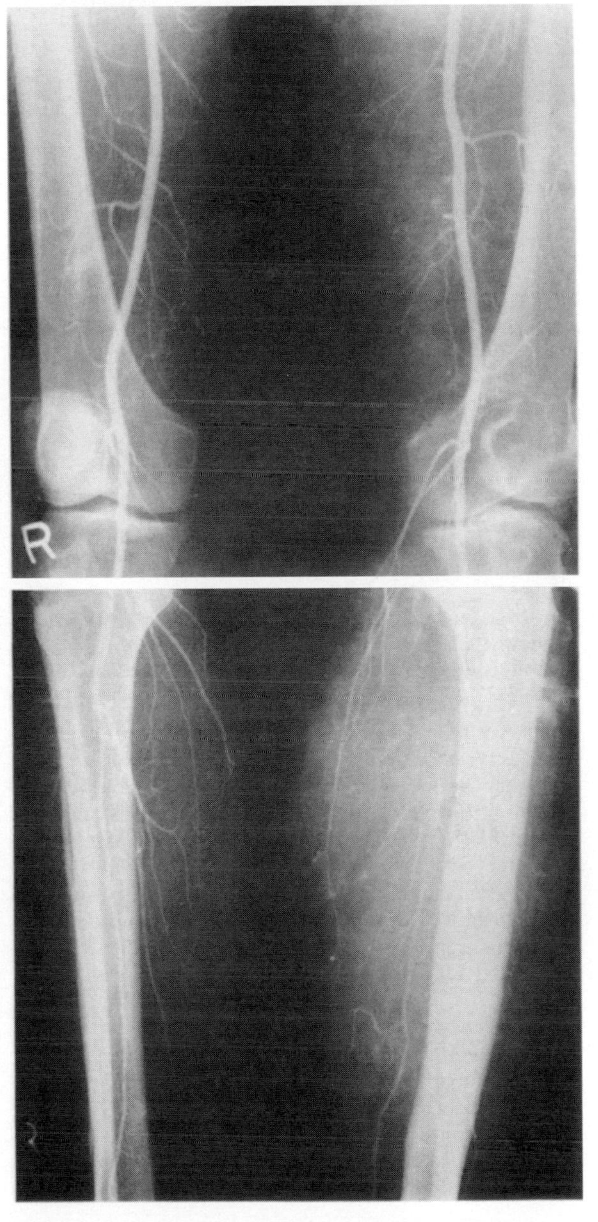

Figure 2. Radiographs from the lower limb arteriogram.

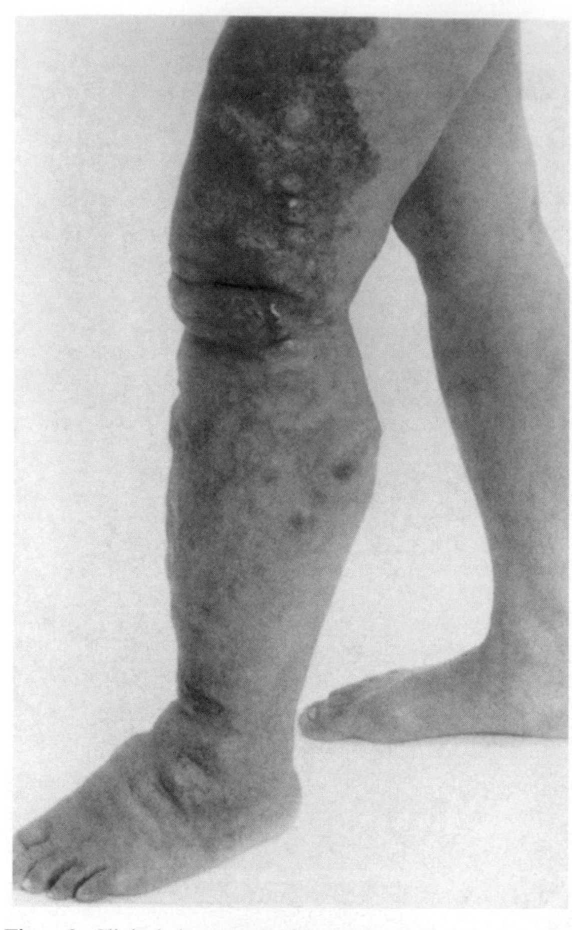

Figure 3. Clinical photograph of the left lower limb demonstrating soft tissue hypertrophy and the cutaneous haemangioma.

The venogram demonstrated multiple venous abnormalities. Varicose veins were seen and there was a venous aneurysm at the level of the left knee. Thrombus was present in the superficial veins. The deep veins appeared patent. The angiogram showed cortical thickening of the tibia and soft tissue hypertrophy, together with multiple small vascular malformations in the left leg. No arteriovenous shunt was seen. On clinical examination, there was a classical port wine stain (Figure 3) and lengthening and soft tissue hypertrophy of the left leg.

The patient has Klippel–Trenaunay Syndrome (KTS). This was first described in 1900 by two French physicians, Klippel and Trenaunay, as the "naevus variqueux osteo-hypertrophique" syndrome. The clinical manifestations are usually monomelic, and consist of venous varicosities, a port wine haemangioma and bone and soft tissue hypertrophy of the affected limb [1]. Parkes-Weber [2] described a similar syndrome in 1907 seen in association with an arteriovenous fistula. It is generally accepted that in KTS there is no clinically apparent or angiographic arteriovenous fistula [3]. Cases that have a significant arteriovenous fistula tend to be classified as Klippel–Trenaunay–Weber Syndrome.

A mesodermal defect which involves angiogenesis in the primitive limb bud has been postulated as a cause for KTS [4]. It is thought that late regression of the vascular reticular network causes persisting arteriovenous connections and venous abnormalities. There are no known hereditary factors, and no sex predeliction.

The syndrome presents at birth with the port wine naevus. The varicose veins become more prominent when the child begins to stand erect. Limb hypertrophy may be gross at birth or may become more noticeable at puberty with the growth spurt. Multiple venous abnormalities are usually present. There may be hypoplasia or aplasia of the deep venous system. A valveless lateral venous channel can be seen in the leg which drains into the pelvic veins, and accompanies the sciatic nerve. Varicosities can be seen in the peroneal and suprapubic areas, and may involve bladder, colon and uterus. The pelvic varicosities can contain phleboliths. Patients may present with haematuria, rectal blood loss or menorrhagia [5]. Superficial thrombophlebitis is not uncommon. Some authors report a high incidence of pulmonary embolus [6].

The manifestations tend to progress until the end of the third decade. Surgery may be indicated for troublesome superficial varicosities. However, generally it should be avoided and only attempted after careful venography. Incisions through the cutaneous haemangioma tend to heal poorly. Epiphysiodesis can be used to correct the leg length discrepancy. Most patients can be managed successfully with elastic stockings. Symptomatic haemodynamically significant arteriovenous malformations may be amenable to embolotherapy.

References

1. Taybi H. Radiology of syndromes and metabolic disorders. Chicago: Year Book Medical Publishers, 1983:210.
2. Parkes-Weber F. Angioma formation in connection with hypertrophy of limbs and hemihypertrophy. Br J Dermatol 1907;19:231–5.
3. Lindenauer SM. Congenital arteriovenous fistula and the Klippel–Trenaunay syndrome. Ann Surg 1971;174:248–63.
4. Baskerville PA, Ackroyd JS, Browse NL. The etiology of the Klippel–Trenaunay syndrome. Ann Surg 1985;202:624–7.
5. Azouz EM. Hematuria, rectal bleeding and pelvic phleboliths in children with the Klippel–Trenaunay syndrome. Pediatr Radiol 1983;13:82–8.
6. Baskerville PA, Ackroyd JS, Lea Thomas M, Browse NL. The Klippel–Trenaunay syndrome: clinical, radiological and hemodynamic features and management. Br J Surg 1985;72:232–6.

"Air-in a view"

[1]R ENGLAND, [2]S M SCHUTZ and [2]J W C LEUNG

[1]Department of Radiology, and [2]Department of Medicine, Division of Gastroenterology, Duke University Medical Center, Durham, North Carolina, USA

A 57-year-old female was referred to Duke University Medical Center (DUMC) for investigation of recurrent pancreatitis. Her first episode of pancreatitis, which had occurred 3 years earlier, manifested as epigastric pain and a markedly elevated serum amylase level which necessitated hospital admission for 9 days. Her history was negative for relevant pancreatic risk factors including alcohol abuse, medications, family history and hyperlipidaemia. Ultrasound (US) of the gallbladder showed no gallstones. CT of the abdomen showed a swollen head of pancreas with peri-pancreatic inflammatory change and fluid, consistent with pancreatitis. The biliary tree was not dilated. She made a complete recovery and was well until 8 months later when she had recurrent epigastric pain of a similar character with elevation of the serum amylase. She was admitted to hospital for 3 days. A repeat US scan showed no cholelithiasis. Following resolution of her symptoms, she underwent endoscopic retrograde cholangiopancreatography (ERCP) to exclude choledocholithiasis or a pancreatic abnormality. The patient's pancreatogram is shown in Figures 1 and 2. The cholangiogram was reported to be normal. She developed post-ERCP pancreatitis and was referred to DUMC for further evaluation.

What does the pancreatogram show? What is the differential diagnosis for this appearance, and what is the cause in this particular case?

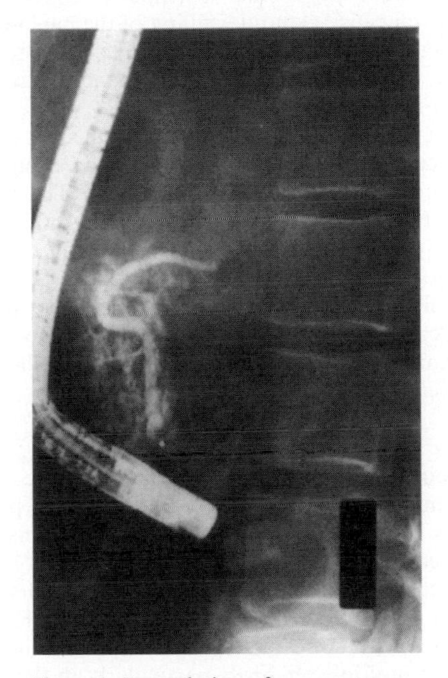

Figure 1. Lateral view of pancreatogram.

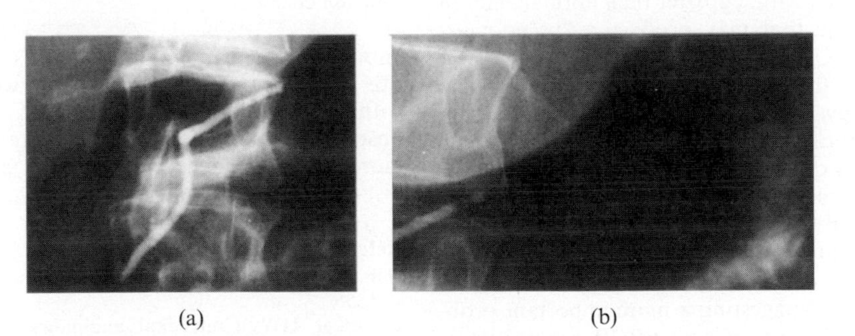

(a) (b)

Figure 2. (a) AP view of pancreatogram. (b) Coned view of pancreatic duct in tail.

Based on the case of the month originally published in Br J Radiol 1996;69:681–2.

The pancreatogram showed abrupt cut-off of the main dorsal duct in the body of the pancreas with glandular filling of the head and body of the gland. Cut-off of the pancreatic duct (PD) may be caused by a neoplasm, a pseudocyst with disruption of dorsal duct continuity, or a calculus. In this case, the pancreatogram showed air in the pancreatic duct (Figures 1 and 2) which is another common cause of this appearance. Air inadvertently injected during ERCP will prevent retrograde filling of the PD with contrast. If air in the PD is not recognized during fluoroscopy, further attempts to inject contrast medium will cause glandular filling of the pancreas. This phenomenon may result in an inadequate study and increase the risk of post-ERCP pancreatitis, which occurred in this instance.

Repeat ERCP and US were performed at DUMC. The pancreatogram (Figure 3) demonstrated duplication of the dorsal duct in the body of the gland. The cholangiogram (Figure 4) showed a cystic dilatation of the common channel at the ampulla—a finding thought to be due to prior impaction of a gallstone. US showed a thick walled gallbladder but no stones. The pancreas was bulky. The patient was referred for cholecystectomy which confirmed chronic cholecystitis and she is currently well at follow-up.

A duplicated dorsal pancreatic duct is a rare congenital variant of pancreatic ductal anatomy. The primitive pancreas is composed of a plexus of small ducts, one of which becomes dominant and assumes the role of the main duct. Alteration of this development results in variations in the number of ducts or their form. Failure to form a main duct results in persistence of the plexus pattern as multiple channels particularly in the head of the gland. Symmetrical duplications, as in this patient, were first described by Barnard [1] and also include ring-like segments or fork-like segments of the duct. The most common symmetrical anomaly is a bifid duct in the tail of the gland [2]. Duplicate variations of all types have been associated with a greater than normal amount of pancreatic tissue that may produce a "pseudomass effect" on US or CT [3]. ERCP is necessary in these cases to delineate the ductal anatomy and exclude significant pathology. These duplication anomalies are otherwise of little clinical significance.

We present this case to highlight two points. Firstly, the importance when performing ERCP of avoiding the injection of air. Air bubbles may be confused with stones and air injected into the pancreatic duct can obstruct the retrograde flow of contrast, causing glandular filling of the pancreas and suggesting a more important problem. In addition, the risk of post-ERCP pancreatitis is higher. Secondly, this is a good example of an unusual congenital pancreatic abnormality, the duplicated pancreatic duct. It is difficult to incriminate this congenital anomaly as the cause of this patient's recurrent pancreatitis as the pancreatogram is otherwise unremarkable, with normal sidebranch filling and no likely areas of obstruction to flow. Cholelithiasis (or microlithiasis) is more likely, particularly given the appearance of her distal common bile duct (CBD).

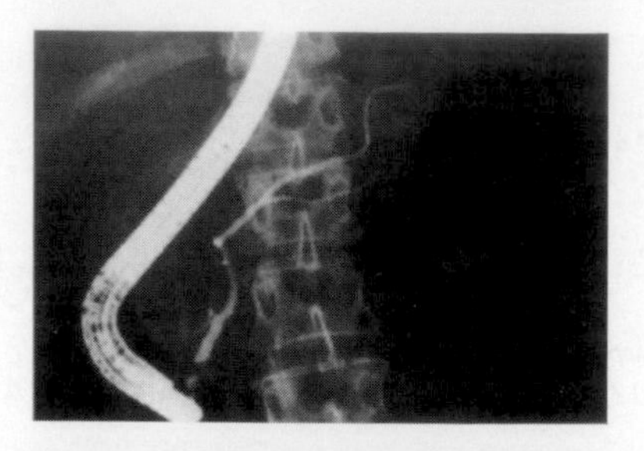

Figure 3. Pancreatogram showing duplicated PD in the body of the gland.

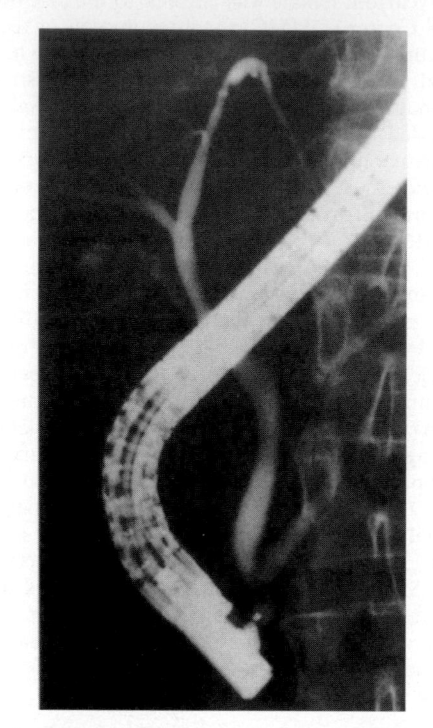

Figure 4. Cholangiogram showing cystic dilatation of the common channel.

References

1. Barnard C. Memoire sur le pancrease. Paris: J B Balliere, 1856.
2. Parker HW. Congenital anomalies of the pancreas. In: Sivak M, editor. Gastroenterologic Endoscopy. Philadelphia: WB Saunders, 1994:770–9.
3. Yatto RP, Siegel J. Variant pancreatography. Am J Gastroenterol 1983;78:115–8.

Did he fall or was he pushed?

C HAMILTON-WOOD

Department of Radiodiagnosis, Bristol Royal Infirmary, Marlborough Street, Bristol BS2 8HW, UK

A 17-year-old male was found unconscious after a road traffic accident and brought to the Casualty Department. On examination he had regained consciousness but exhibited the signs of cerebral irritation; he responded purposefully to pain, and cranial nerve and full neurological assessment of his limbs revealed no localizing signs. He had facial grazes with a haematoma over the right frontal region.

Observation overnight was followed the next morning by radiological examination, and the radiographs taken are shown in Figure 1. What observations can you make?

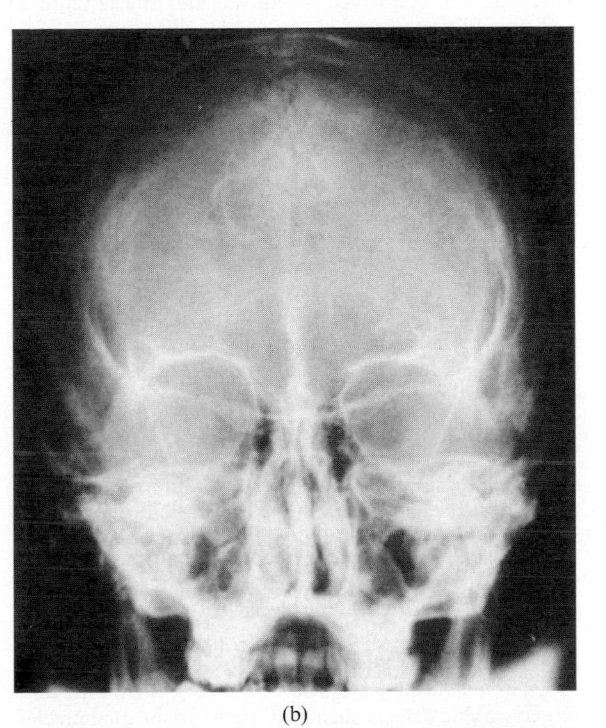

(b)

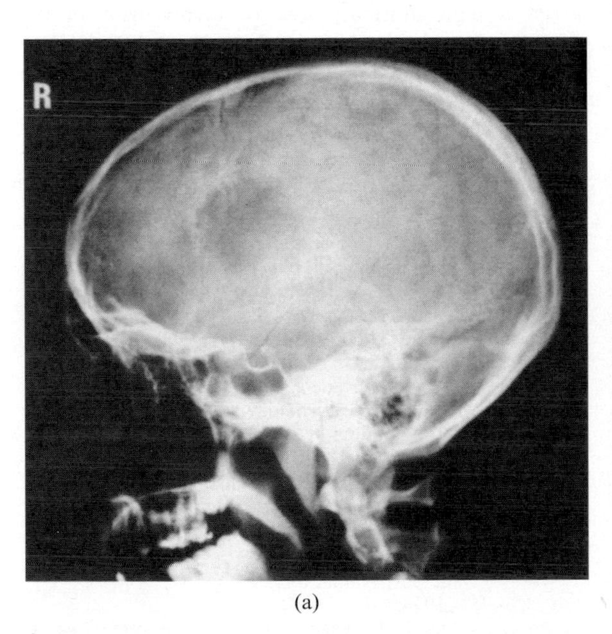

(a)

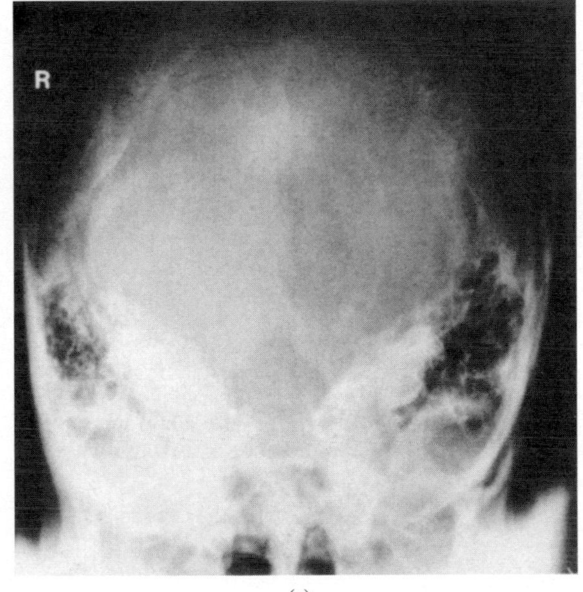

(c)

Figure 1. Radiographs of the skull taken on morning after the accident.

Based on the case of the month originally published in Br J Radiol 1987;60:199–200.

Two linear parietal fractures were shown. In addition, however, there were several areas of abnormal calcification; curvilinear in shape, they were present one on each side of the midline and their full extent was best shown on the Towne's projection. The lateral radiograph also showed an area of unusually low density within the line of calcification.

These features are typical of a lipoma of the corpus callosum. CT confirmed its nature and site (Figure 2) and, in addition, revealed ventricular dilatation.

The patient recovered satisfactorily from his head injury and suffered no subsequent problems. He was referred, however, to the Neurosurgical Department.

It was decided not to intervene surgically, at least initially, but it was considered that a future shunting procedure might be necessary to relieve his hydrocephalus.

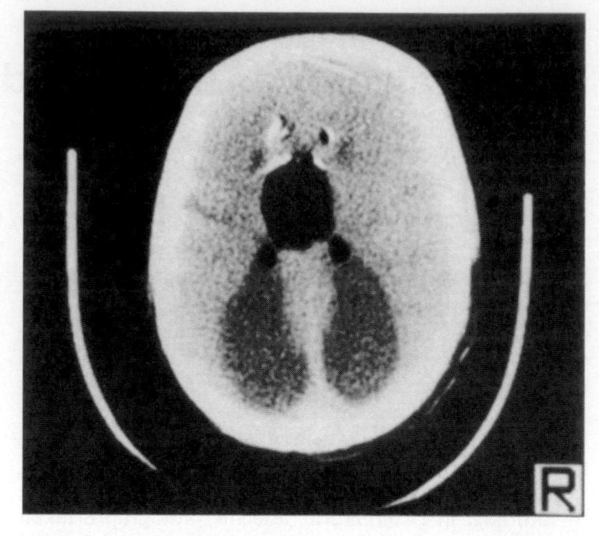

Figure 2. CT (L + 20, W 75), showing central, fat attenuation mass with calcification in its capsule, associated with symmetrical dilatation of the posterior horns of the lateral ventricles.

A lipoma of the corpus callosum is an unusual, benign tumour of the central nervous system, and produces characteristic features on plain radiographs of the skull because of the presence of calcium within its capsule. It occurs in the region of the genu of the corpus callosum, although it may occasionally extend downward into the septum.

Such a tumour produces symptoms in approximately 50% of cases, these varying from fits and hemiplegia to minor disturbances such as headaches, vertigo, vomiting unrelated to raised intracranial pressure, or emotional lability [1]. They are considered to be congenital and about half of the reported cases are associated with agenesis of the corpus callosum itself. In some of these cases, associations have also been recognized with midline dysraphic defects such as hypertelorism, median cleft nose, myelomeningocoele, agenesis of the cerebellar vermis, or spina bifida.

Lipoma of the corpus callosum is sometimes associated with a defect in the frontal bone [2]. Lipomas of the corpus callosum may cause hydrocephalus, as was the case in our patient as shown by dilatation of the posterior parts of the lateral ventricles on CT.

CT clearly defines the lesion and, by assigning it a negative attenuation coefficient, is the most effective and least invasive tool in establishing the diagnosis of a lipoma of the corpus callosum [3].

If angiography is performed, then displacement of the pericallosal arteries is seen to be present; the arteries are either incorporated within or lying on the surface of the tumour [4].

Although relief of hydrocephalus may be indicated if severe, treatment is usually conservative; indeed, surgery carries a high mortality due to involvement of the anterior cerebral arteries in the tumour, and to its great intrinsic vascularity.

References

1. Wallace D. Lipoma of the corpus callosum. J Neurol Neurosurg Psychiatr 1976;39:1179–85.
2. Kushnet MW, Goldman RL. Lipoma of the corpus callosum associated with frontal bone defect. AJR 1978;131:517–8.
3. Harwood-Nash DC. Congenital cranio-cerebral abnormalities and computed tomography. Semin Roentgenol 1977; 12:39–51.
4. Wolpert SM, Carter BL, Ferris EJ. Lipoma of the corpus callosum; an angiographic analysis. AJR 1972;115:92–9.

The misleading pre-operative chest radiograph

J IPINYOMI and I WATT

Department of Radiology, Bristol Royal Infirmary, Bristol BS2 8HW, UK

A 66-year-old man presented to the Accident and Emergency Department with pain in the right hip and difficulty in weight bearing after falling in the street that morning. He smoked about 15 cigarettes a day and had a wheeze which was relieved by Salbutamol. No other relevant history was elicited, apart from a vague story of ill defined upper chest pain in the past.

On examination he was observed to walk with a limp. His right hip was externally rotated, with limitation of movement because of pain. His right lower limb was 2 cm shorter than the left. Radiographs of the pelvis and chest and an apical view are shown in Figures 1 and 2. Frontal tomography of the chest was subsequently performed (Figure 3).

What are the abnormalities demonstrated? What differential diagnosis should be considered and what might skeletal scintigraphy show?

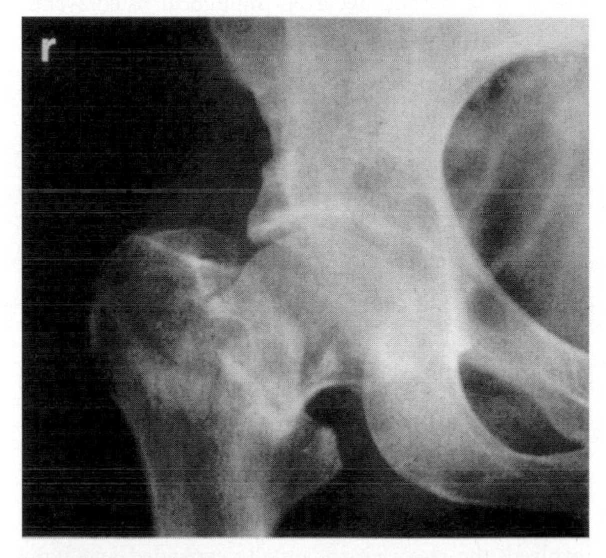

Figure 1. Frontal view of the right hip at presentation to the Accident and Emergency Department.

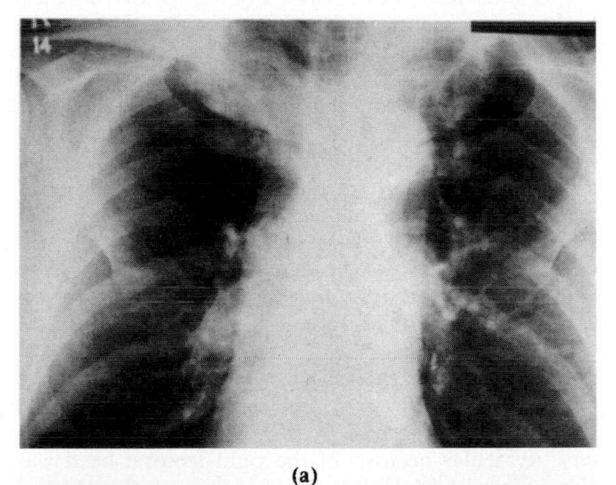

(a)

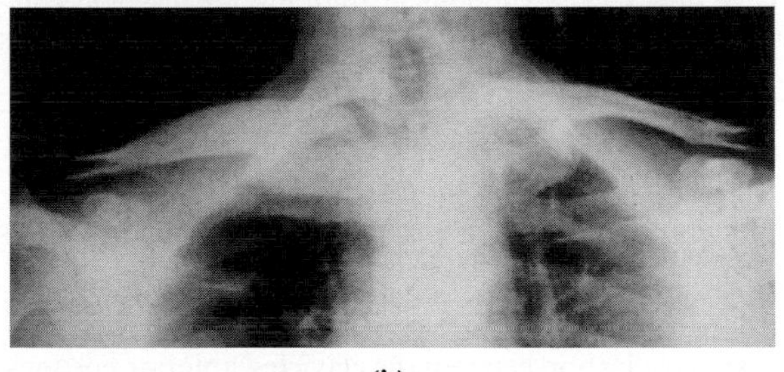

(b)

Figure 2. (a) Frontal and (b) apical views of the chest.

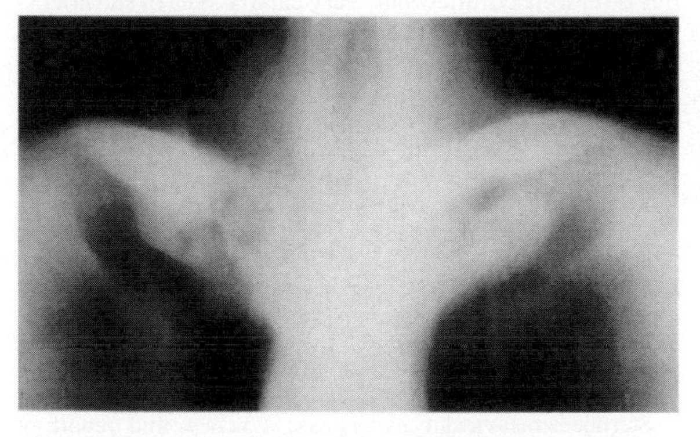

Figure 3. Frontal tomogram of the upper chest.

Based on the case of the month originally published in Br J Radiol 1989;62:279–80.

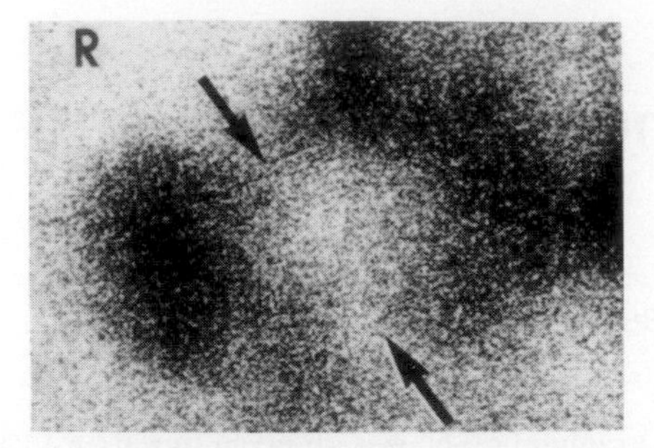

Figure 4. Late phase of an HDP bone scintigram, centred over the right upper femur and hip.

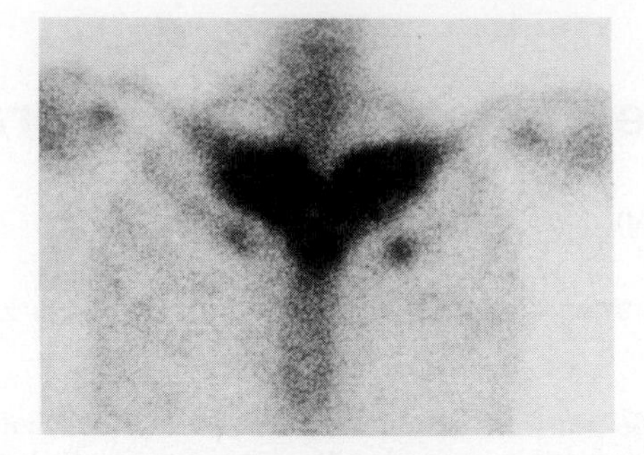

Figure 5. Late phase scintigram centred over the upper anterior chest.

A bone scintigram was performed a few days after admission to hospital. The right femoral head was imaged to assess vascularity (Figure 4). Increased activity was shown at the fracture site but the femoral head was photon deficient. Delayed views of the upper thorax demonstrated marked activity in both clavicles medially, the manubrium and anterior upper ribs (Figure 5).

Post-traumatic avascular necrosis and sternocostoclavicular hyperostosis were diagnosed. The pelvic radiograph showed a transcervical fracture of the femur. The chest radiograph demonstrated no lung or mediastinal lesions but an ill defined opacity overlying the apices. An apical lordotic view confirmed that the apices were normal, the opacities being shown to be bony, corresponding to considerable sclerosis of the clavicles, first ribs and first costal cartilages. This was confirmed on tomography (Figure 3). An initial impression of an apparent apical abnormality raised the possibility of a Pancoast tumour with, possibly, a pathological fracture of the femur, but the subsequent demonstration of sclerotic clavicles opened up a further differential diagnosis, including Paget's disease and prostatic metastases. No abnormality of blood chemistry was found, apart from a slight increase in serum alkaline phosphatase to 15 (normal range 3–13) KA units, consistent with a recent fracture.

The bone scan showed increased activity over the upper chest, confirming considerably increased bone activity in the abnormal areas shown on plain radiography. Avascular necrosis of the right femoral head was also shown. Histological examination of the femoral head and neck at subsequent total hip replacement confirmed recent avascular necrosis and showed no evidence of other pathology.

The sclerotic clavicles, sternum and first ribs result from a disorder known as sternocostoclavicular hyperostosis with no known relevance to the fracture of the femoral neck. Sternocostoclavicular hyperostosis is a benign disorder characterized by hyperostosis and soft tissue ossification between the clavicles, anterior portions of upper ribs and sternum. It was first reported in 1974 [1] and over 50 cases have been described, mainly in the Japanese literature. The aetiology is unknown, but the condition may be more common than presently recognized. Males are affected more than females and patients are usually middle-aged (30–50 years), presenting with chronic upper chest pain of several years duration, local bullous eruptions and some with pustulosis palmaris et plantaris. Similar skin lesions are also described in chronic recurrent multifocal osteomyelitis which affects a younger age group [2]. A few reported cases had psoriasis for several years [3]. The current patient did not present with any of the above symptoms, apart, perhaps, from his vague history of chest pain.

Local complications include bony overgrowth which may lead to a wide, thick sternum and occlusion of subclavian veins. Other associated skeletal disorders have included sacroilitis and abnormalities of the spine similar to diffuse idiopathic skeletal hyperostosis (DISH), ankylosing spondylitis and peripheral inflammatory arthritis [4]. Laboratory findings include raised erythrocyte sedimentation rate, positive C-reactive protein, and elevated $\alpha 2$ globulin. Rheumatoid factors are characteristically absent.

Differential diagnosis includes other sclerosing conditions of the clavicles, in particular osteoblastic metastasis, Paget's disease, chronic sclerosing osteomyelitis and condensing osteitis of the clavicles [5]. Osteoblastic metastases are rarely isolated to the clavicles. Paget's disease may affect the clavicles, but other bones are typically involved; the clavicles are usually expanded and bony fusion with the ribs and sternum is unlikely. Chronic sclerosing osteomyelitis may have similar appearances but is seldom symmetrical. Very early stages of sternocostoclavicular hyperostosis may simulate condensing osteitis of the clavicles. The latter, however, tends to affect a younger age group and is not progressive.

References

1. Sonozaki H, Furusawa S, Seki H, Kurokawa T, Tateishi A, Kabata K. Four cases with symmetrical ossifications between the clavicles and the first ribs of both sides. Kanto J Orthoped Trauma 1974;5:244–7.
2. Cyrlak D, Pais MJ. Chronic recurrent multifocal osteomyelitis (CRMO). Skel Radiol 1986;15:32–9.
3. Colhoun EN, Hayward C, Evans KT. Intersterno-costoclavicular ossifications. Clin Radiol 1987;38:33–8.
4. Sartoris DJ, Schreiman JS, Kerr R, Resnick CS, Resnick D. Sternocostoclavicular hyperstosis: a review and report of eleven cases. Radiology 1986;158:125–8.
5. Franquet T, Lecumberri F, Rivas A, Inaraja L, Idoate MA. Condensing osteitis of the clavicle. Skel Radiol 1985; 14:184–7.

The dry tap

D I BOXER

Department of Radiology, Westminster Hospital, Horseferry Road, London SW1P 2AP, UK

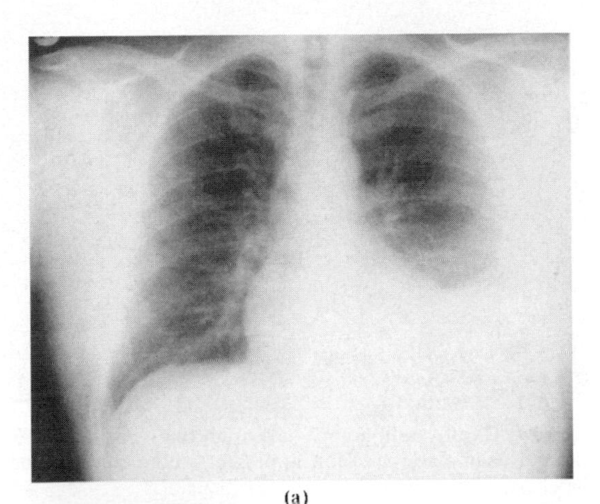

(a)

(b)

Figure 1. (a) Posteroanterior and (b) left lateral chest radiographs on admission.

Based on the case of the month originally published in Br J Radiol 1988;61:267–8.

A 39-year-old man was admitted with discomfort in the left side of the chest. This had started 2 years previously, and it was intermittent and associated with non-specific "flu-like" symptoms. He was generally fit. His only past medical history was a car accident 19 years previously in which he had suffered a fractured clavicle, fractured ribs and crush fractures of the cervical spine which required surgical fusion.

He had been previously investigated for the same symptoms at another hospital where a diagnosis of pneumonia with partial collapse of the left lower lobe and pleural effusion had been made. A number of thoracenteses had failed to produce fluid and bronchoscopy was reported as normal.

Posteroanterior and lateral chest radiography (Figure 1) was performed on admission. In order to confirm the presence of a pleural effusion, a left lateral decubitus radiograph was obtained (Figure 2). A further thoracentesis was attempted, but no fluid was obtained.

What diagnoses should be considered in this situation, and which do you think is most likely?

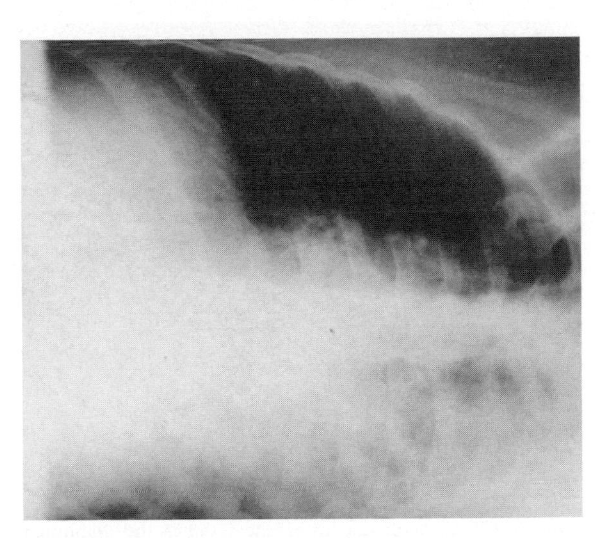

Figure 2. Left lateral decubitus chest radiograph.

Unsuccessful thoracentesis may be due to failure of the technique or to the incorrect diagnosis of a pleural effusion. The former may be due to insertion of the needle too high or too low, or the fluid being too viscous (*e.g.* pus) or loculated. Conditions which may mimic pleural effusion radiologically include pleural thickening, consolidation and herniation of bowel contents through a diaphragmatic defect. In these latter cases the chest radiograph will usually show further abnormalities and should therefore be reviewed whenever thoracentesis fails.

This patient had a traumatic diaphragmatic hernia, presumably sustained during the road traffic accident 19 years previously. CT (Figure 3) demonstrated the rupture and the presence of bowel and omentum within the chest. A barium follow-through examination (Figure 4) showed the herniated bowel to be the splenic flexure of the colon. At operation, the colon and omentum were found to have herniated through a 5 cm × 4 cm defect in the lateral portion of the diaphragm. There was also a left lower lobe collapse.

Traumatic diaphragmatic hernia is a lesion of increasing importance [1]. It may be caused by penetrating or severe blunt injury, most commonly sustained in road traffic accidents. The majority occur on the left side. Presentation may be acute or delayed. In the former, the diagnosis is made during hospitalization for the original injuries which are often multiple. In the latter group, diagnosis may not be made for many years, the patient remaining symptom free and the diagnosis being made incidentally. In these circumstances, presentation may be with chronic chest or abdominal symptoms or as a surgical emergency with obstruction or a strangulated viscus.

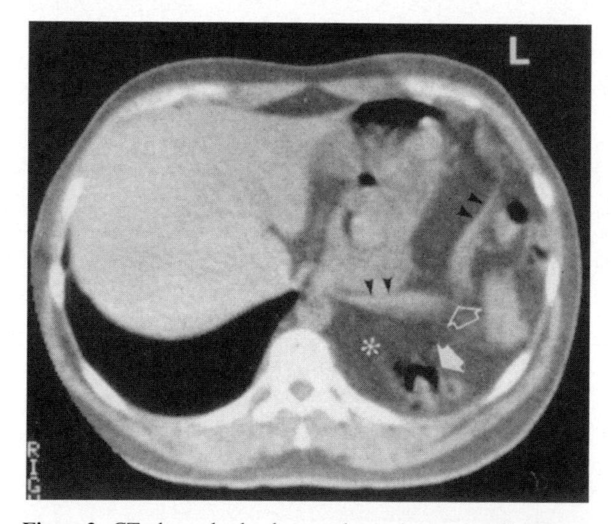

Figure 3. CT through the lower chest shows the diaphragm (arrowheads) and the diaphragmatic defect (open arrow). Bowel (solid arrow) and omentum (*) are present within the chest.

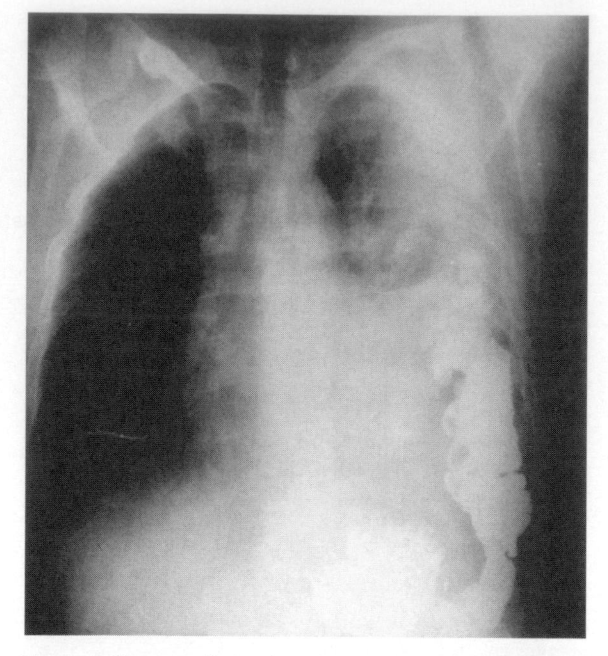

Figure 4. Chest radiograph taken during barium follow-through examination. Colon is present within the left side of the chest.

In this case, diagnosis was delayed because of misinterpretation of the lateral decubitus radiograph. Omental fat within the chest can behave in a fluid manner and simulate pleural fluid by layering along the chest wall in the decubitus view [2]. Cystic lucencies were visible within the area of opacification on the decubitus radiograph and should have indicated the possibility of a gas-containing viscus being present within the chest. Early diagnosis is important in patients with traumatic diaphragmatic hernias because of the risk of bowel strangulation or obstruction. Mortality rates as high as 80% have been reported in the presence of gangrene [3]. Thoracentesis should be avoided because of the risk of fistula formation between the alimentary tract and the pleural space [3].

CT is a simple, reliable method of diagnosing traumatic rupture of the diaphragm [4].

References

1. Adamthwaite DN. Traumatic diaphragmatic hernia. Surg Ann 1983;15:73–97.
2. Gurney J, Harrison WL, Anderson JC. Omental fat simulating pleural fluid in traumatic diaphragmatic hernia: CT characteristics. JCAT 1985;9:1112–4.
3. Hegarty MM, Bryer JV, Angorn IB, Baker LW. Delayed presentation of traumatic diaphragmatic hernia. Ann Surg 1978;188:229–33.
4. Heiberg E, Wolverson MK, Hurd RN, Jagannadharao B, Sundaram M. CT recognition of traumatic rupture of the diaphragm. AJR 1980;135:369–72.

A lytic lesion in bone

V W K NG and D MACVICAR

Department of Radiology, Royal Marsden Hospital, Downs Road, Sutton, Surrey SM2 5PT, UK

A 16-year-old Caucasian male presented with pain in his left leg which he attributed to a footballing injury. A radiograph showed a lesion in the left femoral neck (Figure 1).

An attempt to biopsy the lesion provoked brisk haemorrhage and no useful tissue was obtained. Once haemostasis was achieved, a second biopsy successfully obtained tissue for histological examination. Further investigations at the time included a normal chest radiograph and normal thoracic CT.

On the basis of the histological diagnosis, treatment was started and satisfactory clinical progress was made for 6 months. At a follow-up visit, the patient complained of some pain and "crackliness" in the centre of his chest. A chest radiograph showed bilateral small pneumothoraces.

What is the most likely diagnosis?

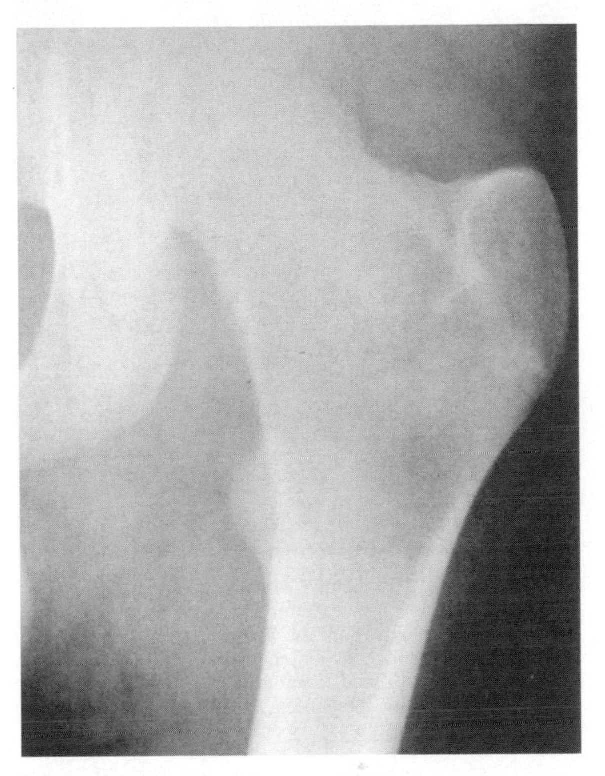

Figure 1. Radiograph of the upper left femur.

Based on the case of the month originally published in Br J Radiol 1996;69:975–6.

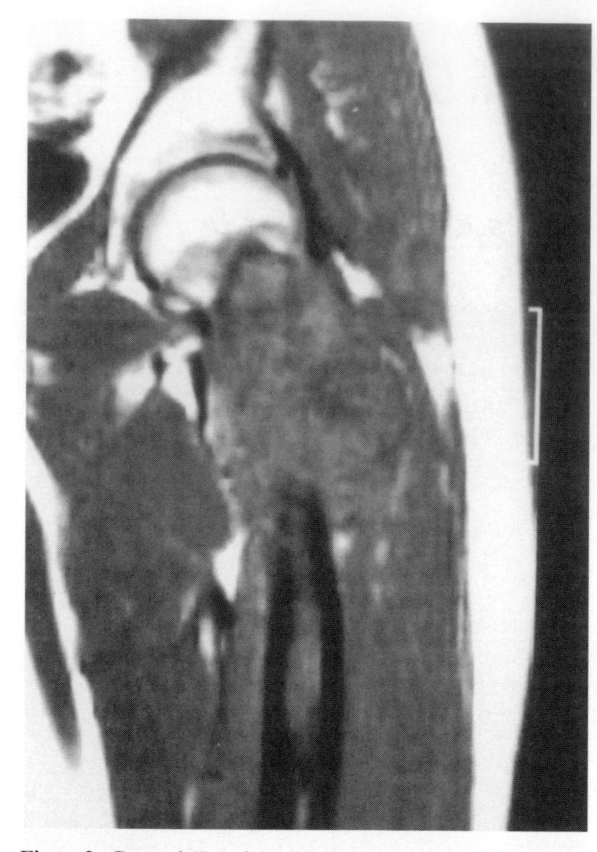

Figure 2. Coronal T_1 weighted MR image of the upper femur. A predominantly low signal tumour is present in the metaphysis. It extends up to and abuts the growth plate of the femoral capital epiphysis and has obliterated the greater trochanter. There is a bulky soft tissue component, although the size of the soft tissue mass may have been exaggerated by spillage of tumour and blood at the biopsy prior to MRI.

The histological diagnosis was telangiectatic osteosarcoma. This rare form of the disease accounts for 2.5–11% of all osteosarcomas [1–3], occurring predominantly in the second and third decade. The usual presenting complaint is of pain and local swelling, the latter sometimes attributable to pathological fracture. Males are affected twice as commonly as females.

Radiographically, telangiectatic osteosarcoma typically affects the metaphyseal region of the growing end of a long bone. Unlike the classical osteosarcoma, it usually presents as a lytic lesion which resembles an aggressive aneurysmal bone cyst. Our patient (Figure 1) demonstrated a typical appearance; namely a lytic lesion with an indistinct zone of transition and "moth-eaten" pattern of bone destruction, but no evidence of new bone formation. Pathologically, the criterion of an osteosarcoma is its ability to form tumour osteoid, but tissues other than bone may be formed, for example, fibrous tissue or cartilage. In telangiectatic osteosarcoma, pleomorphic cells and scanty streamers of osteoid form cyst-like walls around vascular spaces.

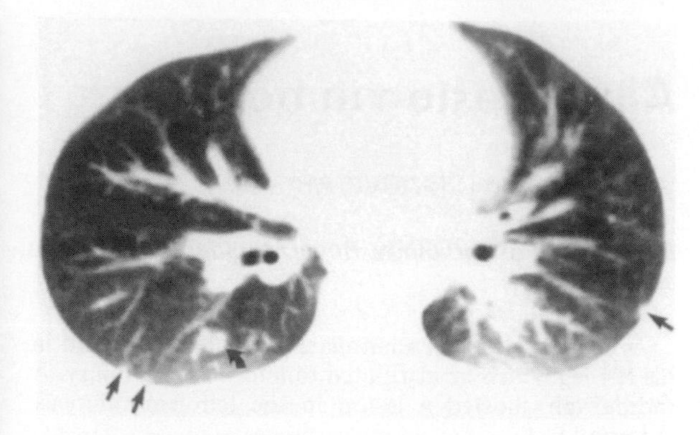

Figure 3. Thoracic CT scan showing very small peripheral pulmonary metastases abutting the pleura (arrows). A larger, more central metastasis is also present (curved arrow).

While plain radiography remains the most useful investigation for the specific diagnosis of bone pathology, MRI is now established as the most accurate method of demonstrating soft tissue masses and the extent of bone marrow involvement. If a bone tumour is suspected, MRI is best performed before biopsy because, as in our case, a post-operative haematoma may cause diagnostic difficulty. Marrow involvement by this tumour was well demonstrated, extending from the growth plate of the femoral capital epiphysis, through the growth plate of the greater trochanter and 17 cm down the shaft, underlining the value of MRI in locoregional staging [4] (Figure 2).

The natural history is for haematogeneous spread to produce pulmonary metastases. The spontaneous bilateral pneumothoraces indicated the development of peripheral pulmonary metastases. Pneumothorax, which may resolve and recur, is a classical, rather than common, presentation of metastatic spread. The underlying deposits may be small or subpleural in location and are frequently not visible on plain radiography. The development of a pneumothorax is therefore an indication for thoracic CT to confirm the presence of metastases (Figure 3).

The prognosis for patients with telangiectatic osteosarcoma has improved recently. Adjuvant chemotherapy is used to salvage those with metastatic disease at presentation, although the survival of those without metastases at presentation is apparently not influenced by neoadjuvant chemotherapy before surgical resection [3].

References

1. Matsuno T, Unni KK, McLeod RA, et al. Telangiectatic osteosarcoma. Cancer 1976;38:2538–47.
2. Huvos AG, Rosen G, Bretsky S, Butler A. Telangiectatic osteosarcoma: a clinicopathological study of 124 patients. Cancer 1982;49:1679–89.
3. Mervak TR, Unni KK, Pritchard DJ, McLeod RA. Telangiectatic osteosarcoma. Clin Orthop 1991;270:135–9.
4. Spina V, Romagnoli R, Manfrini M, et al. La risonanza magnetica nello studio dell'osteosarcoma. Radiol Med 1991; 81:29–37.

A far cry

R JONES and I ZAMMIT-MAEMPEL

Department of Radiology, Freeman Hospital, Freeman Road, Newcastle upon Tyne NE7 7DN, UK

A 39-year-old man attended the Ear, Nose and Throat (ENT) Outpatient Clinic complaining of epiphora and a chronically blocked nose. On clinical examination and anterior rhinoscopy there was some widening of the nasal bridge, a narrowed nasal airway and left septal deviation. The patient denied previous trauma to his nose. Plain radiographs of his sinuses and facial bones were unremarkable.

CT coronal sections through the sinuses (Figure 1) followed by limited transaxial views of the nasal bones (Figure 2) were then performed. What is the abnormality demonstrated on CT? What is the differential diagnosis and what further radiological investigation might aid the diagnosis?

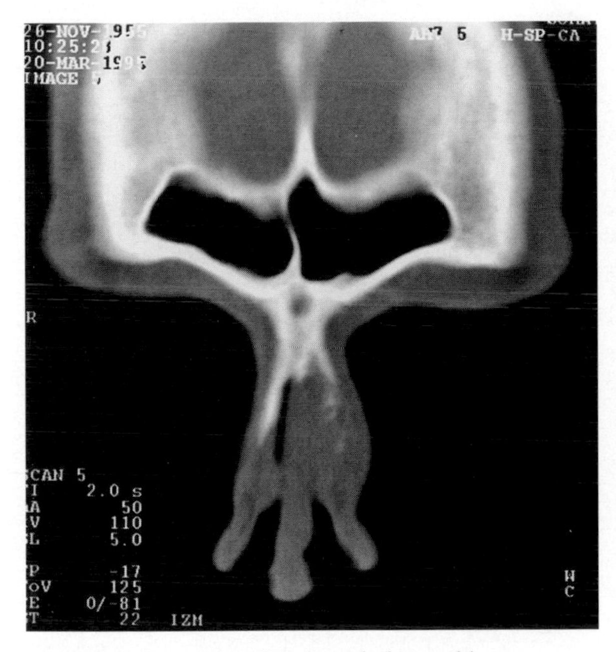

Figure 1. CT coronal section through the nasal bones.

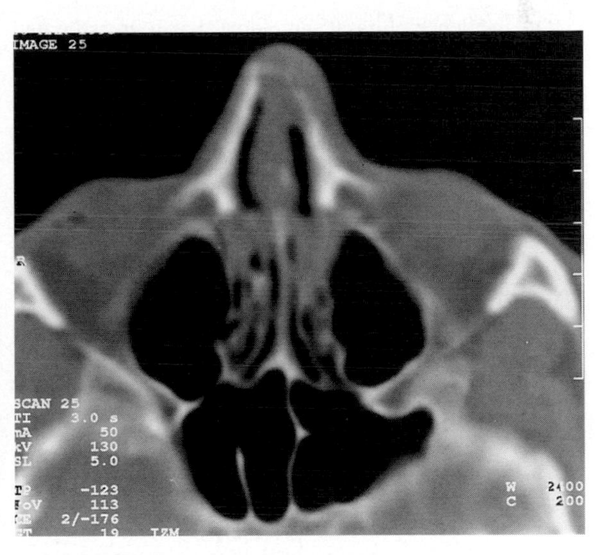

Figure 2. CT axial section of the nasal bones.

Based on the case of the month originally published in Br J Radiol 1997;70:1307–8.

The CT scan showed destruction of the anterior aspect of the left nasal bone with a small associated soft tissue mass. The differential diagnosis would include the granuloma-producing diseases such as Wegener's granulomatosis, sarcoidosis and chronic infections including tuberculosis, actinomycosis and syphilis. In addition, malignant conditions such as lymphoma need to be considered.

A chest radiograph showed bilateral hilar lymphadenopathy with no evidence of interstitial shadowing (Figure 3). The radiological picture strongly suggested sarcoidosis. Examination under anaesthesia and biopsy of the lateral wall, middle meatus and nasal septum showed generalized inflammatory changes with discrete coalescing granulomata. No acid fast bacilli were identified. Serum analysis revealed a marginally raised angiotensin converting enzyme level. The remainder of the biochemical profile was normal, as was the autoantibody screen including ANCA titres.

As there was no evidence of intrapulmonary disease based on normal respiratory function tests, the only medication was betnesol nasal drops. Since the patient's main complaint was epiphora combined with a recurrent left lacrimal gland pyocele, an ipsilateral dacryocystorrhinostomy was performed. He remained well 15 months after diagnosis.

The incidence of nasal sarcoidosis has been estimated as 3–20% of patients with systemic sarcoidosis [1]. In a few isolated cases nasal involvement may be the first and only manifestation of sarcoidosis and usually presents with obstruction and widening of the nasal bridge [2]. CT findings are usually non-specific with nodular soft tissue thickening of the nasal cavity, nasal septum and paranasal sinuses [3].

Destruction of the nasal bones is unusual [4] and is found in association with lupus pernio or, as in this case, disease of the nasal mucosa [5]. Nasal bone lesions are usually small lytic defects on a background of osteoporosis.

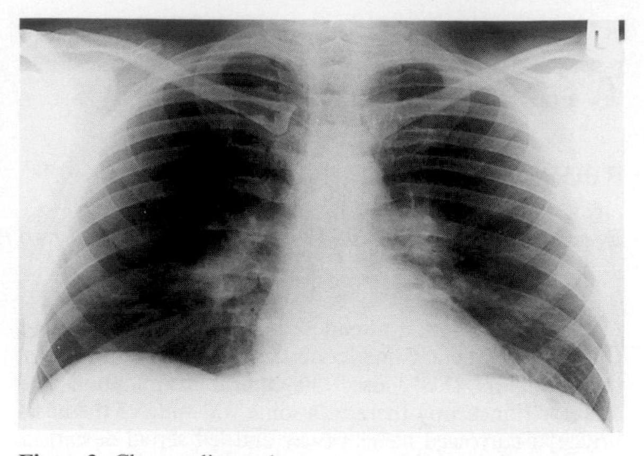

Figure 3. Chest radiograph.

In our case, the associated bone destruction together with the chest radiograph appearance led to a diagnosis of sarcoidosis.

References

1. Gordon WW, Cohn AM, Greenberg SD, et al. Nasal sarcoidosis. Arch Otolaryngol 1976;102:11–14.
2. Munro-Black JL. Sarcoidosis of the nose. Proc Roy Soc Med 1973;66:669–75.
3. Forbes W St C. The paranasal sinuses. In: Gillespie JE, Gholkar A, editors. Magnetic resonance imaging and computed tomography of the head and neck. London: Chapman and Hall, 1994:126.
4. Madoule P, Ellrodt A, Chevrot A, et al. Case report 306. Skel Radiol 1985;13:304–8.
5. Neville E, Carstairs LS, James DG. Sarcoidosis of bone. Q J Med 1977;46:215–27.

There's more to it than meets the eye

S EVANS

Department of Radiology, Walsgrave Hospital, Coventry, UK

A 39-year-old Indian man presented to the Casualty Department with a 3-week history of headaches and nasal congestion, and a 3-day history of a painful swollen right eye. On examination, he was unwell and pyrexial with a sinus tachycardia. He had a tender right eye with a swollen upper eyelid and an obvious sixth nerve palsy with almost complete failure of abduction.

CT of the head was performed (Figure 1). What is the diagnosis? How many abnormalities can you detect? What is the appropriate management?

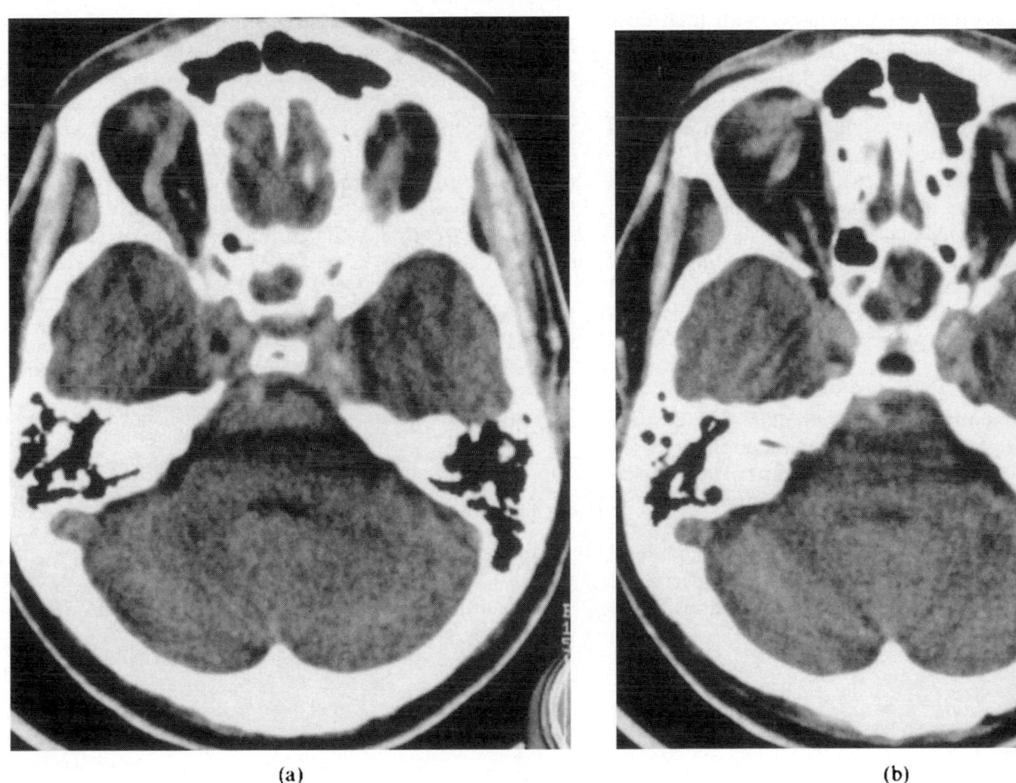

(a) (b)

Figure 1. Post-contrast 3 mm axial CT sections.

Based on the case of the month originally published in Br J Radiol 1991;64:279–80.

High resolution slices 3 mm thick were obtained before and after administration of intravenous contrast medium, in an axial plane of section parallel to the orbitomeatal line. No reformatting was considered necessary.

A right-sided cavernous sinus thrombosis was shown. There was enlargement and asymmetry of the right cavernous sinus with irregular filling defects within it, representing thrombus formation. Smaller regular filling defects were also seen in the left cavernous sinus and these represented normal structures and/or fat within the sinus [1]. In addition, there was a marked engorgement of the right superior ophthalmic vein containing several thrombi. The sphenoid sinus was opaque and contained material of soft tissue density which denotes a sphenoid sinusitis.

The patient had opacification of the right maxillary antrum and sphenoid sinus on admission which, taken together with his clinical presentation, suggested a tentative diagnosis of cavernous sinus thrombosis, duly confirmed by CT.

The patient was treated immediately with high dose intravenous antibiotics and nasal decongestants but had still not improved significantly after 48 h. He then underwent bilateral sphenoid sinoscopy and washout, and right maxillary antrostomy. The right sphenoid sinus contained much purulent debris, and had a very hyperaemic mucosa and a blocked ostium. The left sphenoid sinus was clear. Culture of the pus yielded a heavy growth of *Streptococcus pneumoniae*.

The patient had dramatically improved within 24 h of the procedure. His symptoms settled after a further 4 days of intravenous antibiotics, and by Day 10 his sixth nerve palsy had completely resolved.

The cavernous sinus is a large, circular venous space which allows free drainage between the right and left compartments [2]. It contains several important vessels and nerves: the horizontal portion of the internal carotid artery running forward through the sinus, and the sixth cranial nerve passing between the artery and the lateral wall of the sinus. The third, fourth and fifth nerves lie within the lateral wall, separated from the venous blood by a thin fibrous sheath [1]. Thus, the likeliest structures to be affected by thrombosis are the internal carotid artery and the sixth nerve. In severe cases of septic cavernous sinus thrombosis, third and fourth nerve palsies also occur. These may be unilateral, bilateral, or progress from one eye to the other [2].

Septic cavernous sinus thrombosis is an uncommon condition, and can be life-threatening unless diagnosed and treated early [3]. The commonest predisposing factors are paranasal sinus, nasal or skin infection. The mechanism of spread from the paranasal sinuses to the cavernous sinus is attributed to thrombophlebitis. More seriously, meningitis may develop with or without generalized septicaemia.

This case highlights several important features of cavernous sinus thrombosis. First, the diagnosis is essentially a clinical one and is generally straightforward when clinical features are severe. Where orbital signs are mild or absent, high resolution CT is invaluable for confirming the diagnosis as it can actually show the thrombus within the sinus [4].

Secondly, having established the diagnosis of cavernous sinus thrombosis complicating acute sphenoid sinusitis, early and aggressive treatment with intravenous antibiotics should be instituted. Prompt surgical intervention is indicated if symptoms continue or complications arise [5]. Thirdly, cavernous sinus thrombosis remains a serious condition that is infrequently encountered and vigilance is required to ensure early diagnosis and rapid treatment. If left untreated, morbidity and mortality are high.

References

1. Kline LB, Acker JD, Post MJD, Vitek JJ. The cavernous sinus: a computed tomographic study. Am J Neuroradiol 1981;2:299–305.
2. Harrington PC. Complications of sinusitis. Ear Nose Throat J 1984;63:163–7.
3. Yarrington CT. Cavernous sinus thrombosis revisited. Proc Roy Soc Med 1977;70:456–9.
4. Clifford-Jones RE, Ellis CJK, Stevens JM, Turner A. Cavernous sinus thrombosis. J Neurol Neurosurg Psychiatr 1982;45:1092–7.
5. Urqhuart AC, Fung G, McIntosh WA. Isolated sphenoiditis: a diagnostic problem. J Laryngol Otol 1989;103:526–7.

Dense bones

[1]S VINNICOMBE, [1]C HERON and [2]M WANSBROUGH-JONES

Departments of [1]Radiology and [2]Infectious Diseases, St George's Hospital, Blackshaw Road, London SW17, UK

A 39-year-old Asian woman was investigated for a 4 year history of generalized aches and pains and more recent malaise, fevers and cervical adenopathy. On admission, her erythrocyte sedimentation rate (ESR) was 62 and there was a mild polyclonal gammopathy. Mantoux and Kveim tests were negative and screening cultures of urine and sputum (including for acid and alcohol fast bacilli) were also negative. The chest radiograph is shown in Figure 1. At this time, radiographs of the skull, pelvis and hands were normal.

The patient received a 6 month trial of antituberculous chemotherapy, but this resulted in minimal symptomatic improvement and her lymphadenopathy persisted. In addition, she complained of increasing pelvic pain. A pelvic radiograph was obtained, followed by isotope scintigraphy with $^{99}Tc^{m}$-methylene diphosphonate (Figures 2 and 3, respectively).

What investigation(s) would you do next? What diagnoses would you consider?

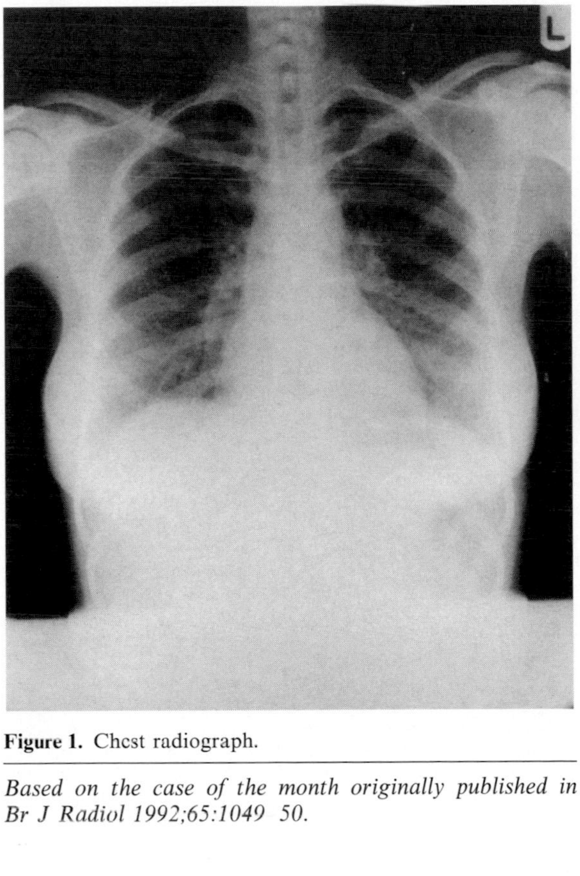

Figure 1. Chest radiograph.

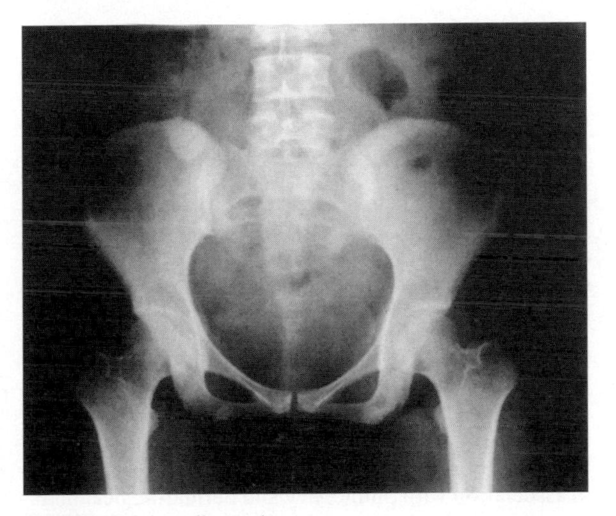

Figure 2. Pelvic radiograph.

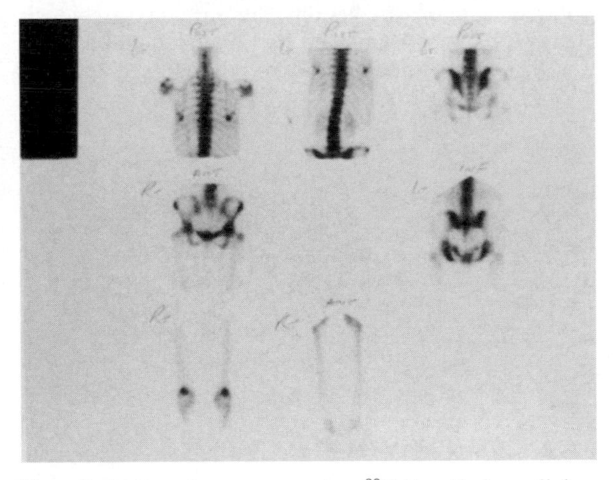

Figure 3. Isotope bone scan using $^{99}Tc^{m}$-methylene diphosphonate; views of the axial skeleton.

Based on the case of the month originally published in Br J Radiol 1992;65:1049 50.

The chest radiograph showed mild nodularity in the lungs, particularly in the midzones. There was also some prominence of the hila, especially on the left, and a suggestion of right paratracheal adenopathy. In the pelvis, there were areas of sclerosis, without expansion, around the sacroiliac joints, ischial tuberosities and iliac blades bilaterally. The radioisotope bone scan showed a small area of increased uptake around the right ischial tuberosity and in the posteromedial part of the right iliac crest.

A bone biopsy was performed under CT guidance and one of the cervical lymph nodes was also biopsied. Non-caseating granulomata were found on histological examination of both specimens. A diagnosis of sclerosing sarcoidosis of bone was made and treatment with steroids commenced. Over the next 6 months the patient improved symptomatically and her ESR slowly fell to 30.

The differential diagnosis of sclerotic bone lesions is large and includes metastatic carcinoma (notably of prostate and breast), lymphoma (particularly Hodgkin's disease) and Paget's disease. Other rarer causes include systemic mastocytosis and osteopetrosis. Most of these are readily excluded, either radiologically or clinically, but this may be difficult in the case of lymphoma even after bone biopsy. The clinical course in the two conditions is of value, as sclerotic sarcoidosis tends to be indolent in nature [1].

Sarcoidosis is a chronic granulomatous condition of unknown aetiology. The reported incidence of bony involvement varies from 6 to 26% of cases [2]. The usual pattern is of osteolytic lesions, predominantly in the small tubular bones of the hands and feet. The vertebrae are occasionally affected. The lesions tend to occur in association with pulmonary and dermatological manifestations of the disease and they are strongly predictive of chronicity of disease.

Purely osteoblastic lesions are rare in sarcoidosis. They were first documented in 1971 by Bonakdarpour et al [3] and a small number of reports have appeared since then. Certain features are common to all the cases described. Firstly, sclerotic lesions have a marked tendency to involve the axial skeleton, in particular the pelvis, spine and occasionally the ribs and skull. The bones of the hands and feet are nearly always spared. This is in contrast with the more usual osteolytic sarcoidosis. The involvement is often strikingly symmetrical and there is little evidence of bony destruction. Patients frequently experience bone pain, unlike those with osteolytic sarcoid of the extremities. Sclerotic lesions may antedate or postdate other manifestations of the disease and skin involvement need not be present. However, lymphadenopathy is a frequent accompaniment. Finally, all the patients reported except one have been middle-aged and of negroid extraction.

Isotope scintigraphy in this patient seriously underestimated the extent of bony involvement. This, again, contrasts with osteolytic sarcoidosis, where it has been shown that bone scintigraphy with $^{99}Tc^{m}$-diphosphonate is much more sensitive than plain radiography [4] with avid uptake [5].

The fact that patients may present with symptomatic sclerotic lesions before the development of the more obvious manifestations of sarcoidosis may pose a diagnostic difficulty. This diagnosis should always be considered in the differential of sclerotic bone especially in patients of an appropriate age and racial background.

References

1. Weston M, Duffy P. Osteosclerosis in sarcoidosis. Austr Radiol 1975;XIX:191–3.
2. Lin SR, Levy W, Go EB, Lee I, Wong WK. Unusual osteosclerotic changes in sarcoidosis, simulating osteoblastic metastases. Radiology 1973;106:311–2.
3. Bonakdarpour A, Levy W, Aegerter EE. Osteosclerotic changes in sarcoidosis. Am J Roentgenol Radiol Therapeut Nucl Med 1971;113:646–9.
4. Rohatgi PK. Radioisotope scanning in osseous sarcoidosis. AJR 1980;134:189–91.
5. Abdelwahab IF, Norman A. Osteosclerotic sarcoidosis. AJR 1988;150:161–2.

"The Dormouse is asleep again" said the Hatter, and he poured a little hot tea upon its nose (*Lewis Carroll*)

S C WARD and V P L HORNSBY

Department of Radiology, Hull Royal Infirmary, Anlaby Road, Kingston upon Hull, UK

A woman aged 31 years presented acutely to her general practitioner with left sided pleuritic chest pain of short duration. She had no significant past medical history and was otherwise asymptomatic. On examination, her doctor found no abnormality in the chest, but discovered a large ill defined mass in the left upper abdomen.

He requested a plain radiograph of the abdomen (Figure 1) and an upper abdominal ultrasound (Figure 2) before referring the patient to hospital where CT of the abdomen was performed (Figure 3).

What is the diagnosis and how should the patient be managed?

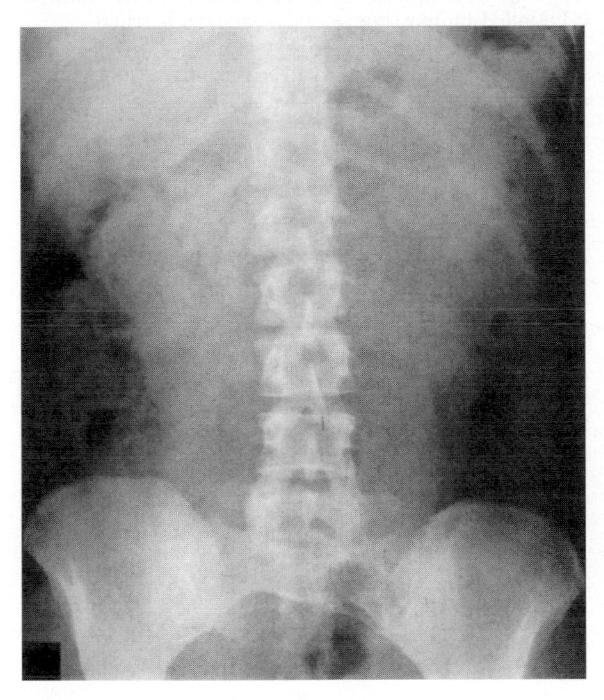

Figure 1. Plain abdominal radiograph.

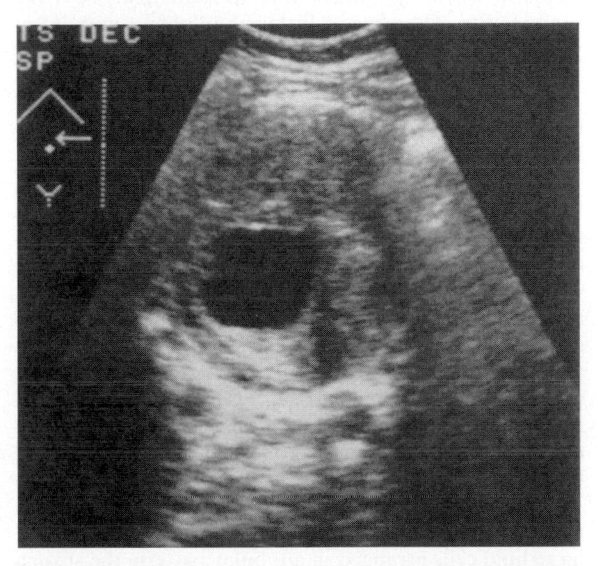

Figure 2. Longitudinal scan through the left upper abdomen (3.5 MHz probe).

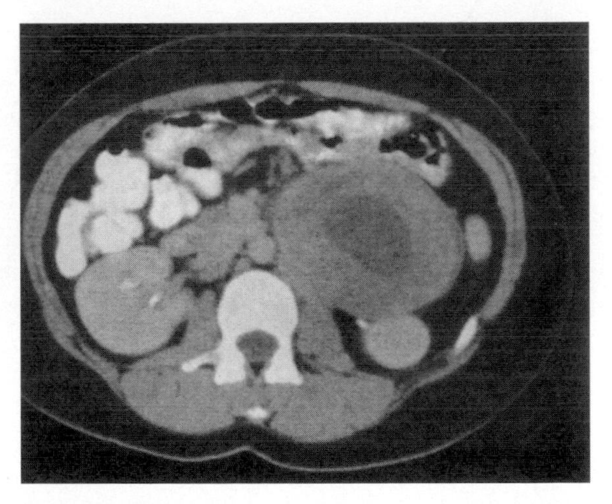

Figure 3. CT through the mid-abdomen, with oral and intravenous contrast medium.

Based on the case of the month originally published in Br J Radiol 1990;63:733–4.

The plain abdominal radiograph confirmed the presence of a large rounded mass of soft tissue density in the left upper quadrant. The psoas shadow was seen distinctly through the mass; there was some bulging of its outline, suggesting the close proximity of the tumour to the belly of the muscle. Ultrasonically, the mass was of mixed echogenicity and CT further delineated its margins and demonstrated attenuation values similar to those of fat, with a cystic area at its centre. The tumour was separate from spleen, pancreas, liver, bowel and both kidneys and all margins were well defined, except posteromedially where the mass was indistinguishable from psoas major. There was a little enhancement with intravenous contrast medium.

Radiologically, the appearances are those of a retroperitoneal connective tissue tumour. Desmoid tumours may arise from muscle fascia but are more commonly found in the anterior abdominal wall. Similarly, fibrosarcomata may arise from aponeuroses and deep fascia but are rare in the trunk. Leiomyosarcomata may grow to a large size but are found most often in the retroperitoneal spaces of the elderly.

CT attenuation values suggested a tumour composed, at least partly, of fat. Lipomata are common tumours but usually occur more superficially. Fibrolipomata and angiolipomata are rarer and are composed of fatty tissue mixed with fibrous and capillary vascular tissue, respectively. The latter generally show more marked enhancement with contrast media [1]. The diagnosis of liposarcoma must also be considered. Laparotomy was carried out and a 10 cm diameter, fatty, encapsulated tumour was removed. Histological examination showed large lipid cells arranged in a lobular pattern, the stroma being of granular Sudanophilic type.

The diagnosis is that of a retroperitoneal hibernoma.

There are two types of adipose tissue: white fat, which is widely distributed in the human body, and brown fat, which is usually found in hibernating animals but may also be found in man. Tumours of brown fat were first described by Merkel in 1905 and were later named hibernomas because of their resemblance to the fat pads laid down by hibernating animals [1].

Hibernomas may occur wherever brown fat is found: between the scapulae, in the axilla, neck [2, 3], mediastinum, groin, thigh [1, 4] and retroperitoneum. The retroperitoneum is a rare site.

The tumour may present at any age but is rare in childhood. There is a slight female preponderance [2]. Hibernomas may produce local discomfort—or other symptoms of mass effect owing to their large size—but they are otherwise asymptomatic.

Hibernomas are extremely slow growing but they may suddenly undergo a period of rapid growth [2]. The tumour is generally regarded as benign but a malignant case has been reported in rats [5]. In man, some local infiltration may occur [1] but complete excision is usually curative.

Ultrasound typically demonstrates an inhomogeneous lesion; CT shows a mass of fat density with slight contrast enhancement [1]. Angiographic studies show a typical tumour blush with early venous return [4]. Whilst the radiological appearances may suggest the diagnosis of hibernoma, the latter may be distinguished from a well differentiated liposarcoma only with difficulty [1]. Histological diagnosis may be made by ultrasound or CT guided biopsy, but surgical excision is usual.

Hibernoma should be considered as a rare cause of a slow growing soft tissue mass in an otherwise asymptomatic patient.

References

1. Coblentz C, Roberts JT, Fitzgerald E. Hibernoma: a patient examined by CT. J Canad Assoc Radiol 1986;37:110–1.
2. Kristensen S. Cervical hibernoma. Review of the literature and a new case. J Laryngol Otol 1985;99:1055–8.
3. Abermayor E, McClean PH, Cobb CJ, Hashimoto CH. Hibernomas of the head and neck. Head Neck Surg 1987;9:362–7.
4. Rossi P, Francone A, Martini S, Pavone P. Multiple imaging modalities in a case of hibernoma. Eur J Radiol 1988;8:125–7.
5. Stefanski SA, Elwell MR, Yoshitomi K. Malignant hibernoma in a Fischer 344 rat. Lab Anim Sci 1987;37:347–50.

Unfit to sit

P S SIDHU, N D JONKER and A M PETERS

Department of Diagnostic Radiology, Hammersmith Hospital, Du Cane Road, London W12 0HS, UK

A 50-year-old male on haemodialysis for end-stage renal failure was admitted with severe retrosternal pain and breathlessness. There was a history of septic arthritis of hip and knee, a sigmoid colectomy for a perforated diverticulum, and three failed renal transplants. Haemoglobin was 6 g dl^{-1}, faecal occult bloods were positive and endoscopy showed severe lower oesophageal ulceration. This was treated appropriately, following which there was an improvement in the retrosternal pain. The breathlessness continued and was accompanied by right sided discomfort. A ventilation/perfusion (V/Q) lung scan was performed using $^{81}Kr^{m}$ and $^{99}Tc^{m}$ labelled macroaggregated albumin (MAA). Because of his general condition, the patient was imaged supine (Figures 1a, b).

What does this supine V/Q scan show? How may the study be modified to gain further information about the clinical status of the patient?

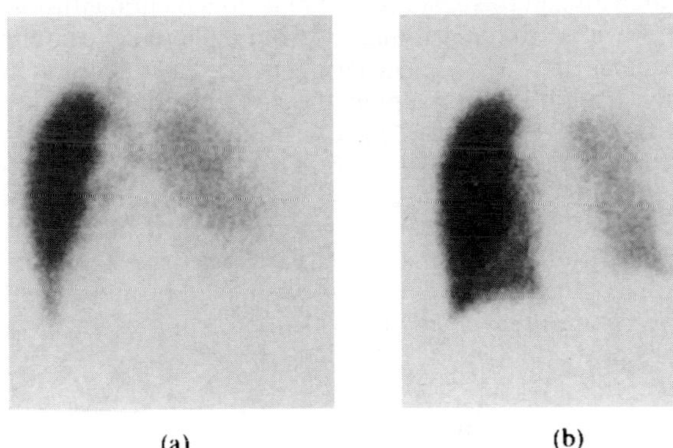

Figure 1. Posterior views in the supine position. (a) Ventilation and (b) perfusion.

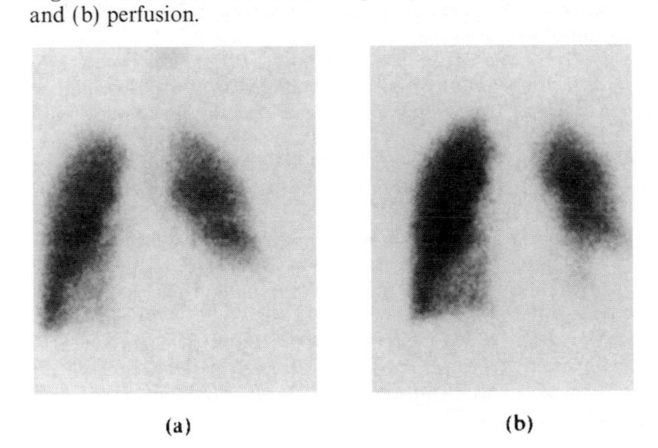

Figure 2. Posterior views in the erect position. (a) Ventilation and (b) perfusion.

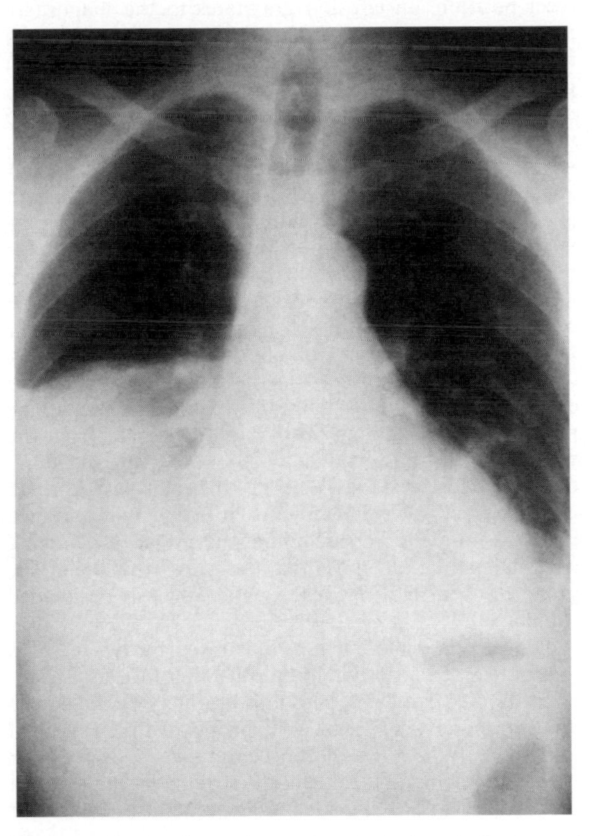

Figure 3. Chest radiograph showing right pleural effusion and enlarged heart.

Based on the case of the month originally published in Br J Radiol 1994;67:411–2.

The posterior supine V/Q images showed an apparent global reduction in perfusion and ventilation to the right lung. On the left, there was absent ventilation to the left lower lobe, but a normal appearing perfusion scan. Further information was gained by imaging the patient in the erect position (Figures 2a, b). In this position, there were focal reductions in both ventilation and perfusion in the right lower zone, corresponding to a pleural effusion seen on the chest radiograph (Figure 3), but the remainder of this lung now looked normal. The previously non-ventilated left lower zone was seen to be normally ventilated on the erect image. An echocardiogram confirmed the cardiomegaly which was apparent on the chest radiograph.

It is important to appreciate in V/Q lung scanning that the perfusion images "capture" the distribution of blood flow at the instant of injection, while the $^{81}Kr^{m}$ images continuously reflect the distribution of ventilation during the inhalation of the agent.

This case illustrates two phenomena, awareness of which is important in the interpretation of V/Q lung scans. The first is the effect of a pleural effusion. In the erect position, an effusion gravitates to the diaphragm and compresses the lower lobe. The ventilation in the right lower lobe is lost because of this lung compression present at the time of $^{81}Kr^{m}$ inhalation. The perfusion, on the other hand, although reduced, is not lost because in the supine position (the position in which the MAA was injected) flow is relatively maintained to the right lower lobe, wherein the MAA is fixed at the time of injection. In the erect position, fluid attenuates the perfusion signal from the right lower lobe, accounting for the apparent reduction in perfusion, although this reduction is not as marked as that of ventilation. The result is a reverse mismatch, *i.e.* an apparently greater loss of ventilation than of perfusion. The right lower lobe, which is compressed in the erect position by the effusion, must have partially re-expanded in the supine position since, although both V and Q signals from the whole lung are attenuated by the now dispersed fluid, there is no longer a focal defect at the right base as there is on the erect views. The practical message of importance is that a lung should not be misinterpreted as showing a global reduction in ventilation and perfusion in the presence of an effusion if the patient has to be imaged supine.

The second phenomenon, illustrated by this case, is that of loss of ventilation in the left lower lobe as a result of cardiomegaly. This could appropriately be called the scintigraphic Ewart's sign. William Ewart first described this sign at the turn of the century as a dullness to percussion below the angle of the scapula by a distended sack in pericardial effusions. Compression of the major airways by an enlarged heart may result in the same clinical findings. Compression by an enlarged left atrium has been shown to occur in infants [1]. Indeed, it has been suggested that bronchial compression with hypoxic vasoconstriction in these instances may lead to hyperinflation of the affected lobe [2].

Ventilation to the left lower lobe and its relationship to cardiomegaly and posture was investigated in adults by Alexander et al [3], who suggested that the partial loss of ventilation in the left lower lobe results from cardiomegaly and is related to posture. A further study into this phenomenon demonstrated that this reduction in left lower lobe ventilation was indeed present in the supine, but not in the prone, position [4]. These authors attributed this to the mass of the heart compressing the lung and leading to airway and/or alveolar closure. Support for this hypothesis has come from further work by Alexander et al [5]. Using inhaled $^{81}Kr^{m}$ and intravenous ^{133}Xe they demonstrated that the mechanism of postural left lower lobe hypoventilation in cardiomegaly is predominantly a regional loss of alveolar volume as a result of compression by the heart in the supine position.

Cardiomegaly, therefore, also produces a reverse mismatch and, in this respect, is similar to a pleural effusion. However, cardiomegaly differs from a pleural effusion in that the MAA (pre-injected) signal remains the same in the left lung in both supine and erect positions because a large heart does not "disperse" like a pleural effusion; in other words, the loss of ventilation signal in cardiomegaly is not due to lung displacement with resulting signal attenuation by the heart. The second practical message of importance illustrated by the case is that cardiomegaly is one of the causes of reversed mismatching, and should not be misinterpreted as evidence of, for example, a consolidated lobe.

References

1. Cochran ST, Gyepes MT, Smith LE. Obstruction of the airways by the heart and pulmonary vessels in infants. Paediatr Radiol 1977;6:81–7.
2. Corr L, McCarthy PA, Lavender JP, Hallidie-Smith KA. Bronchial compression by an enlarged left atrium in infants: a cause of hypovascularity of the left lung. Paediatr Radiol 1988;18:459–63.
3. Alexander MSM, Arnot RN, Lavender JP. Left lower lobe ventilation and its relation to cardiomegaly and posture. Br Med J 1989;299:94.
4. Wiener CM, McKenna WJ, Myers MJ et al. Left lower lobe ventilation is reduced in patients with cardiomegaly in the supine but not the prone position. Am Rev Resp Dis 1990;141:150–5.
5. Alexander MSM, Peters AM, Cleland J, Lavender JP. Impaired left lower lobe ventilation in patients with cardiomegaly. An isotope study of mechanisms. Chest 1991;101:1189–93.

A single diagnosis: that is the question

[1]G R AVERY and [2]A J CHIPPINDALE

Departments of Radiology, [1]Hull Royal Infirmary, Anlaby Road, Hull, and [2]Newcastle General Hospital, Westgate Road, Newcastle upon Tyne NE4 6BE, UK

A 3-month-old boy presented with a 6 week history of persistent cough, general malaise and increasing pallor. On examination he was noted to have hepatosplenomegaly and his chest radiograph demonstrated miliary shadowing. The diagnosis was confirmed on liver biopsy and urine culture. However, despite appropriate therapy the patient's condition slowly deteriorated.

This chest radiograph was taken 2 months after therapy had been introduced (Figure 1).

What is the diagnosis?

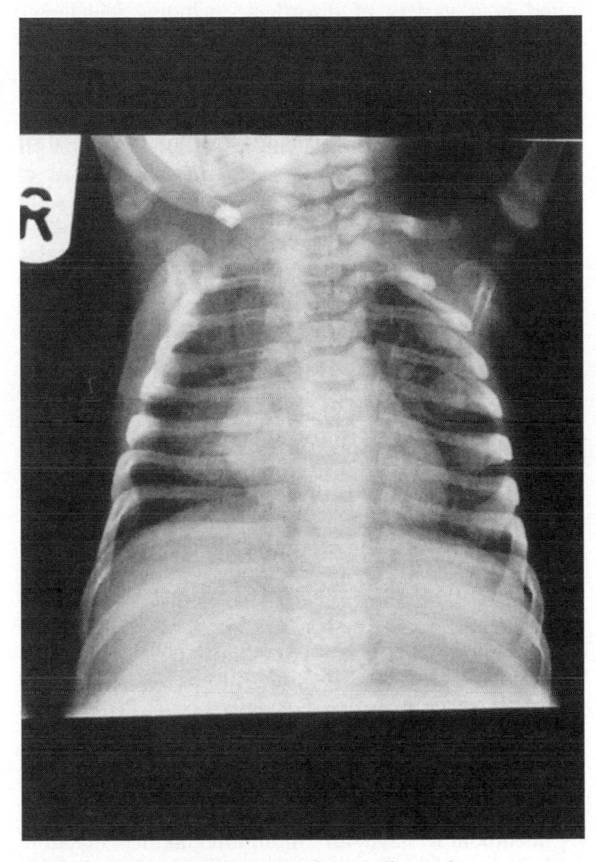

Figure 1. Posteroanterior erect chest radiograph.

Based on the case of the month originally published in Br J Radiol 1995;68:665–6.

A firm diagnosis of tuberculosis had been made at presentation on liver biopsy which showed large numbers of granulomata, some caseating and occasional acid fast bacilli. Mycobacterium tuberculosis was subsequently grown on urine cultures.

Figure 1 shows right midzone consolidation with associated right paratracheal lymphadenopathy. These features had appeared since the initial radiograph.

In addition, there were now radiolucent bands in the humeral metaphyses with adjacent dense bands which were not present on the presentation film. These may be found in a variety of disorders, including leukaemia, metastatic neuroblastoma and hypervitaminosis D. The serum calcium at this time was 3.6 mmol l^{-1}. A renal ultrasound scan showed hyperechoic renal pyramids compatible with nephrocalcinosis (Figure 2) and an abdominal radiograph calcification along the liver biopsy tract.

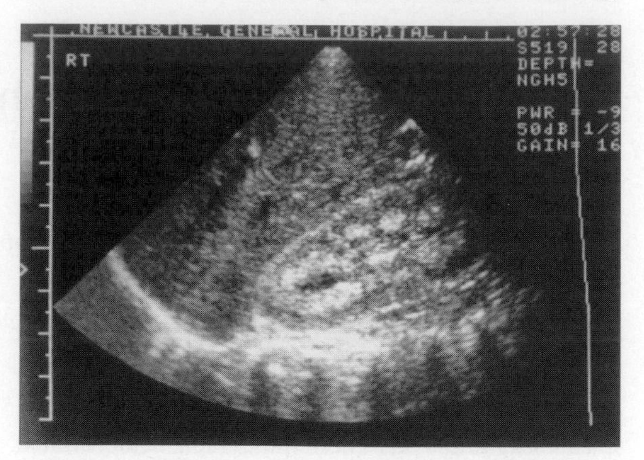

Figure 2. Longitudinal ultrasound scan of the right kidney, demonstrating hyperechoic renal pyramids.

A diagnosis of hypervitaminosis D secondary to tuberculosis was made. Serum calcium returned to normal on a low vitamin D diet. The bone changes also resolved although the nephrocalcinosis persisted at follow-up 6 months later.

Whilst the commonest presentation of paediatric tuberculosis is hilar lymphadenopathy with a small parenchymal focus, more marked consolidation can occur. Miliary tuberculosis is also not uncommon, particularly in infants, and some of these patients have additional areas of focal consolidation at presentation [1].

Despite prompt and appropriate therapy one-third of paediatric patients demonstrate radiographic progression of pulmonary tuberculosis within 3 months of initial presentation. The features noted are extension of consolidation and enlargement or development of lymphadenopathy. This is thought to be due to a hypersensitivity reaction which normally occurs 2–10 weeks after the initial infection [2]. This phenomenon probably explains the change in the radiographic appearances in the present case.

As well as their role in calcium metabolism vitamin D_3 metabolites have an immunoregulatory function. Activated monocytes and macrophages can convert $25(OH)D_3$ into the more active $1,25(OH)_2D_3$ and $24,25(OH)_2D_3$. Monocytes incubated with these metabolites inhibit the growth of mycobacterium tuberculosis [3]. The levels in granulomata are regulated locally by T cells and are independent of parathyroid hormone. Generally, these vitamin D metabolites have no systemic sequelae. However, if sufficient quantities are produced "overspill" can occur into the circulation resulting in hypercalcaemia [4]. Hypercalcaemia is an uncommon but recognized complication of tuberculosis. A similar case of hypercalcaemia in a 21-month-old boy due to miliary tuberculosis has been reported [5].

References

1. Stansberry SD. Tuberculosis in infants and children. J Thorac Imaging 1990;5:17–27.
2. Leung AN, Muller NL, Pineda PR, Fitzgerald JM. Primary tuberculosis in childhood: radiographic manifestations. Radiology 1992;182:87–91.
3. Rook GAW, Steele J, Fraher L et al. Vitamin D_3, gamma interferon, and control of proliferation of mycobacterium tuberculosis by human monocytes. Immunology 1986; 57:159–63.
4. Rook GAW. The role of vitamin D in tuberculosis. Am Rev Respir Dis 1988;138:768–70.
5. Gerritsen J, Knol K. Hypercalcaemia in a child with miliary tuberculosis. Eur J Pediatr 1989;148:650–1.

The pre-operative chest radiograph

S A THOMPSON and J S HARPER

Radiology Department, Princess Alexandra Hospital, Brisbane, Australia

A 50-year-old woman presented with iron deficiency anaemia and bleeding per rectum. Sigmoidoscopy and barium enema were negative at that time and she underwent sclerotherapy and banding of rectal haemorrhoids.

She returned 30 months later with lethargy due to recurrent anaemia and a recent episode of blood loss per rectum. There was no weight loss or alteration in bowel habit. Colonoscopy 1 month later showed a sessile mass at the ileocaecal valve. Biopsy of the mass confirmed invasive, moderately differentiated carcinoma.

A chest radiograph showed a lesion in the left lung (Figure 1). CT of the abdomen and chest (Figure 2) was performed to stage the caecal tumour accurately. This showed no other intraabdominal disease. A dynamic scan was performed through the centre of the lesion following a rapid intravenous bolus injection of contrast medium, and time–density curves were generated (Figure 3).

The patient underwent a right hemicolectomy, with a left lower lobectomy 2 months later.

What do you expect the diagnosis of the pulmonary lesion to be?

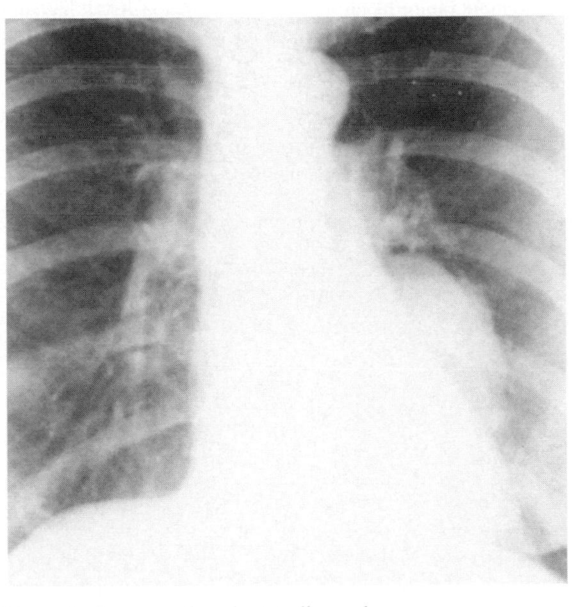

Figure 1. Pre-operative chest radiograph.

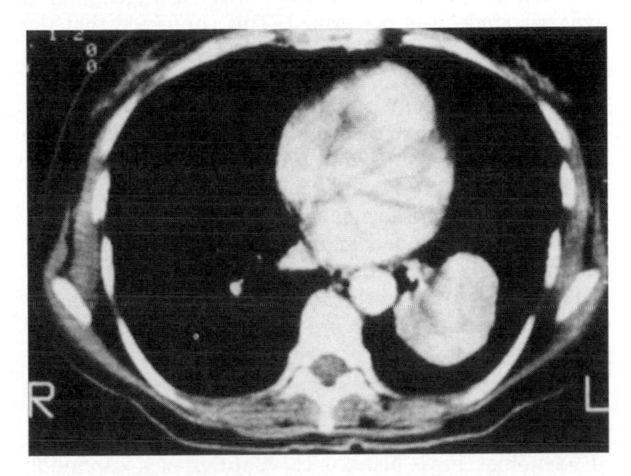

Figure 2. CT scan through the pulmonary lesion.

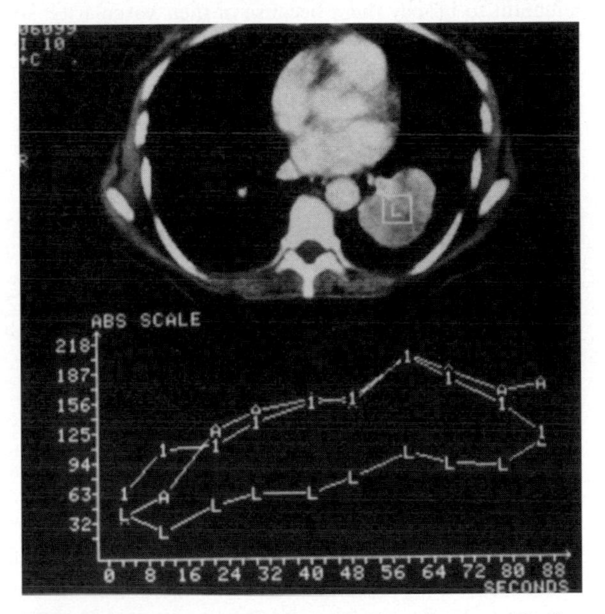

Figure 3. Dynamic scan showing density changes with time following injection of contrast medium (L, pulmonary mass; A, descending aorta; 1, ascending aorta).

Based on the case of the month originally published in Br J Radiol 1987;60:597–8.

The plain radiographic finding of a well defined, centrally located single lesion is unusual for a secondary deposit, and secondaries in the lung from a primary caecal lesion without liver involvement are rarely seen. This raised the possibility that the pulmonary lesion was a second primary tumour.

For this reason contrast enhanced CT was performed. Because of the close relationship of the mass to the lower lobe bronchus (Figure 2) and its enhancement post-contrast, a bronchial adenoma was suspected and a dynamic study was performed. This confirmed that the mass enhanced more than normal soft tissue but less than vascular structures such as the aorta (Figure 3). This excluded lesions such as pulmonary artery aneurysm or an arteriovenous malformation (AVM), which had also been considered.

At this stage, bronchial adenoma was considered most likely and endoscopic biopsy was thought unwise. Percutaneous fine-needle biopsy confirmed bronchial carcinoid.

The histology of both the caecal and the pulmonary specimens confirmed the pre-operative diagnosis.

The characteristic features of bronchial adenoma on CT have been described by Aroncheck et al [1]. 80–90% of adenomas have histological features of a carcinoid. They are smooth surfaced, well defined lesions of bronchial origin which often extend into the surrounding lung. They are characteristically very vascular and have a typical endoscopic appearance. Endoscopists have been reluctant to biopsy them because of their vascularity, so that knowledge of their characteristic features on CT is useful prior to percutaneous biopsy or surgery.

The characteristic location of these tumours and the association with distal atelectasis and pneumonitis have been described [2]. The enhancement characteristics present in our patient allowed differentiation from primary bronchogenic tumour and separation of tumour from distal atelectasis/pneumonitis [3]. Confusion with vascular lesions (aneurysm/AVM) may occur in some cases of marked enhancement but the use of dynamic scanning with plotting of time–density curves, as in this case, will allow differentiation in most cases [4].

MR is said to have an accuracy comparable with CT in the detection of hilar and mediastinal masses. Bronchial carcinoid tumours appear light on T_2 weighted and STIR sequences but cannot be distinguished from other hilar masses [5]. However, ultrafast contrast enhanced MR, as with CT, shows marked signal enhancement reflecting the high degree of vascularity in these tumours [6].

References

1. Aroncheck JM, Wexler JA, Christen B, Miller W, Epsten D, Gefter W. Computed tomography of bronchial carcinoid. JCAT 1986;10:71–4.
2. Naidich DP, McCauley DI, Siegelman SS. Computed tomography of bronchial adenomas. JCAT 1982;6:725–32.
3. Webb WR, Gamsu G, Birnberg FA. CT appearances of bronchial carcinoid with recurrent pneumonia and hyperplastic hilar lymphadenopathy. JCAT 1983;7:707–9.
4. Godwin JD, Webb WR. Dynamic computed tomography in evaluation of vascular lung lesions. Radiology 1981; 138:629–35.
5. Doppman JL, Pass HI, Nieman LK, et al. Detection of ACTH-producing bronchial carcinoid tumors. MR imaging *vs* CT. AJR 1991;156:39–43.
6. Douek PC, Simoni L, Revel D, et al. Diagnosis of bronchial carcinoid tumor by ultrafast contrast-enhanced MR imaging. AJR 1994;163:563–4.

The warm and tender hip

S H LEE

Department of Imaging, The Middlesex Hospital, Mortimer Street, London W1, UK

An 18-year-old white woman presented with left-sided low back pain of 9 months duration. Physical examination showed a warm, tender area over the left sacroiliac joint. There was wasting of the ipsilateral quadriceps femoris muscle and limitation of hip movements because of pain. The patient was apyrexial. Investigations revealed a haemoglobin of 12.4 g dl^{-1}, a white cell count of $7.9 \times 10^9\ l^{-1}$, an erythrocyte sedimentation rate (ESR) of 33 mm h^{-1} and an alkaline phosphatase of 341 iu l^{-1}. A radiograph of the pelvis (Figure 1) and CT (Figure 2) were performed.

What is the abnormality and the differential diagnosis? How would one proceed with further management?

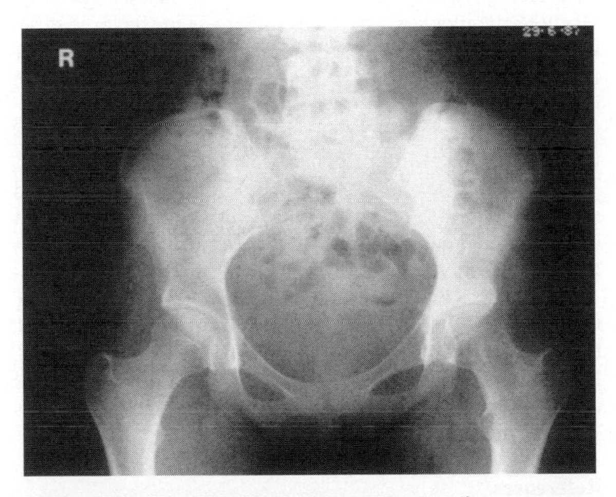

Figure 1. Radiograph of the pelvis on presentation.

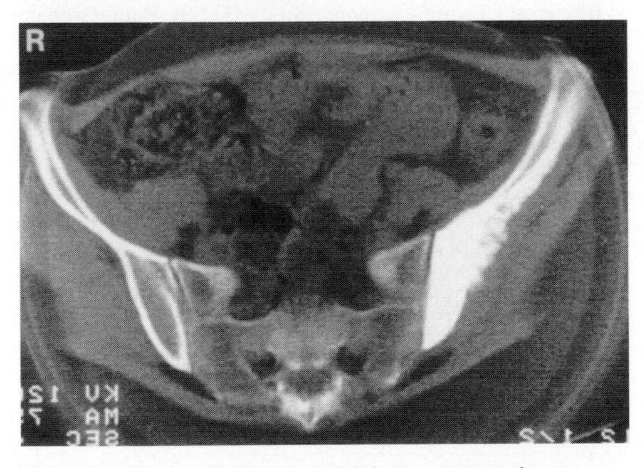

Figure 2. CT scan of the upper pelvis on presentation.

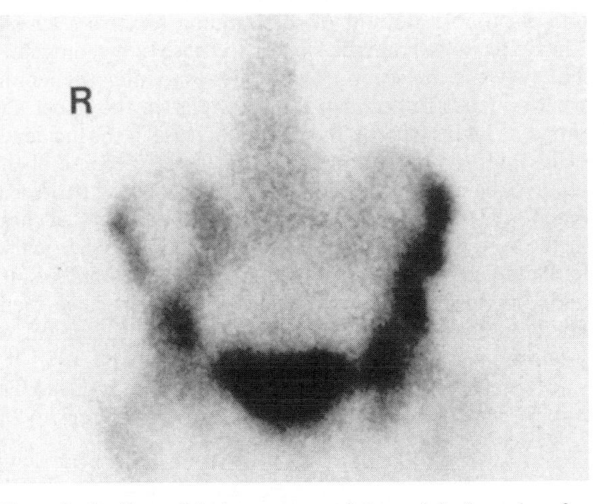

Figure 3. Radionuclide bone scan of the pelvis 8 weeks after CT scan. Supine view showing increased uptake over left anterior iliac bone.

Based on the case of the month originally published in Br J Radiol 1989;62:495–6.

The plain radiograph showed diffuse sclerosis adjacent to the left sacroiliac joint. CT also showed widespread sclerosis, a spiculated periosteal reaction and wasting of the left iliopsoas and gluteal muscles. These appearances could be caused by a Brodie's abscess, primary bone tumour or a lymphoma. There was no evidence elsewhere of lymphadenopathy, and the patient was apyrexial, so that a primary bone tumour seemed most likely. An open bone biopsy was performed, and it was noted that there was new bone completely replacing the medullary cavity and extensive periosteal new bone. Bacteriology showed no growth of organisms.

Histological examination with haematoxylin and eosin stain showed marrow replacement with malignant round cells, the majority of which had undergone necrosis. Glycogen granules positive to periodic acid-Schiff stain were present in some cells, which helped confirm the diagnosis of Ewing's sarcoma. Lymphoma markers were not detectable.

A radionuclide bone scan was done to look for other lesions or metastases. A chest radiograph should also be done with CT of the chest if no metastases are seen. The bone scan was performed 8 weeks following the initial CT and showed an increased uptake of $^{99}Tc^{m}$ on the left side of the pelvis on the supine view (Figure 3), and the postero-inferior aspect of the right ilium on the prone view (Figure 4). A further radiograph of the pelvis at that time showed a sclerotic area in the right side of the pelvis conforming to the area of increased uptake on the bone scan. There were no other abnormalities present. MRI confirmed the bilateral iliac bone involvement and soft tissue extension on the left side, but added no other useful information.

Ewing's sarcoma represents 10% of all primary malignant bone tumours and is seen in patients aged 3–25 years. It typically presents with an area of permeative destruction and a variable amount of surrounding reactive sclerosis. The appearances may be similar to those of osteomyelitis. The pelvis is the second commonest site after the femur, where it tends to occur in the diaphysis. In the upper age range, as in this patient, there is an increase in the incidence of Ewing's tumour occurring in flat bones because of the relative increase in red marrow in these sites. A periosteal reaction is present in most cases. In the series of 372 cases in the Intergroup Ewing's Sarcoma Study (IESS), 56.6% had a laminated periosteal reaction and 27.7% had a spiculated periosteal reaction, the latter being vertically orientated and unlike the "sunburst" appearance typical of osteosarcoma [1].

Diffuse sclerosis in Ewing's sarcoma is a recognized feature. It was found in 10% of cases in an early series [2].

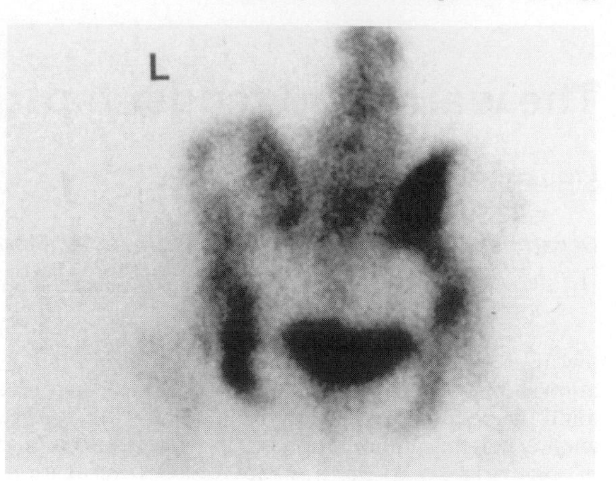

Figure 4. Prone view showing increased uptake in the metastasis over the right posterior sacroiliac joint.

In a later series it was seen in 27% of cases [3]. More recently, the incidence of diffuse sclerosis in the large series collected by the IESS was 37.6%, with 57% of pelvic tumours showing this feature. Sclerosis alone was seen in only two cases out of a total of 210.

Systemic symptoms occur as a result of necrosis within the tumour, resulting in general malaise and raised ESR. There may be fever, normochromic anaemia and raised white cell count. CT of the primary lesion shows the extent of periosteal new-bone formation, tumoral reactive sclerosis, cortical invasion and tumour infiltration into soft tissues [4]. MRI is superior to CT for showing marrow infiltration and soft tissue extension and has replaced CT for the assessment of operability [5]. However, unlike CT, MRI cannot show cortical destruction, and both periosteal new bone and reactive sclerosis are more difficult to assess with this technique.

References

1. Reinus WR, Gilula KA. Radiology of Ewing's sarcoma: Intergroup Ewing's Sarcoma Study (IESS). RadioGraphics 1984;6:929–44.
2. Sherman RS, Soong KW. Ewing's sarcoma: its roentgen classification and diagnosis. Radiology 1956;66:529–39.
3. Lombardi F, Gasparini M, Gianni C, Petrillo R, Tesoro-Tess JD, Volterrani F, et al. Ewing's sarcoma: an approach to radiologic diagnosis. Tumori 1979;65:389–99.
4. Vanel D, Contesso G, Couanet D, Pilkarski JD, Sarazin D, Masselot J. Computed tomography in the evaluation of 41 cases of Ewing's sarcoma. Skel Radiol 1982;9:8–13.
5. Boyko OB, Cory DA, Cohen MD, Provisor A, Mirkin D, de Rosa GP. MR imaging of osteogenic and Ewing's sarcoma. AJR 1987;148:317–22.

Diffuse skeletal hyperostosis in a young patient

M HAMMOUDEH and A R SIAM

Division of Rheumatology, Department of Medicine, Hamad General Hospital, PO Box 3050, Doha, Qatar, Arabian Gulf

A 27-year-old male patient was referred to a rheumatology clinic because of mild pain in the neck of 3 years duration. The pain was mainly present in the morning and after a rest, associated with 10–20 min stiffness, subsiding with activity. He also noticed that he had had some limitation of neck motion. More recently, he complained of shoulder pain bilaterally upon raising his arms. The patient denied any history of neck, low back or joint pain in his childhood. He gave no history of any drug ingestion. He had mild acne at a younger age which required no treatment. Examination disclosed a healthy looking individual with no psoriatic or other skin lesions. Neck movement showed slight limitation of flexion, extension and lateral rotation. Radiographic examination revealed calcification of the anterior longitudinal ligament extending between C2 and C5, bridging of the pubis symphysis and bony outgrowth from the iliac crest and lower border of the acetabula on both sides (Figures 1 and 2). These changes were present when the patient was aged 24 years. Shoulder radiographs revealed large bony outgrowths from the coracoid process bilaterally and from the lower rim of the glenoid in the left side (Figures 3 and 4). The sacroiliac joints and lumbar and dorsal spines were normal. HLA B 27 was negative. Complete blood count and erythrocyte sedimentation rate were normal. Calcium, phosphate, blood urea, creatinine and fasting blood sugar were all at normal levels.

What is the diagnosis?

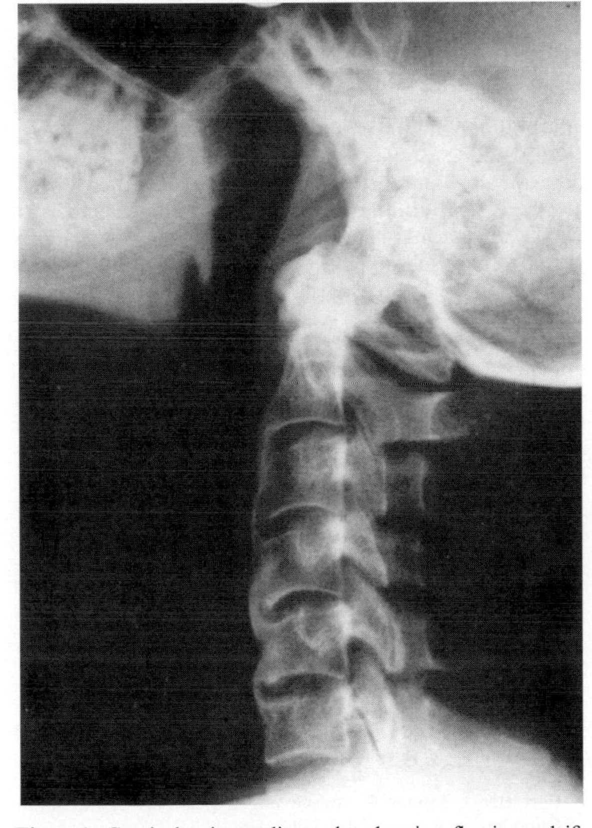

Figure 1. Cervical spine radiography showing flowing calcification of the anterior spinal ligament between C2 and C5 with preservation of disc space.

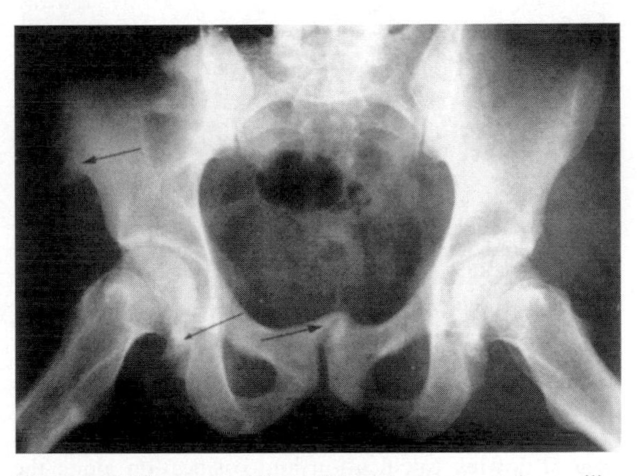

Figure 2. Radiograph of the pelvis showing normal sacroiliac joints with bony outgrowth from the ileum, lower border of the acetabulum and bridging of the pubic symphysis.

Based on the case of the month originally published in Br J Radiol 1994;67:609–10.

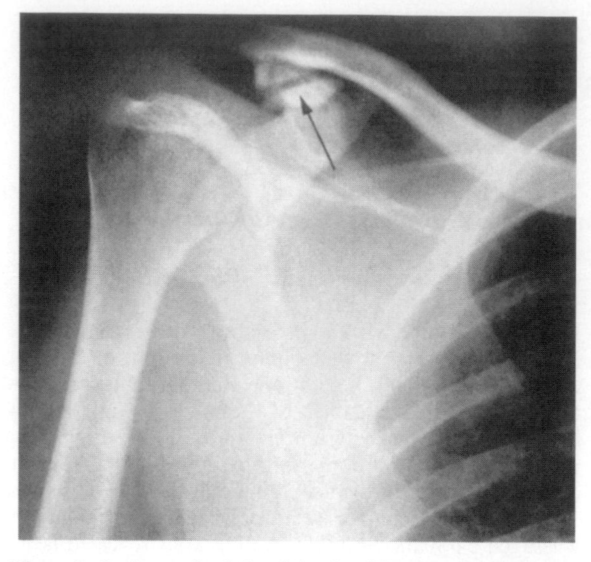

Figure 3. Radiograph of the right shoulder showing bony outgrowth from the coracoid process.

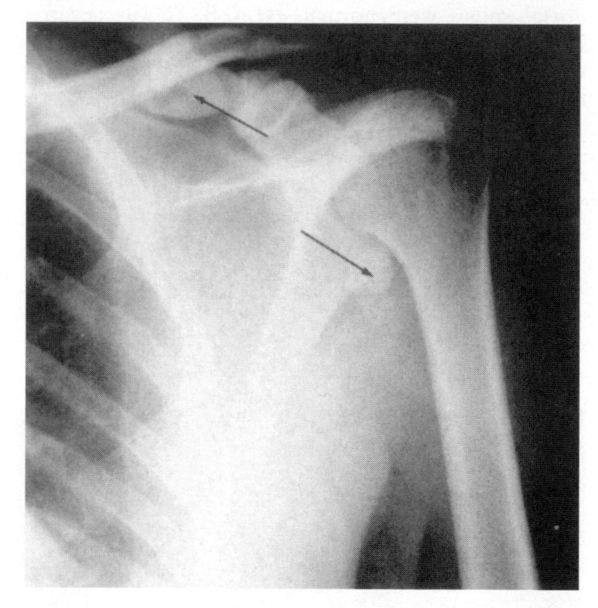

Figure 4. Radiograph of the left shoulder showing large bony outgrowth from the coracoid process and from the inferior border of the glenoid.

The patient discussed here was 24 years of age when he was found to have radiographic changes meeting the proposed criteria for the diagnosis of diffuse idiopathic skeletal hyperostosis (DISH). These included the presence of flowing calcification and ossification along the anterolateral aspects of at least four contiguous vertebral bodies, relative preservation of intervertebral disc height in the involved vertebral segment and absence of intraarticular bony ankylosis of the sacroiliac and apophyseal joints [1, 2].

The cause of this disorder is unknown. Changes associated with DISH may be seen in fluorosis, hypervitaminosis A, ankylosing spondylitis, Reiter's syndrome, psoriasis, hypoparathyroidism, acromegaly and etretinate therapy, but, in most cases of DISH, there is no convincing evidence to link hyperostosis to any of these disorders [3].

Our patient did not have any of the disorders normally associated with DISH-like changes, at no time did he consume Vitamin A or etretinate, and he had no past history to suggest a diagnosis of end stage inflammatory spondylitis.

It is hard to speculate at what age the patient developed the calcification of the anterior spinal ligament of the cervical spine, the large bony outgrowth in the shoulder area and changes in the pelvis. However, during the 3 years prior to presentation there were only minimal changes of the cervical spine which indicate that the process may have started at a much younger age than 24 years.

DISH occurs in middle-aged and elderly individuals. In a series by Resnick and Niwayama, the age ranges from 48 to 85 years [1]. This is similar to the age ranges in other large series [4, 5]. The frequency of occurrence of DISH in patients over 65 years of age is approximately 5–10% [3]. Some younger patients (20–40 years) occasionally demonstrate radiographic features which, although not fulfilling the criteria for the diagnosis of DISH, are strongly suggestive of this entity. A lengthy period of time is necessary before spinal abnormalities progress to such a degree that they fulfil the radiographic criteria [1] of DISH.

We believe that DISH may occur at a younger age and it should be considered as part of the differential diagnosis in this age group if the X-ray findings meet the proposed criteria for diagnosing DISH and after excluding disorders known to be associated with DISH-like changes.

References

1. Resnick D, Niwayama G. Diffuse idiopathic skeletal hyperstosis (DISH)—ankylosing hyperostosis of Forestier and Rotes-Querol. In: Diagnosis of bone and joint disorders. Philadelphia: WB Saunders, 1988:1563–1600.
2. Resnick D, Niwayama G. Radiographic and pathologic features of spinal involvement in diffuse idiopathic skeletal hyperstosis (DISH). Radiology 1976;119:559–68.
3. Resnick D. Diffuse idiopathic skeletal hyperstosis. In: Primer of Rheumatic Diseases. Georgia: Arthritis Foundation, 1988:251–3.
4. Forestier J, Lagier R. Ankylosing hyperstosis of the spine. Clin Orthop Rel Res 1971;74:65–83.
5. Harris J, Carter AR, Glick EN, Storey GO. Ankylosing hyperstosis. I. Clinical and radiological features. Ann Rheum Dis 1974;33:210–8.

Differential calculus

[1]D J ROEBUCK and [2]L M MACDONALD

Departments of Radiology, [1]The Children's Hospital, Camperdown, NSW 2050, Australia, and [2]St Thomas' Hospital, London SE1 7EH, UK

A previously well 8-year-old girl presented to a casualty department with a 3-week history of urinary frequency, dysuria and nocturia associated with intermittent abdominal pain. She had also had 10 days of watery diarrhoea following antibiotic treatment given by her general practitioner.

Examination revealed only mild generalized abdominal tenderness. Urinalysis showed protein "+" but no haematuria.

A provisional diagnosis of urinary tract infection with antibiotic-associated diarrhoea was made and a plain abdominal radiograph was obtained (Figure 1). The casualty doctor interpreted this as showing a right renal calculus and referred the patient for renal ultrasound.

What features are shown on this radiograph and was the casualty doctor right?

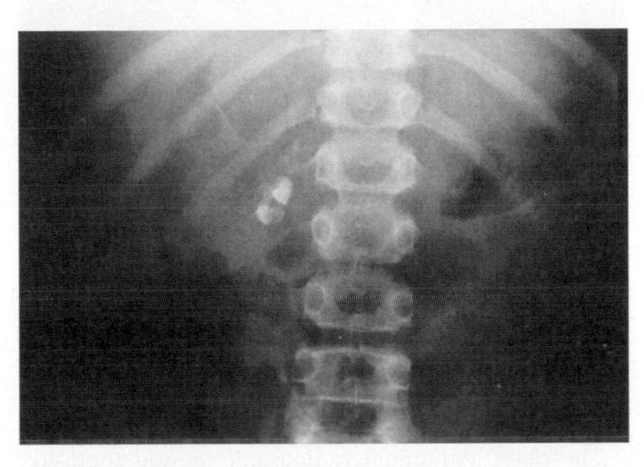

Figure 1. Plain abdominal radiograph.

Based on the case of the month originally published in Br J Radiol 1995;68:1037–8.

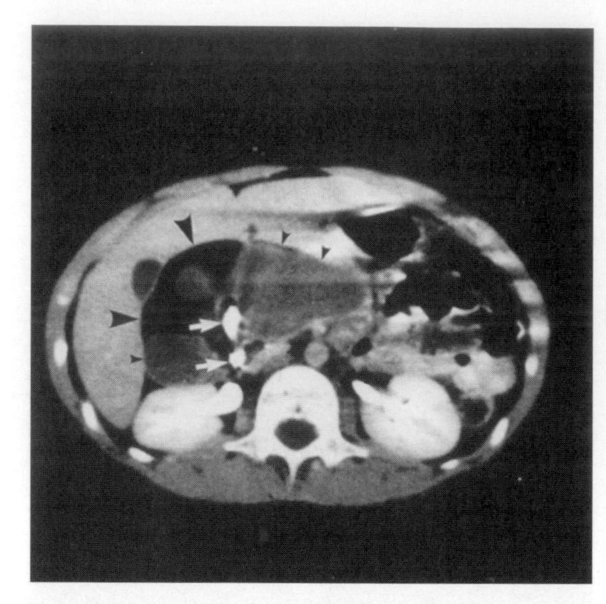

Figure 2. Abdominal CT showing a large lobulated retroperitoneal tumour with fat (—108 Hounsfield units (HU), large arrowheads), soft tissue (33 HU, small arrowheads) and calcific (white arrows) attenuation components.

The plain abdominal radiograph showed tooth-like structures and areas of more diffuse calcification in the right upper quadrant. The visceral surface of the liver was clearly outlined by a region of fat density which did not have the characteristics of any normal structure. These are the features of a teratoma.

Ultrasound (not shown) demonstrated a partly solid mass lying in the region of the head of the pancreas which contained echogenic areas with acoustic shadowing consistent with teeth or bone. There was also a large area containing only low-level echoes representing sebaceous material. The paediatric surgeons requested CT (Figure 2) and a barium meal (Figure 3) to help them plan their operation.

At laparotomy a large lobulated retroperitoneal tumour was found posterior to the lesser sac, extending behind the epiploic foramen to reach the anterior surface of the right kidney. It was successfully excised.

The tumour was a 110 × 100 × 80 mm benign dermoid cyst containing hair, smooth muscle, bone, cartilage, adipose tissue and respiratory, gastrointestinal, salivary and pancreatic epithelial elements.

Teratomas are tumours which contain elements derived from more than one germ layer. Mature retroperitoneal teratoma is a rare benign neoplasm. It is more common in females and is usually diagnosed in childhood [1]. In mature teratoma all the elements are differentiated and there is no evidence of malignancy. Dermoid cysts are a type of mature teratoma in which there is predominantly ectodermal differentiation. The cyst is lined by tissue similar to skin with adnexal structures including hair and sebaceous glands. It is impossible to be certain that a teratomatous lesion is benign on radiological grounds [2]. Even if the tumour is benign it may cause death due to relentless growth and should always be removed.

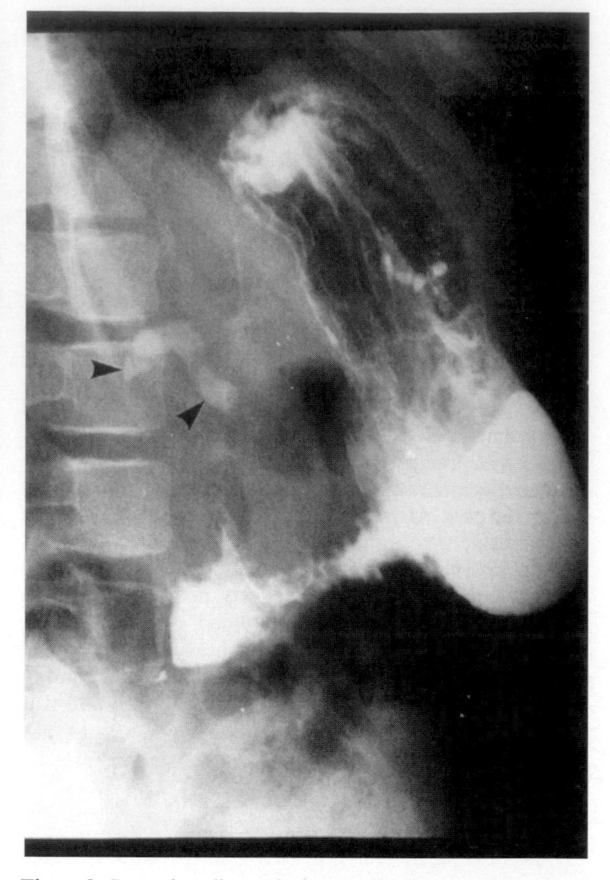

Figure 3. Lateral radiograph from a barium study showing teeth (arrowheads) within a retroperitoneal mass which displaces the stomach anteriorly.

In our case the plain film findings of fat attenuation and apparent tooth formation were present. Bone and teeth are not commonly seen in retroperitoneal teratoma (although they are common in ovarian teratoma) but the combination of one or both of these with the presence of fat is probably pathognomonic.

Not unexpectedly, CT is superior to plain radiography and ultrasound in the demonstration of both fat and calcium [1].

References

1. Davidson AJ, Hartman DS, Goldman SM. Mature teratoma of the retroperitoneum: radiologic, pathologic and clinical correlation. Radiology 1989;172:421–5.
2. Billmire DF, Grosfeld JL. Teratomas in childhood: analysis of 142 cases. J Pediatr Surg 1986;21:548–51.

The lateral cervical spine in major trauma

P M LOGAN, D L JANZEN and D G CONNELL

Department of Radiology, University of British Columbia and the Vancouver Hospital and Health Sciences Centre, 855 W. 12th Avenue, British Columbia, Canada V5Z 1M9

A 17-year-old male cyclist was struck by a speeding car. Upon arrival at the scene, the paramedics found the patient to have no cardiac output. Following intubation and successful resuscitation the patient was transferred to the Emergency Department.

On admission the patient was hypotensive and had a heart rate of 40 beats min^{-1}. Neurological examination showed a left pupil fixed at 7 mm and a sluggishly reactive right pupil. Corneal and gag reflexes were absent as were all deep tendon reflexes. The only spontaneous movements were twitching of the right thumb and index finger, and eyelid blinking, although not in response to verbal commands.

Radiographs revealed fractures of many of the bones in the left hand and a fractured right clavicle. The lateral cervical spine radiograph, obtained at that time, is shown in Figure 1. What is the diagnosis? What is the best method of radiographic assessment of this injury on plain films? What are the implications of the diagnosis?

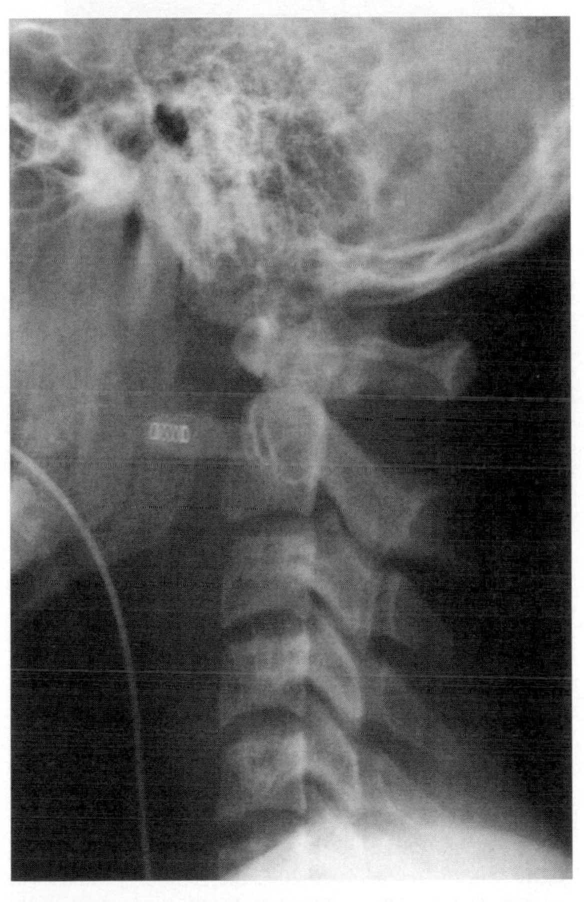

Figure 1. Lateral cervical spine radiograph.

Based on the case of the month originally published in Br J Radiol 1996;69:1197–8.

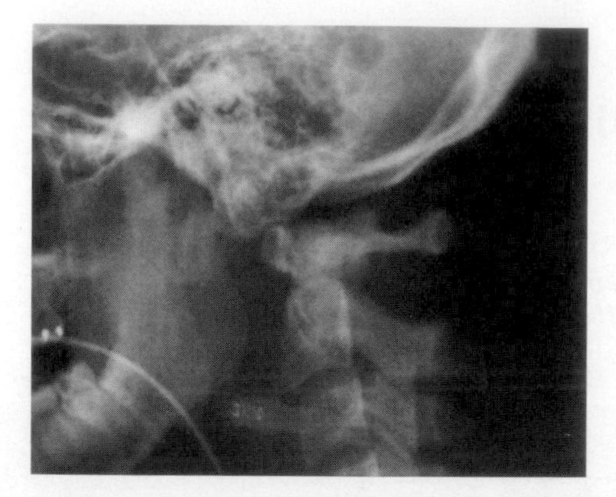

Figure 2. Further lateral spine radiograph taken with the patient supine, but with a slightly different craniocaudal tube angulation. Atlanto-occipital separation is clearly visible.

The lateral cervical spine radiograph (Figure 1) demonstrated normal alignment of the cervical vertebrae in relation to each other with no fracture evident. The atlanto-occipital alignment, however, was markedly abnormal. There was anterior dislocation of the occiput relative to the first cervical vertebra. Furthermore, the soft tissues anterior to the upper cervical spine were increased in thickness; this sign was less conspicuous after the patient had been intubated. A further lateral cervical spine radiograph taken a short time later (Figure 2), at a slightly different craniocaudal angulation, clearly demonstrated atlanto-occipital distraction with dislocation. The patient was quadriplegic. CT of the brain revealed extensive closed head injury. He died 2 days later as a result of cardiac arrest.

Many methods of assessing the occipitovertebral relationship have been proposed. However, it has been suggested that these methods are frequently difficult to apply and unreliable because of "the number of reference points and landmarks required for each, the difficulty in detecting the opisthion, the frequency and variety of anomalies of the posterior arch of C1 and the variable relationship of the dens to the body of the axis" [1]. Harris et al describe a simple yet accurate method of assessing this region [1, 2]. Using the basion–axial interval (BAI) and basion–dental interval (BDI) they detected 100% of 31 patients with clinically established atlanto-occipital dislocation [2].

The posterior axial line (PAL) is defined as a line which coincides exactly with the posterior cortex of the body of the atlas. The basion is defined as the midpoint on the anterior margin of the foramen magnum, and on the lateral cervical spine is at the point where the base of the clivus meets the skull base. The basion is normally 12 mm, or less, anterior to the PAL (the BAI), when measured at a point perpendicular to the upward extension of the PAL. The BAI reflects anterior or posterior dissociation injuries. In our case the basion is 30 mm anterior to the PAL (Figure 3).

The basion–dens interval (BDI) is defined as the distance between basion and the rostral cortex of the dens. This interval should not exceed 12 mm. The application of the BDI is to identify distracted dissociation. In the case reported here, the BDI measured 22 mm.

Atlanto-occipital dislocation occurs most commonly as part of a fatal spinocraniofacial injury complex. Considered to be a rare injury by some authors [3], atlanto-occipital dislocations have been demonstrated in up to 26% of road traffic accident fatalities with cervical spine injuries [4]. The increasing number of patients reported as surviving with this injury [3, 5] serves to reinforce the importance of making the diagnosis, which will usually be on the basis of the horizontal beam lateral cervical spine radiograph performed as part of an initial work-up in an emergency department. A review of 24 reported survivors by Lee et al revealed a 63% long-term survival rate and a complete recovery rate of 25% [5]. It has been suggested that a significant number of survivors will have associated carotid or vertebral arterial injuries and that the neurological deficits which can result from these vascular injuries are potentially reversible.

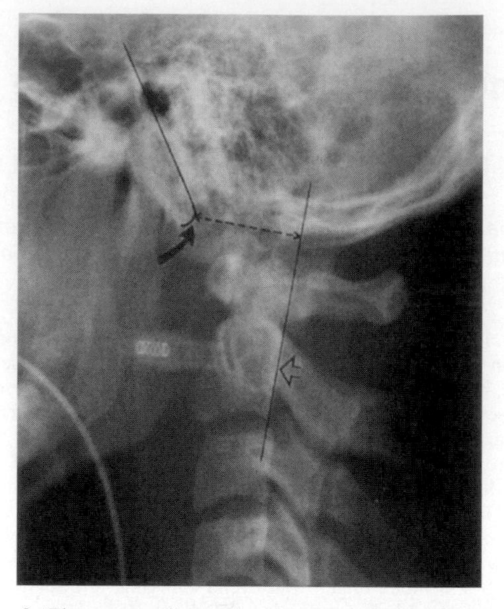

Figure 3. The same radiograph as in Figure 1. The basion-axial interval (broken line), i.e. basion (curved arrow) to posterior axial line (hollow arrow), is demonstrated to be 30 mm, indicating atlanto-occipital dislocation.

References

1. Harris JH, Carson GC, Wagner LK. Radiologic diagnosis of traumatic occipitovertebral dissociation: 1. Normal occipitovertebral relationships on lateral radiographs of supine patients. AJR 1994;162:881–6.
2. Harris JH, Carson GC, Wagner LK, Kerr N. Radiologic diagnosis of traumatic occipitovertebral dissociation: 2. Comparison of three methods of detecting occipitovertebral relationships on lateral radiographs of supine subjects. AJR 1994;162:887–92.
3. Matava MJ, Whitesides TE, Davis PC. Traumatic atlanto-occipital dislocation with survival. Spine 1993;18:1897–1903.
4. Alker GJ, Young SO, Eugene VL et al. Postmortem radiology of head and neck injuries in fatal traffic accidents. Radiology 1975;114:611–7.
5. Lee C, Woodring JH, Walsh JW. Carotid and vertebral artery injury in survivors of atlanto-occipital dislocation: case reports and literature review. J Trauma 1991;31:401–7.

Double and nothing

J D HUNTER, M P CALLAWAY and C J WAKELEY

Directorate of Imaging, Bristol Royal Infirmary, Marlborough Street, Bristol BS2 8HW, UK

A 35-year-old male noticed a hard lump in his right testis after listening to a radio programme on testicular self examination. An ultrasound examination confirmed a 2 cm diameter hypoechoic mass in the right testis. The patient was referred directly to a urologist who arranged urgent admission for a right orchidectomy. The staging CT scan of the abdomen and pelvis is shown (Figure 1), together with an MR image at the same level (Figure 2).

What is the abnormality? What is the differential diagnosis? What course of action would you recommend?

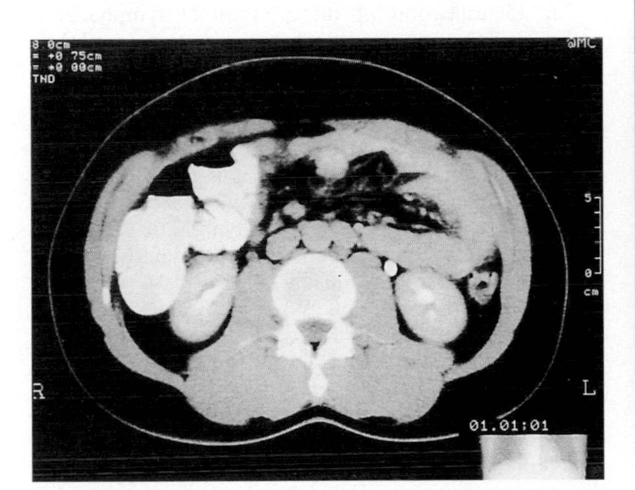

Figure 1. Staging CT scan. Axial slice through lower abdomen.

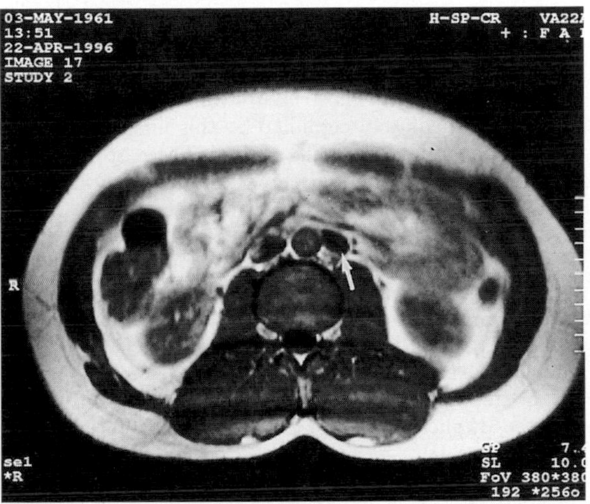

Figure 2. Axial T_1 weighted MRI scan which corresponds to Figure 1.

Based on the case of the month originally published in Br J Radiol 1998;71:99–100.

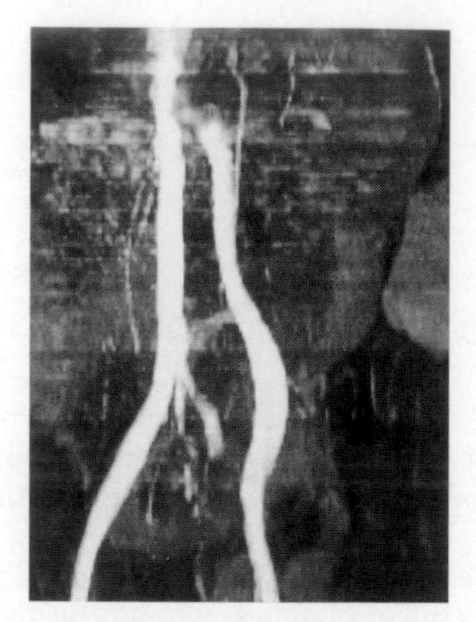

Figure 3. MRV demonstrating duplication of the IVC and draining of the left sided IVC into the left renal vein.

The axial CT scan through the lower abdomen following intravenous contrast medium (Figure 1) demonstrated that, in addition to the inferior vena cava (IVC) and aorta, there was a third round structure anterior to the vertebral body. This structure was identified on both the slice immediately cephalad to this image and on a number of the images more caudad. These appearances are likely to represent either paraaortic lymphadenopathy or left sided anomalous venous drainage.

An axial T_1 weighted MRI scan of the lower abdomen (Figure 2) illustrated that the previously identified abnormal structure has a similar signal flow void (arrow) to the IVC. On more cephalad axial images this structure could be followed up to the level of the left renal vein where it terminated abruptly.

A magnetic resonance venogram (MRV) demonstrated that the duplicated left IVC drained into the left renal vein (Figure 3).

Congenital anomalies of the IVC are uncommon but can have important clinical implications [1]. The radiologist must be aware of these anomalies and be able to distinguish these variants from pathological processes such as paraaortic lymphadenopathy.

The development of the IVC is a complex and continually evolving process from conception through the embryonic period which ends 56–60 days later. There is a vast network of communicating veins, the most important of which are three pairs of parallel veins. The postcardinal veins appear first and eventually regress to form the iliac bifurcation. The subcardinal veins appear next, the right forming the suprarenal IVC while the left subcardinal vein regresses. The supracardinal veins are the last to appear, the right persisting to form the infrarenal IVC while the left sided portion completely regresses in fetal life. Both the subcardinal and supracardinal veins contribute to the formation of the renal veins. This complex development provides the potential for a great variation in intraabdominal venous drainage but in clinical practice six common anomalies are seen (retroaortic left renal vein, circumaortic left renal vein, retrocaval right ureter (pre-ureteric vena cava), interrupted IVC with azygos continuation, transposition of the IVC and duplication of the IVC) [2].

Duplication of the IVC has an incidence of 0.2–3.0% [2]. The size of both vessels is variable. Typically, the left vena cava crosses to join the right at the level of the renal veins which are commonly short. Duplication has been associated with other anomalies. In the case we describe, a second large calibre left sided vein was identified cephalad to the kidney crossing in front of the aorta to drain into the IVC at the level of the hepatic venous confluence. Duplication of the IVC has also been associated with cloacal extrophy and horseshoe kidney.

The identification of intraabdominal lymphadenopathy is of the utmost importance in patients with testicular tumours, allowing the distinction between stage 1 and stage 2 disease. The spread of testicular tumours is mainly through lymphatic vessels, initially to the lymph nodes of the ipsilateral retroperitoneum. When contralateral lymphadenopathy is present, it is more often as a result of right to left cross-over than *vice versa* [3]. However, despite the occurrence of lymphatic cross-over in the retroperitoneum, lymphadenopathy on the contralateral side alone is very unusual [4]. The case we present raises exactly this question. While contralateral disease alone is very rare, the finding of a duplicated IVC in a patient with a testicular tumour is also unusual. Ultrasound may well have given the correct diagnosis in this case but, in view of the additional left sided paravertebral abnormality cephalad to the kidney, we chose MRI. Proceeding to MRI and MRV allowed us confidently to diagnose the left sided IVC, identify the anomalous left suprarenal venous drainage and exclude intraabdominal lymphadenopathy in this patient.

References

1. Giordano JM, Trout HH. Anomalies of the inferior vena cava. J Vasc Surg 1986;3:924–8.
2. Freidland GW, de Vries PA, Nino-Murcia M, et al. Congenital anomalies of the inferior vena cava: Embryogenesis and MR features. Urol Radiol 1992;13:237–48.
3. Dixon AK, Ellis E, Sikora K. Computed tomography of testicular tumours: Distribution of abdominal lymphadenopathy. Clin Radiol 1986;37:519–23.
4. Lee JKT, Maclennan BL, Stanley RJ, Sagel SS. Computed tomography in the staging of testicular neoplasms. Radiology 1979;130:387–90.

A pearl of wisdom

J RAWLINSON, C L COBLENTZ and S FRANIC

Department of Radiology, McMaster University Medical Centre, 1200 Main Street West, Hamilton L8N 3Z5, Ontario, Canada

An 8-year-old girl presented with progressive unsteadiness on her feet over a 2-year period. She was otherwise fit and well. No neurological deficit was found on examination, but movements of the lumbar spine were reduced. Conventional radiographs of the lumbar spine, myelogram and CT myelographic findings are demonstrated in Figures 1, 2 and 3 respectively.

What is your differential diagnosis? What further information would you seek to clarify the diagnosis?

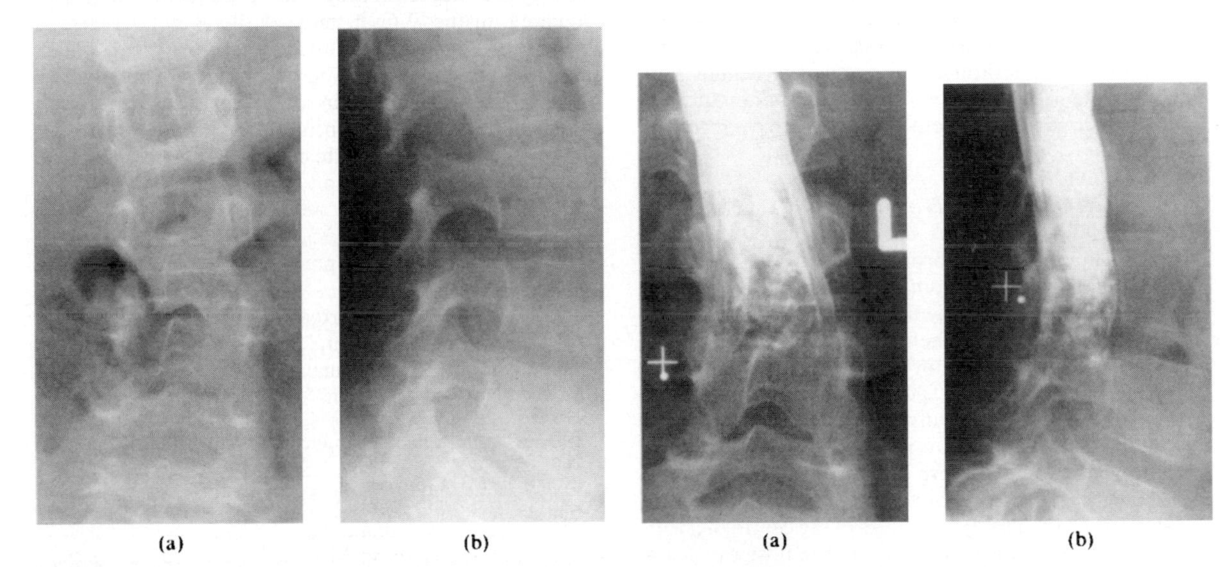

(a) (b) (a) (b)

Figure 1. (a) Anteroposterior and (b) lateral conventional radiographs of the lumbar spine.

Figure 2. Myelogram: (a) anteroposterior and (b) lateral views of the lumbar region.

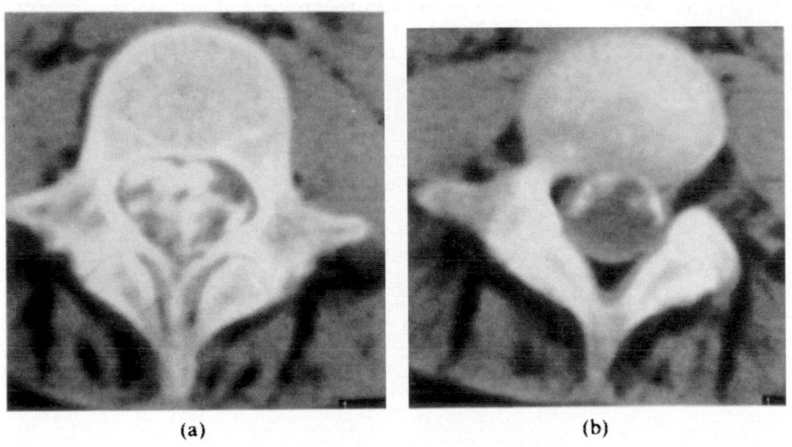

(a) (b)

Figure 3. Post-myelography CT: axial sections (a) through the body of L3 and (b) at the level of the L3/4 disc.

Based on the case of the month originally published in Br J Radiol 1991;64:473–4.

The plain radiographs of the lumbar spine showed a scoliosis concave to the right and subtle scalloping of the posterior aspects of the lumbar vertebral bodies 3–5. On the anteroposterior view there was some flattening of the medial side of both L4 pedicles. There was no evidence of bone destruction, disc space narrowing or expansion of the exit foramina.

The myelogram demonstrated an intradural mass composed of conglomerate nodules embedded within the cauda equina. This mass had expanded the theca and obstructed the flow of contrast medium in a caudal direction from the level of L3. Post-myelography CT showed the intradural lesion intimately related to the cauda equina. The mass was low in density and could not be easily differentiated from the nerve roots.

An intradural "pearly grey" mass was found at surgery. This was loosely adherent to the nerve roots of the cauda equina from which it was easily peeled. Histological examination of the excised tissue showed abundant keratin composed of stratified squamous epithelium with characteristic features of an epidermoid tumour. Following surgery the patient made a complete recovery.

The differential diagnosis of an intradural mass at this site in childhood includes ependymoma of the filum terminale, lipoma, neurofibroma, metastases (*e.g.* medulloblastoma, neuroblastoma), dermoid/epidermoid tumour and teratoma; meningiomas may also rarely occur in childhood [1]. The plain radiographic findings and the length of the history suggest a slow growing, relatively benign lesion. Lipomas and dermoid/epidermoid tumours are usually associated with spinal dysraphism, for which there is no evidence here; neurofibromas commonly involve the exit foramina and are associated with other stigmata of neurofibromatosis.

Epidermoid or "pearly" tumours of the central nervous system are rare and usually found in the posterior fossa; they are even less common in the spinal canal where they tend to occur in the lumbosacral region. In a review of 90 intraspinal epidermoid tumours [2], all were located in the lumbar region and most were in children. It is notable that 39 (43%) of these patients had been subjected to lumbar puncture in periods ranging from 6 months to 10 years prior to their presentation.

Lumbar punctures in children, particularly infants, are sometimes performed using a "butterfly" infusion needle [3, 4]. Such unstiletted needles may collect a core of epithelial tissue during their passage through the skin [5]; furthermore, this tissue can implant and grow within the theca [6]. There is good presumptive evidence, therefore, that intraspinal epidermoid tumours may be a late complication of lumbar puncture. Normal myelograms prior to lumbar puncture in at least four of the reported cases support the hypothesis of iatrogenic implantation of epithelial cells.

The relevant information which should be sought to clarify the diagnosis is a history of lumbar puncture. Our patient had undergone two lumbar punctures at the age of 4 months to investigate a neurological reaction to metoclompramide, administered for vomiting. A full recovery was made and she was subsequently well until becoming unsteady on her feet at the age of 7 years.

While the incidence of iatrogenic intraspinal epidermoid tumours appears to be declining [7], a survey in 1985 [3] showed that 32% of paediatricians routinely use an unstiletted needle for lumbar puncture in neonates and small children. Sporadic cases are therefore likely to occur in the future.

References

1. Peacock WJ, Lazareff JA. Spinal tumours of childhood. S Afr Med J 1986;70:668–70.
2. Manno NJ, Uhlein A, Kernohan JW. Intraspinal epidermoids. J Neurosurg 1962;19:754–65.
3. Halcrow SJ, Crawford PJ, Craft AW. Epidermoid spinal tumours after lumbar puncture. Arch Dis Childhood 1985;60:978–9.
4. Ersbak V, Hobolth N. Iatrogenic intraspinal epidermoid tumour (Short communication). Acta Paediatr Scand 1988;77:759.
5. Gibson T, Norris W. Skin fragments removed by injection needles. Lancet 1958;ii:983–5.
6. Van Gilder JC, Schwartz HG. Growth of dermoids from skin implants to the nervous system and surrounding spaces of the newborn rat. J Neurosurg 1967;26:14–20.
7. Visciani A, Savoiardo M, Balestrini MR, Solero CL. Iatrogenic intraspinal epidermoid tumour: myelo-CT and MRI diagnosis. Neuroradiology 1989;31:273–5.

No way out

P J GUEST, A MCLEAN and N GRAHAM

Department of Diagnostic Radiology, St Bartholomew's Hospital, London EC1A, UK

A 51-year-old man presented with a 2-week history of painless haematuria following which he had experienced severe pain in the right groin. Examination was unremarkable. The control radiograph of an intravenous urogram is shown (Figure 1). Intravenous contrast medium demonstrated diffuse parenchymal loss of the right kidney with partial obstruction of the right ureter. A spot radiograph taken during screening of the lower right ureter is also shown (Figure 2). CT of the pelvis was subsequently performed (Figure 3).

What is the diagnosis? Is there a differential?

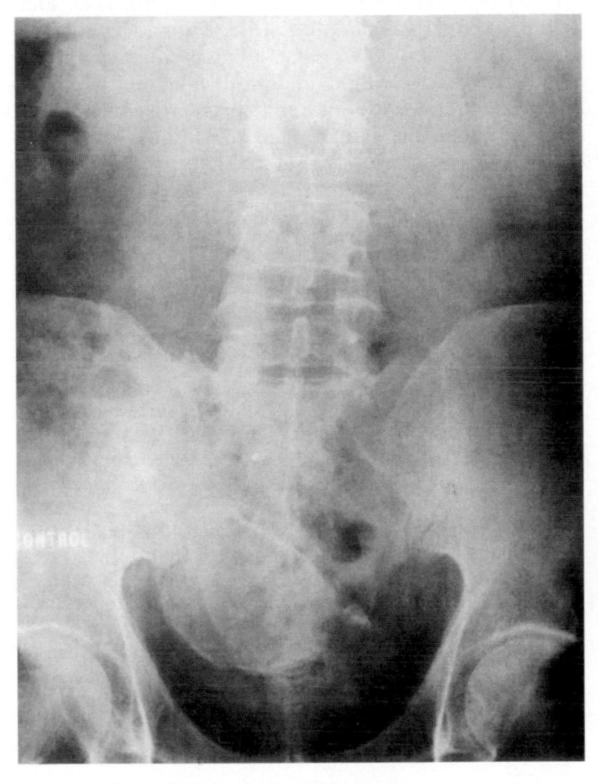

Figure 1. Control abdominal radiograph.

Based on the case of the month originally published in Br J Radiol 1989;62:629–30.

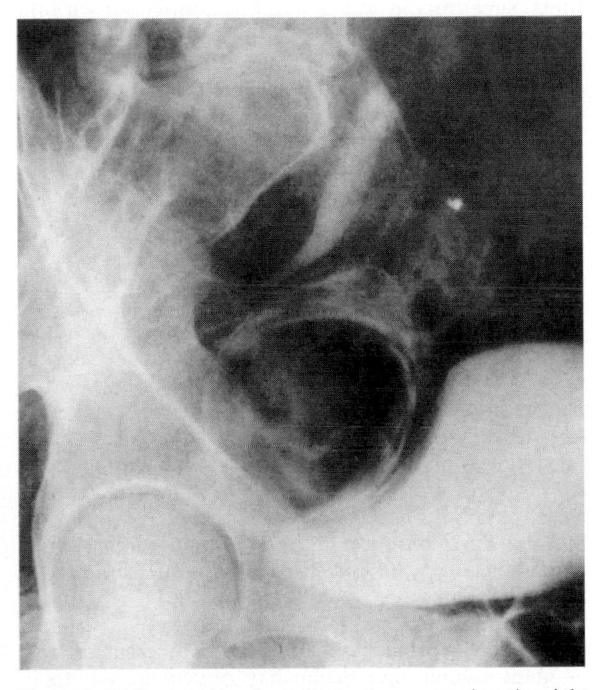

Figure 2. Right anterior view obtained on screening the right hemipelvis.

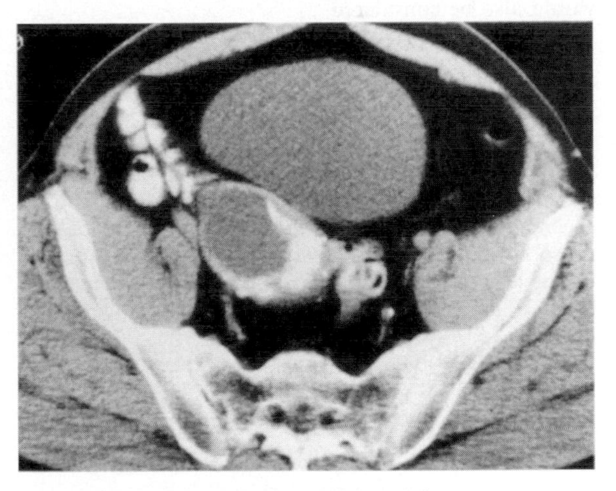

Figure 3. Unenhanced CT through the pelvis.

The control radiograph showed a soft tissue mass with a curvilinear rim of calcification measuring 8 cm in diameter. The oblique view showed that the ureter passed posteriorly to the mass and that the mass itself was separate from, but indenting, an otherwise normal bladder. CT confirmed the presence of a cystic mass in the right hemipelvis with calcification in its rim. It appeared separate from the bladder and of homogeneous texture with a higher attenuation than urine. It was related to, but distinct from the seminal vesicles and vascular structures. Superiorly, it was apparently contiguous with the caecum.

Laparotomy, undertaken in view of the ureteric obstruction, demonstrated an adherent appendix mucocoele with an associated polypoid mass in the caecum. This proved to be a carcinoid tumour of the caecum. The appendiceal wall had been replaced by fibrous tissue with patchy bone formation.

Radiographically, the lesion showed several features suggestive of an appendix mucocoele as discussed below. Iliac artery aneurysms may present with curvilinear calcifications in the pelvis, but in this case the mass lay anterior to the ureter, which rendered this possibility unlikely. It may be noted that appendix mucocoele may present as a pulsatile mass [1]. Chronic abscess or haematoma may develop calcification. Fish and Smulewicz [2] described an appendiceal abscess with similar appearances on CT, including mural calcification which was causing ureteric obstruction. Similar appearances were seen in another case described by Fish and Smulewicz [2] but the additional feature of solid components suggested the correct diagnosis of an appendix adenocarcinoma.

In addition, abscesses and tumours are likely to have less well defined margins. Duplication or mesenteric cysts or giant colonic diverticula may present as soft tissue masses and may have calcification in their walls. In women, uterine fibroids or tubo-ovarian pathology would also be considered.

This uncommon finding is rarely diagnosed preoperatively. Certain radiological findings may suggest the diagnosis [3]. An appendix mucocoele appears as a well defined, globular, soft tissue mass, on occasion with calcification in its wall, attached to and displacing the caecum (usually laterally or cephalad). While its location is usually in the right iliac fossa, large masses may present on the left. Non-filling of the appendix on barium enema is usual and, rarely, intussusception of the appendix or mucocoele may be seen. Its location is usually in the right iliac fossa but large masses may present on the left.

On ultrasound, the mass appears cystic with posterior acoustic enhancement. An echogenic wall may signify mural calcification. The contents may be anechoic or have a variable echo pattern with gravity dependence and occasionally septations [1, 4]. Internal echoes are presumably due to inspissated mucus.

Findings on CT are those of a cystic mass with or without calcification or septation. Attenuation values usually lie between those of water and soft tissue [2, 4]. CT may also demonstrate the associated condition of pseudomyxoma peritonei.

The exact pathological nature of appendix mucocoeles is debated. The term describes distension of the lumen of the appendix with sterile mucus, which may be associated with obstruction secondary to an inflammatory stricture, carcinoid tumour, carcinoma, appendolith, endometriosis or occasionally extrinsic compression. This, however, is a relatively uncommon situation and more often no obstructing lesion is found. Higa et al [5] considered that the condition should be regarded as a primary proliferative process: mucinous neoplasms, analogous to epithelial tumours of the colon. They defined three distinct entities, namely, mucosal hyperplasia, associated with only mild dilatation of the lumen, mucinous cystadenoma with some epithelial atypia and marked distension of the lumen, and mucinous cystadenocarcinoma. In their series, mucosal hyperplasia was usually an incidental finding in appendicectomy specimens and obstruction of the lumen rare. The latter two categories accounted for the majority of lesions diagnosed as mucocoele and were usually indistinguishable clinically, radiologically and on direct inspection at surgery.

References

1. Athey PA, Hacken JB, Estrada A. Sonographic appearance of mucocoele of the appendix. J Clin Ultrasound 1984; 12:333–7.
2. Fish B, Smulewicz JJ. Role of computer tomography in diagnosis of appendiceal disorders. New York State Med J 1981;81:900–4.
3. Euphrat EJ. Roentgen features of mucocoele of the appendix. Radiology 1947;48:113–7.
4. Dachmann AH, Lichtenstein JE, Friedman AC. Mucocoele of the appendix and pseudomyxoma peritonei. AJR 1985;144:923–9.
5. Higa E, Rosai J, Pizzimbono CA, Wise L. Mucosal hyperplasia, mucinous cystadenoma, and mucinous cystadenocarcinoma of the appendix: a re-evaluation of appendix mucocoele. Cancer 1973;32:1525–41.

The case of the missing calcified disc

J WARDLAW and I BEGGS

Department of Radiology, Edinburgh Royal Infirmary, Lauriston Place, Edinburgh EH3 9YW, UK

A 39-year-old male, with chronic renal failure following a failed renal transplant, presented with acute back pain. His previous history included crystal arthropathy, tertiary hyperparathyroidism and parathyroidectomy.

He had initially presented with tuberculosis of the L5 region and associated psoas and gluteal abscesses 1 year previously. The abscesses had been drained and he had been on apparently adequate chemotherapy ever since. Radiographs of the lower lumbar spine at the time of the original presentation (Figure 1) showed well defined calcification of the nucleus of the D12/L1 disc.

At the time of re-presentation he was afebrile and was tender at the dorsolumbar junction, but clinical and laboratory examinations were otherwise unremarkable. Radiographs of the lumbar spine (Figure 2) showed that the dense D12/L1 nuclear calcification had disappeared, although faint streaks of calcification were present at the periphery of several intervertebral discs adjacent to the vertebral end-plates. An isotope bone scan (Figure 3) showed increased activity in the body of L1.

What are the causes of intervertebral disc calcification? What had happened to the disc calcification in this case?

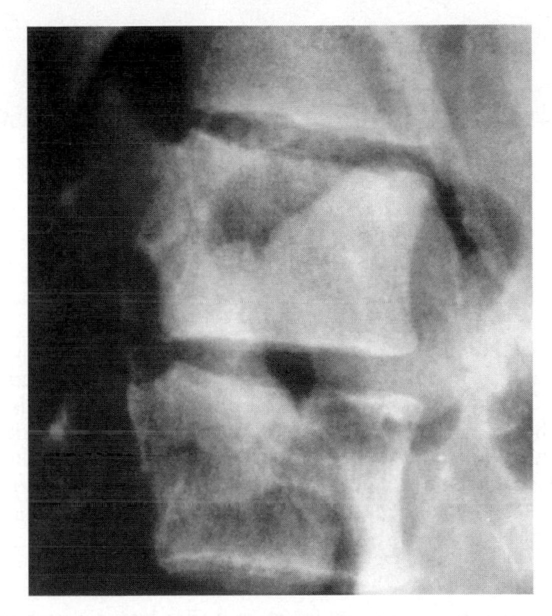

Figure 2. Radiograph of the thoracolumbar junction 1 year later.

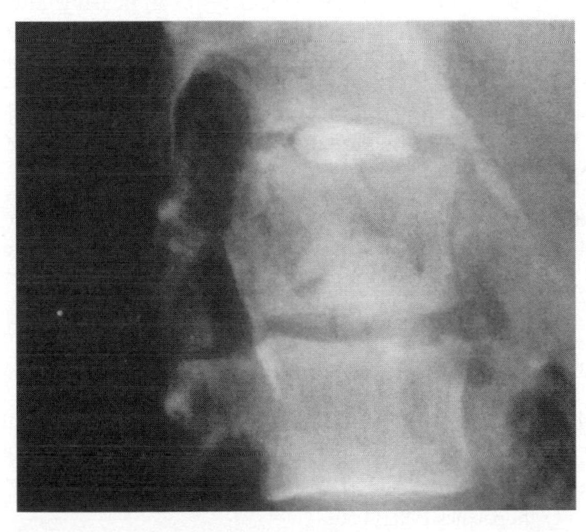

Figure 1. Radiograph of lumbar spine.

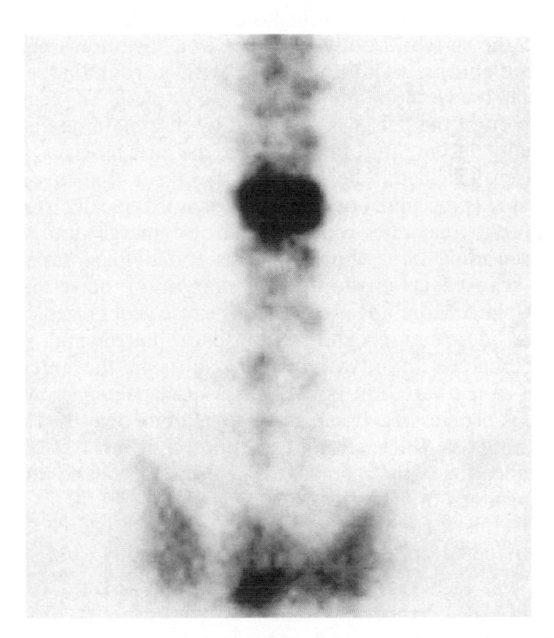

Figure 3. Isotope bone scan taken at the same time as Figure 2.

Based on the case of the month originally published in Br J Radiol 1993;66:89–90.

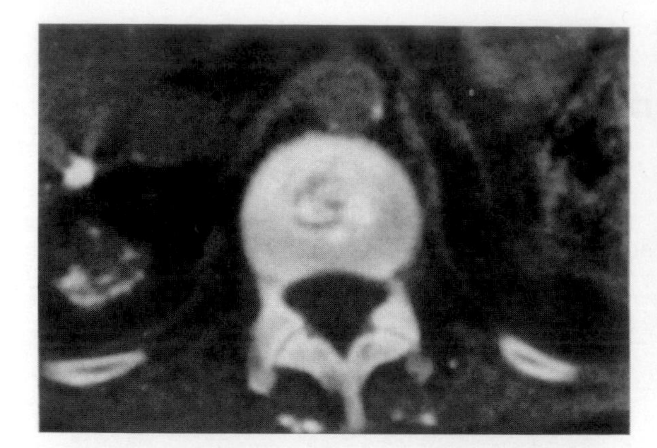

Figure 4. Axial CT image through superior aspect of L1, taken at the same time as Figure 2.

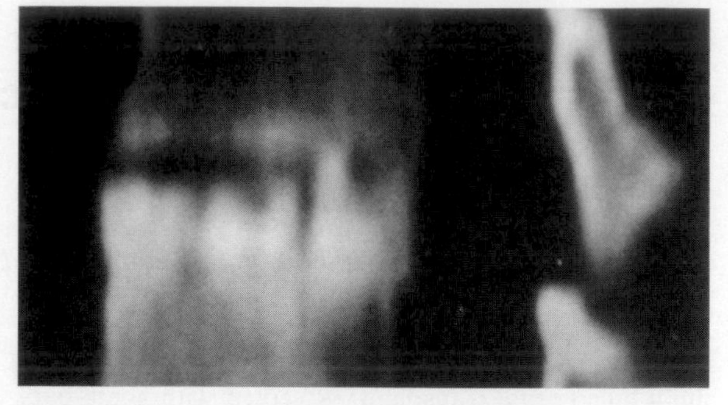

Figure 5. Sagittal reconstruction of the CT images of T12/L1, taken at the same time as Figure 2.

CT (Figure 4) of the dorsolumbar spine showed a lucent defect in the superior end-plate and adjacent body of L1. The defect contained extensive central calcification and had an irregular sclerotic margin which merged into the surrounding bone. A sagittal reconstruction (Figure 5) showed that the intravertebral calcification was continuous with calcification in the adjacent disc. These appearances closely resemble Schmorl's nodes except for the central calcification. It was assumed that the calcified disc nucleus had acutely herniated into the vertebral body, causing the localized back pain, which rapidly resolved spontaneously.

Herniation of an intervertebral disc into a vertebral body is a recognized complication of hyperparathyroidism [1]. Subchondral bone resorption at the discovertebral junction weakens the bone. Disc material herniates into the vertebral body, resulting in a "Schmorl's node" which appears as a lucent defect with surrounding sclerosis in the vertebra adjacent to the end-plate. The central portion of the defect is occupied by disc material and is usually lucent, but in this case the disc nucleus was densely calcified. The sclerotic margin is due to compressed trabecular bone. The sclerosis is typically irregular, but may be well defined, or merge into the surrounding bone. Early dialysis spondyloarthropathy may cause focal erosions at the margins of the vertebral end-plate. More advanced lesions cause generalized end-plate destruction and disc space narrowing [2]. Tuberculous spondylitis usually starts in the anterior part of the vertebral body, causes disc space narrowing and is progressive. It can cause focal bony defects, which do not have thick sclerotic margins, and intravertebral calcification which tends to be less dense and more amorphous than in this case.

In this case, the herniated defect was large and extended deeply into the vertebral body and this probably accounts for the involvement of the whole of the body of L1 seen on the isotope scan.

Calcification in the intervertebral discs of adults arises from a variety of causes. Aetiologies which predominantly affect the nucleus pulposus include degenerative spondylosis, ankylosing spondylitis, juvenile chronic arthritis (JCA) and diffuse idiopathic skeletal hyperostosis (DISH). Those predominantly affecting the annulus fibrosis include alkaptonuria, calcium pyrophosphate dihydrate deposition disease (CPDDD), haemochromatosis and hyperparathyroidism, although considerable overlap in the site of calcification occurs [3]. In none of these does the calcification usually resolve.

Calcification in intervertebral discs is a relatively common finding in the thoracic spine. It most commonly affects the T9/10 disc, with peak incidence in 40–50 year old males, it may prolapse, and it is inconsistently related to symptoms. It may be a passive phenomenon secondary to acute nuclear necrosis.

In children, a syndrome of acute febrile illness and pain, associated with disc calcification appearing after several weeks, is described, usually affecting cervical discs. It may be triggered by minor trauma or viral infection. Usually the calcification disappears over several months, after the symptoms have subsided [4, 5]. A similar syndrome occurs in young adults, but the disc calcification persists.

References

1. Resnick D, Niwayama G. Diagnosis of bone and joint disorders. Philadelphia: WB Saunders, 1988:2230–9.
2. Naidich JB, Mossey RT, McHeffey-Atkinson B, et al. Spondyloarthropathy from long-term hemodialysis. Radiology 1988;167:761–4.
3. Weinberger A, Myers AR. Intervertebral disc calcification in adults: a review. Semin Arthritis Rheum 1978;19:69–75.
4. Sonnabend DH, Taylor TKF, Chapman GK. Intervertebral disc calcification syndromes in children. J Bone Joint Surg 1982;64B:25–31.
5. Hayes M, Yngve DA, Herndon WA. Disc space calcification. Orthopaedics 1988;11:501–3.

That's torn it!

M S MOSS and J P WINGATE

Department of Diagnostic Radiology, Dudley Road Hospital, Birmingham B18 7QH, UK

A 7-year-old male victim of a road traffic accident was admitted to hospital. On examination he was drowsy with a bruise on the left side of his forehead and a clinically obvious fracture of his right femur. He was described as being "completely flaccid" and unresponsive to painful stimuli. No physical signs were found in the chest, abdomen or central nervous system. Plain radiographs of the cervical spine, skull and pelvis were interpreted as normal. The chest radiograph is shown in Figure 1. What is the abnormality? How may it have arisen?

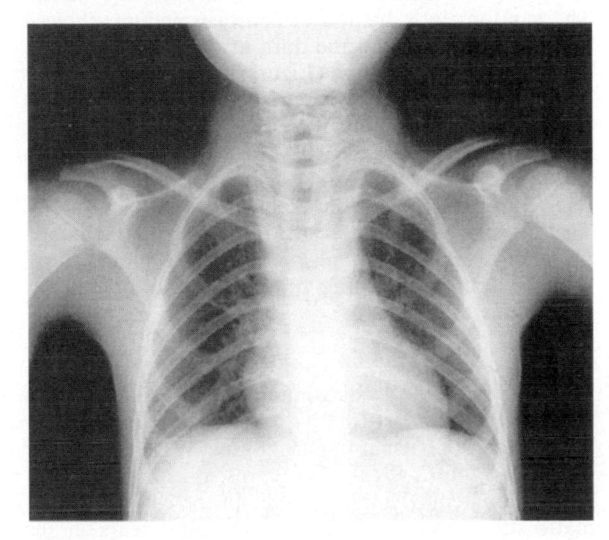

Figure 1. Chest radiograph.

Based on the case of the month originally published in Br J Radiol 1996;69:479–80.

The chest radiograph showed widening of the superior mediastinum, extending laterally into a thick rim over the apices of both lungs. In addition there was an impression of soft tissue swelling in the neck.

As the patient's conscious level improved over the next few hours, it became apparent that he had a T2 sensory level with weakness of the hands and paraplegia. No fractures could be identified on radiographs of the thoracic and cervical spine. At myelography, cerebrospinal fluid (CSF) would not flow back through the needle. The cautious introduction of contrast medium showed anterior indentation of the dura at the D1/2 disc level, causing cord compression (Figure 2a). A paucity of subarachnoid space was apparent below the level of this block. Contrast medium was seen to leak through the right C7 and C8, and left T1 nerve root foramina (Figure 2b). A smaller leak was shown at the right C5 level. No nerve roots could be identified at these points. The appearances are those of traumatic subarachnoid–pleural fistulae due to avulsion of brachial plexus roots. The mediastinal widening on the chest radiograph is largely due to CSF.

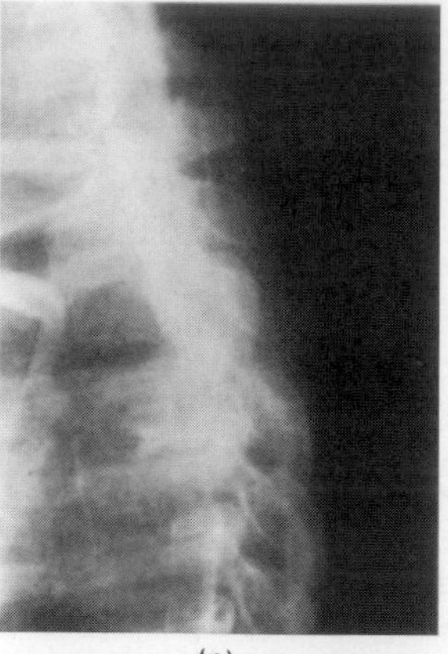

(a)

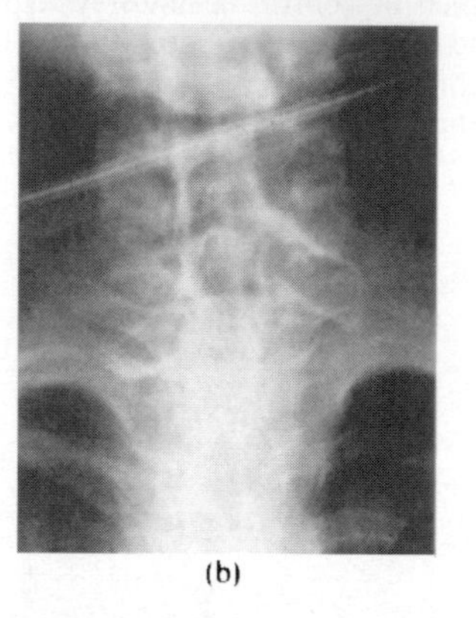

(b)

Figure 2. Myelogram showing lower cervical and upper thoracic region. (a) Lateral and (b) frontal projections.

Widening of the mediastinum is an ominous sign in the immediately post-trauma chest radiograph. It may be the result of haematoma from great vessel rupture or vertebral fracture. It can also represent leakage of oesophageal contents, lymph or CSF. In the case of a traumatic subarachnoid–pleural fistula, dural tears in the thoracic region permit the egress of CSF into the pleural space and mediastinum. These tears may result from fractures, nerve root avulsion, penetrating injury or surgery. After a period of time the leaks tend to wall-off, giving the more familiar appearance of a pseudomeningocele. These are wide-necked, blind-ending sacs of variable size containing CSF and, in the case of nerve root avulsion, extending through their respective neural foramina. Occasionally, a persistent fistula may cause a symptomatic pleural effusion. Congenital pseudomeningoceles are a recognized feature of neurofibromatosis [1].

Nerve root avulsion injury within the spinal theca has been appreciated since the early part of this century [2]. The term traumatic meningocele was coined in 1947 after its serendipitous demonstration during Pantopaque myelography to rule out a traumatic cervical disc prolapse [3]. The injury may initially be overlooked since the patients have often suffered multiple trauma and the subsequent symptoms may be confused with peripheral nerve lesions [4].

In a series of 60 myelograms performed in brachial plexus traction injuries, CSF leakage rather than discrete pseudomenigoceles were seen in the six cases performed during the first 10 days post-injury. Blood and protein were found in the CSF in these early cases [5].

MRI has considerable advantages over conventional myelography, more clearly demonstrating nerve root avulsions and any associated spinal cord damage. MRI can also differentiate collections of CSF from both blood and lymph, as well as giving useful information about the surrounding soft tissues [4]. It virtually eliminates the need for exploratory laminectomy and helps to determine the need for surgical intervention, as well as giving a better guide to prognosis [1].

References

1. Cook DA, Heiner JP, Breed AL. Pseudomeningocele following spinal fracture: A case report and review of the literature. Clin Orthop 1989;247:74–9.
2. Frazier CH, Skillern PG. Supraclavicular subcutaneous lesions of the brachial plexus not associated with skeletal injuries with the report of a case of avulsion of the anterior and posterior spinal roots. JAMA 1911;57:1957–63.
3. Murphey F, Hartung W, Kirklin JW. Myelographic demonstration of avulsing injury of the brachial plexus. AJR 1947;58:102–5.
4. Freedy RM, Miller KD, Eick JJ, Granke DS. Traumatic lumbosacral nerve root avulsion: evaluation by MR imaging. JCAT 1989;13:1052–7.
5. Yeoman PM. Cervical myelography in traction injuries of the brachial plexus. J Bone Joint Surg 1968;50B:253–60.

A case of forgetfulness?

[1]P C TONG, [2]L MCLEAN and [1]S P BAILLIE

[1]*Department of Medicine (Geriatrics), North Tyneside General Hospital, North Shields NE29 8NH and*
[2]*Department of Radiology, Newcastle General Hospital, Newcastle upon Tyne NE4 6BE, UK*

An obese 24-year-old man was admitted following a road traffic accident, during which he crashed into several cars and a shop. He had not been drinking alcohol, yet did not recall the incident. The family had noticed recent odd behaviour, episodic aggression and a glazed look at times. Apart from a minor whiplash injury, he was uninjured and clinically normal. CT head scan and encephaloelectrography were both normal. Routine investigations were unremarkable apart from a fasting glucose of 0.9 mmol l^{-1}.

In view of the presenting symptoms and fasting hypoglycaemia, CT of the abdomen was performed (Figure 1). What does this show?

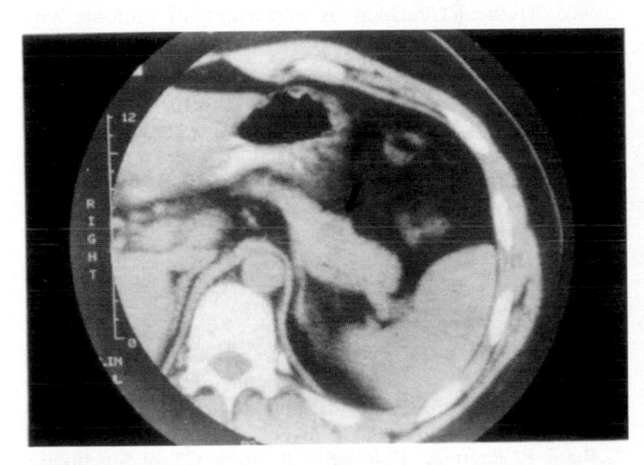

Figure 1. CT of the abdomen.

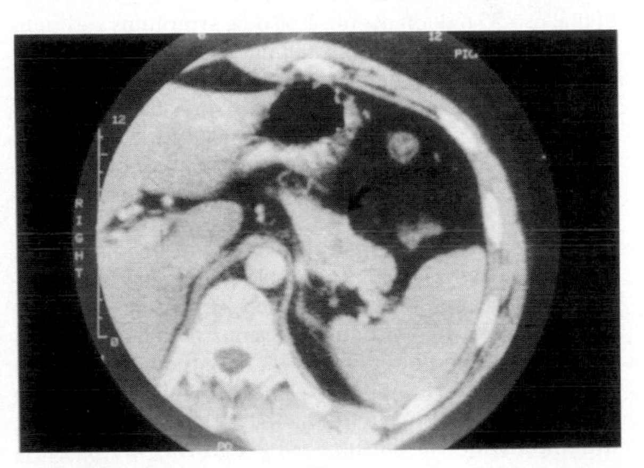

Figure 2. CT of the abdomen after iv contrast medium.

Based on the case of the month originally published in Br J Radiol 1994;67:215–6.

The pre-contrast CT of the abdomen showed a localized bulge on the anterior aspect of the tail of the pancreas, where there was a small 1.5 cm low attenuation mass which did not enhance after intravenous injection of contrast medium (Figure 2). Selective angiography failed to show the blushing of the pancreatic mass although there was displacement of the artery within the tail of the pancreas, corresponding with the mass seen on the CT scan (Figure 3). Surgical exploration showed a nodule about 2 cm × 1 cm in size present in the corresponding site in the tail of the pancreas. Left pancreatectomy was performed. Histology of the resected specimen confirmed the presence of the islet cell tumour which contained insulin secreting cells and somatostatin cells.

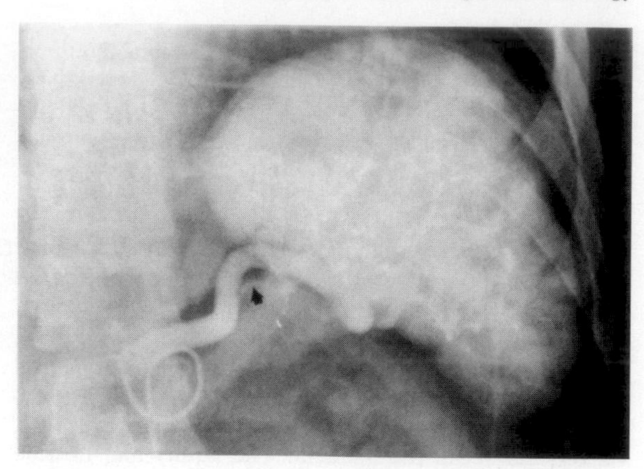

Figure 3. Selective angiography of the pancreas showing displacement of the artery within the tail of the pancreas (arrow).

Insulinomas are usually very vascular, and usually have a homogeneous well defined blush on the capillary phase of the angiogram. On the CT, after intravenous contrast is given, a well circumscribed enhancing mass is usually identified.

In this case, the radiological features are unusual as the insulinoma is identified as a low attenuation mass on the CT which does not enhance, and there is no characteristic blushing on the selective angiography. The displacement of the artery in the tail of the pancreas is very subtle and difficult to visualize, but the mass was seen in the exact position at operation.

Insulinoma is an uncommon tumour with an incidence of one in 1.25 million people. Episodic symptoms and signs of hypoglycaemia are the hallmark of the insulinoma, although the presentation is variable and neurological symptoms tend to predominate. When insulinoma is suspected, the determination of the fasting glucose, insulin and C-peptide should be made. Once the presence of the insulinoma has been confirmed biochemically, the next step is to locate the tumour.

Until recently, the diagnostic procedure of choice for the localization of the insulinoma was selective pancreatic angiography. The reported rates for successful localization vary from 63 to 90% [1]. In doubtful lesions, digital subtraction angiography can be very helpful. CT of the pancreas with either single or multiple intravenous boluses of contrast medium has been shown to be as accurate as angiography, with the additional benefit of being less invasive [2]. Early poor results reported with CT are probably owing to slow scan machines and the method of giving contrast medium. Ultrasound is not sensitive as a primary tool for investigation of insulinomas, as it depends heavily on the skills and experience of the operator. Intraoperative ultrasonography appears to be a promising modality with an 84% sensitivity reported for solitary insulinomas. When combined with surgical palpation, localization of solitary insulinomas increases to 100% [3]. Recently, considerable progress has been made using endoscopic ultrasonography in evaluating the pancreas. Small (less than 2 cm) islet cell neoplasms such as insulinoma and gastrinoma can be identified, allowing accurate location of these difficult-to-detect lesions. However, the availability of instrumentation and expertise and the degree of invasiveness prohibits the use of endoscopic ultrasound as a screening procedure [4]. When both CT and angiography are negative, transhepatic pancreatic venous sampling may offer additional sensitivity [5], although the procedure is more invasive and the results can be difficult to interpret. To date, MRI has no advantage over CT for evaluation of the pancreas as it is technically difficult to image both the normal and the diseased pancreas.

Surgical resection of the tumour is the treatment of choice. Medical treatment is important for patients with extensive metastatic tumour, in those who are unfit for surgery, with persistent post-operative symptoms and for those who are undergoing pre-operative localization. Diazoxide is an effective agent in reducing pancreatic insulin secretion. Streptozotocin is useful in metastatic disease and long acting somatostatin analogues, such as octreotide acetate, have also been used with some success.

[While MR is becoming the non-invasive technique for imaging endocrine tumours of the pancreas [6], interoperative ultrasound yields good results in the often small insulinomas, ED]

References

1. Rossi P, Allison DJ, Bezzi M. Endocrine tumors of the pancreas. Radiol Clin North Am 1989;27:129–61.
2. Rossi P, Baert A, Passariello R, et al. CT of functioning tumours of the pancreas. AJR 1985;144:57–60.
3. Galiber AK, Reading CC, Charboneau JW, et al. Localization of pancreatic insulinoma: comparison of pre- and intraoperative US with CT and angiography. Radiology 1988; 166:405–8.
4. Lux G, Heyder N. Endoscopic ultrasonography of the pancreas—technical aspects. Scan J Gastroenterol (Supplement 123) 1986;21:112–8.
5. Roche A, Raissonier A, Gillion-Savouret MC. Pancreatic venous sampling and arteriography in localizing insulinomas and gastrinomas: procedure and results in 55 cases. Radiology 1982;145:621–7.
6. Moore NR, Rogers E, Britton BJ. Magnetic resonance imaging of endocrine tumours of the pancreas. Br J Radiol 1995;68:341–7.

A bulging eye

J GHOLKAR, J P R JENKINS and T SEKIYA

Department of Diagnostic Radiology, University of Manchester, Oxford Road, Manchester M13 9PT, UK

A 27-year-old man presented with a long history of left-sided proptosis. Decreased vision in this eye was detected at a school eye-test at the age of 5 years. The patient reported further deterioration of vision over recent years, increasing proptosis and pain in the affected eye.

On examination, there was 4 mm of axial proptosis on the left. The vision in the left eye was 6/24 compared with 6/6 in the right eye. Full ocular movements were noted. Visual field testing showed no significant abnormality and formal examination of the central nervous system was otherwise normal. Radiographs of the skull and orbits were performed; the 20° occipitofrontal view is illustrated (Figure 1).

What does the radiograph show and what is your differential diagnosis?

What would be your next investigation?

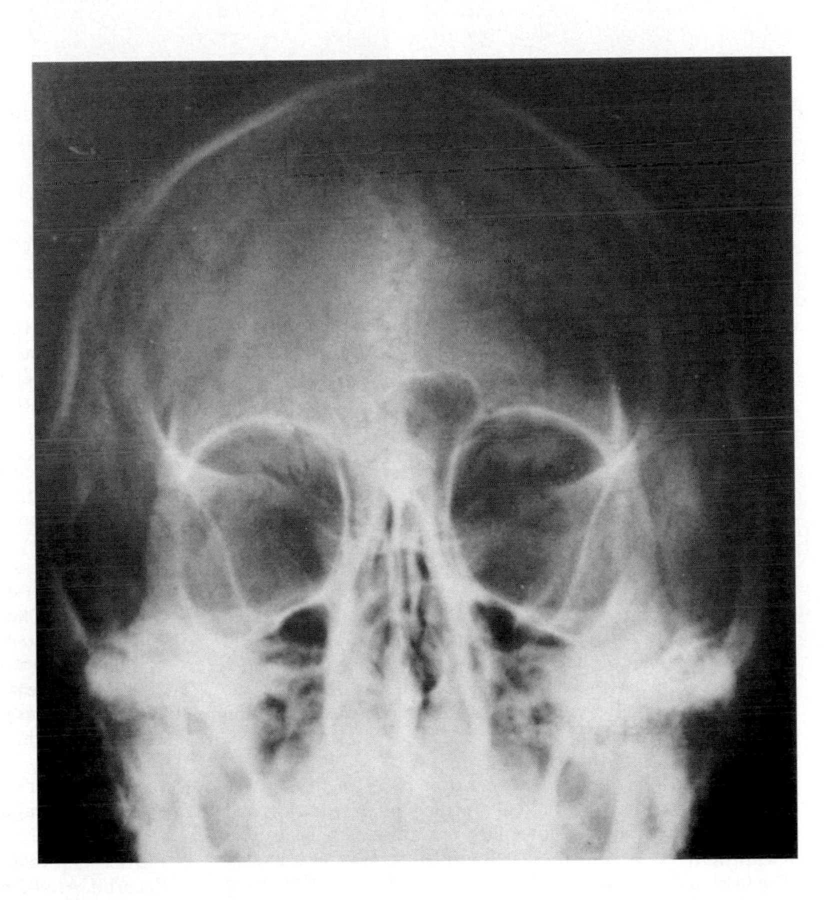

Figure 1. Plain radiograph taken at presentation.

Based on the case of the month originally published in Br J Radiol 1986;59:1047–9.

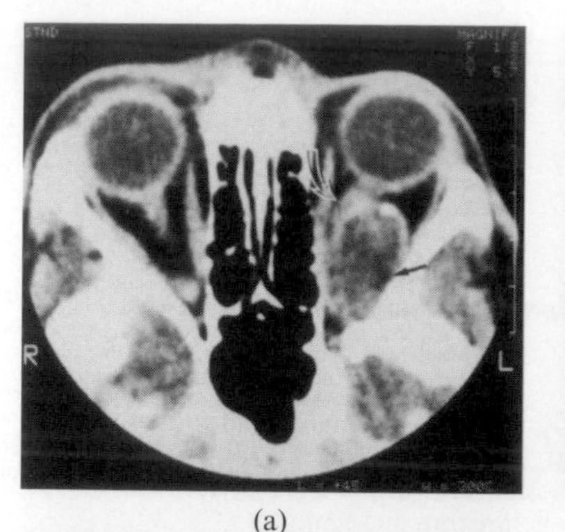

(a)

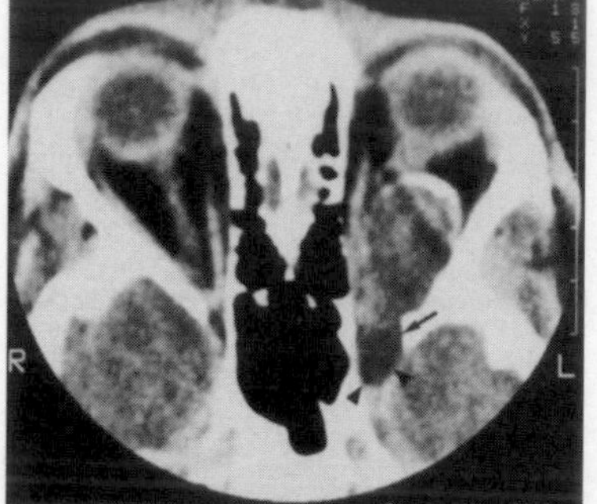

(b)

Figure 2. CT through the orbits, (a) 3 mm inferior to (b). Note the large left intraconal tumour with calcification in its anterior wall and areas of low attenuation in keeping with fat (straight arrows). The medial displacement of the optic nerve (curved arrow in (a) and the posterior extension of the tumour through the superior orbital fissure (arrowheads in (b)) are shown.

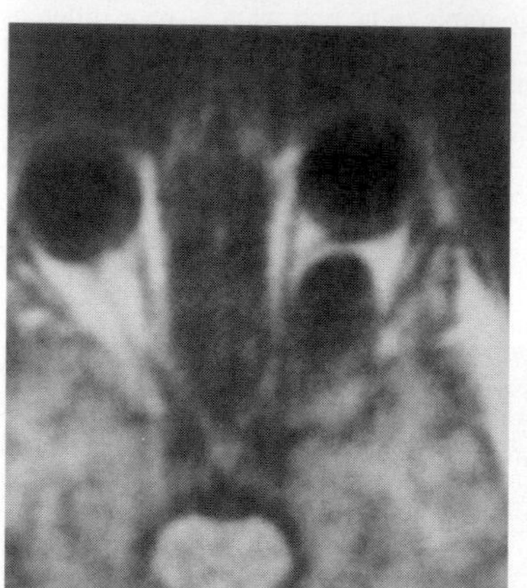

(a)

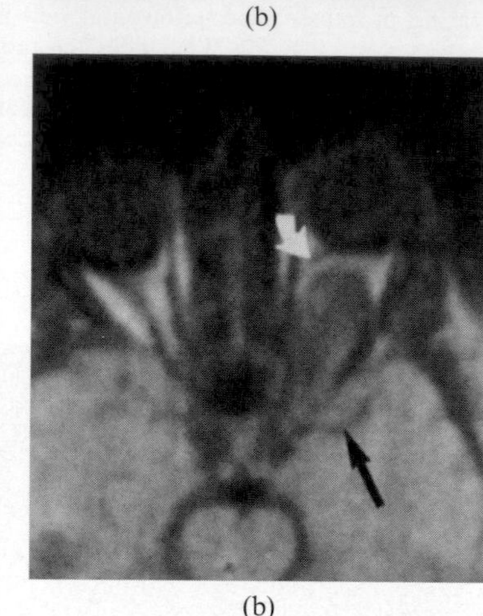

(b)

Figure 3. Two transverse MR images at the same anatomical level through the orbit and tumour. (a) T_1 weighted (inversion recovery 1500/500) and (b) T_2 weighted (spin echo 1000/60). In (a) the tumour gives a low signal anteriorly (very long T_1) in keeping with a cyst. The posterior extent of the tumour through the superior orbital fissure has a shorter T_1 due to more solid elements. The medial displacement of the optic nerve is shown (curved arrow). The middle cerebral artery is undisplaced (straight arrow).

The radiograph showed widening of the left superior orbital fissure, which had a well defined rounded sclerotic margin. The pathological causes of this include [1]: (1) neurofibromatosis; (2) metastasis to the wing of sphenoid; (3) extension of orbital lesions, *e.g.* arteriovenous malformations, haemangioma, meningioma, dermoid; and (4) extension of an intracranial lesion, *e.g.* meningioma, infraclinoid aneurysm, parasellar chordoma.

The long history and sclerotic margin in this case make a primary or secondary malignancy extremely unlikely and there were no other manifestations of neurofibromatosis.

CT of the orbits showed a well defined tumour lying within the muscle cone of the left orbit, measuring approximately 4 cm × 2 cm × 2 cm. The tumour had a thin, partially calcified wall, contained areas of low attenuation (0 to −20 Hounsfield Units) compatible with fat, and showed heterogeneous enhancement after intravenous contrast. The lesion was displacing the optic nerve medially (Figure 2a; posteriorly it was expanding the superior orbital fissure and extended intracranially for approximately 1 cm (Figure 2b).

MRI was also performed, at one anatomical level, through the orbits using a variety of T_1 and T_2 weighted pulse sequences and a back-projection method for image reconstruction. The site of the intraconal mass and associated displacement of surrounding structures were displayed. The lesion was well demarcated from surrounding retrobulbar fat on all sequences (Figure 3). It had a well defined capsule and appeared cystic, with a very long T_1 relaxation time. The calcification within the wall of the lesion was not delineated on MRI because of poorer resolution for the detection of calcification compared with CT, and MRI added no extra useful information.

The diagnosis was made of an intraconal dermoid because of the well defined nature of the lesion, calcification in its rim and areas of fat. The tumour was excised and was shown to be an epidermoid cyst on histology.

Sequestration dermoids and epidermoids are formed when dermal or epidermal elements become pinched off along one of the lines of fusion in the course of embryonic development. They contain varying amounts of keratin and cholesterol. In the skull, these lesions are usually situated either in the intradiploic spaces or subperiosteally. Dermoids and epidermoids account for approximately 4% of all cases of exophthalmos [2] and are usually sited extraconally. Their characteristic CT appearance has been described [3, 4]. Intraconal dermoids are rare but should be considered when the plain radiographic appearances suggest the presence of a slowly expanding benign lesion.

References

1. Lloyd GAS. Radiology of the orbit. London: WB Saunders, 1975:7–29.
2. Pfeiffer RL, Nicholl RJ. Dermoid and epidermoid tumours of the orbit. Arch Opthalmol 1948;40:639–64.
3. Wende S, Aulich A, Nover A, Lanksch W, Kazner E, Steinhoff H, et al. Computed tomography of orbital lesions. Neuroradiology 1977;13:123–34.
4. Blei L, Chambers JT, Liotta LA, Di Chiro G. Orbital dermoid diagnosed by computed tomographic scanning. Am J Ophthalmol 1978;85:58–61.

APPENDIX

Distribution of cases in relation to body systems

Body System	*Page no.*
Alimentary tract	11, 27, 35, 39, 61, 73, 79, 95, 121, 141, 143, 147, 153, 155, 179, 185, 189, 231
Liver and biliary tract	3, 19, 101, 161
Pancreas	25, 171, 195, 237
General abdomen	55, 77, 103, 109, 151, 157, 211, 223, 227, 231
Urinary tract	21, 69, 83, 91, 103, 113
Obstetrics and gynaecology	37, 47, 187
Head and neck	5, 43, 97, 105, 129, 131, 133, 205, 239
Brain	59, 87, 115, 145, 165, 181, 183, 197, 207
Spine	9, 31, 49, 65, 123, 139, 149, 159, 169, 177, 191, 225, 229, 233, 235
Respiratory system	7, 29, 53, 71, 75, 107, 201, 213, 215, 217
Heart and mediastinum	15, 41, 45, 89, 93, 111, 119, 125, 137, 163, 167, 175, 217, 235
Bone and joints	13, 23, 33, 51, 57, 67, 81, 85, 99, 117, 127, 199, 203, 209, 215, 219, 221
Paediatrics	19, 29, 41, 53, 153, 215
Vascular system	1, 17, 63, 135, 193, 227

INDEX